CASE STUDIES
IN PEDIATRIC SURGERY

CASE STUDIES IN PEDIATRIC SURGERY

EDITOR

R. Lawrence Moss, MD

Assistant Professor of Surgery and Pediatrics
Stanford University School of Medicine
Stanford, California

CONTRIBUTORS

Erik D. Skarsgard, MD

Assistant Professor of Surgery and Pediatrics
Stanford University School of Medicine
Stanford, California

Ann M. Kosloske, MD

Professor of Surgery and Pediatrics
Texas Tech University Health Sciences Center
Lubbock, Texas

Baird M. Smith, MD

Assistant Professor of Surgery and Pediatrics
Stanford University School of Medicine
Stanford, California

McGraw-Hill
MEDICAL PUBLISHING DIVISION

New York   St. Louis   San Francisco   Auckland   Bogotá   Caracas
Lisbon   London   Madrid   Mexico City   Milan   Montreal
New Delhi   San Juan   Singapore   Sydney   Tokyo   Toronto

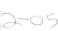
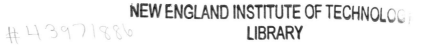

McGraw-Hill

*A Division of The **McGraw·Hill** Companies*

Case Studies in Pediatric Surgery

Copyright © 2000 by the **McGraw-Hill Companies,** Inc. All rights reserved.
Printed in the United States of America. Except as permitted under the
United States Copyright Act of 1976, no part of this publication may
be reproduced or distributed in any form or by any means, or stored
in a data base or retrieval system, without the prior written permission
of the publisher.

1 2 3 4 5 6 7 8 9 0   QWKQWK   0 9 8 7 6 5 4 3 2 1 0

ISBN 0-8385-1548-7

This book was set in Minion by Rainbow Graphics, Inc.
The editors were Michael Medina, Kathleen McCullough, and Karen Davis.
The production supervisor was Rick Ruzycka.
The cover designer was Aimee Nordin.
The interior designer was Joan O'Connor.
The index was prepared by Editoral Services.
Quebecor World/Kingsport was printer and binder.

This book is printed on acid-free paper.

Cataloging-in-Publication Data is on file for this title at the Library of Congress.

CONTENTS

* The letters in parentheses are the initials of the contributor responsible for the case study.

Color plates fall between pages 340 and 341.

PREFACE

The inspiration for the creation of this book comes from the inquisitive minds of our students and residents of pediatric surgery. While there are several outstanding comprehensive textbooks in the field, there is very little "problem-based" material available. We have also been asked by our colleagues in neonatology and other pediatric specialities, "Where can I read about the evaluation of bilious vomiting?" or "How should I work up an abdominal mass?"

We referred these students to a fine text edited by the late Dr. John Lilly entitled, *Case Studies in Pediatric Surgery,* published over 20 years ago. With the input of one of the original authors of that text, Dr. Ann Kosloske, we have attempted to provide an up-to-date, colorful, stimulating, and even provocative problem-oriented text for the field. We do not intend this book to be a comprehensive review of pediatric surgery. Rather, we carefully selected the most common and relevant clinical problems encountered by the clinician. The book is organized and built around these clinical problems when the diagnosis is not known. The emphasis of the text is to teach the reader to manage the problem. Thus, it covers initial clinical management, appropriate diagnostic evaluation, differential diagnosis, and surgical or medical management.

The authors recognize the management of clinical problems is frequently the subject of lively debate and disagreement among pediatric surgeons. In this text we have suggested management algorithms which have proven to be effective in the hands of the authors and colleagues. We do not suggest that our approach is the only correct one.

We would like to acknowledge the invaluable administrative assistance of Monique Aguirre and Anita Nunez in preparation of the manuscript.

We hope that the option of obtaining Continuing Medical Education (CME) credit will increase the work's usefulness to practicing professionals who may care for children with surgical problems. Most of all, we hope that this book will help the reader provide excellent care to his or her patients.

R. Lawrence Moss

A 3-DAY-OLD BOY WITH ABDOMINAL DISTENTION AND VOMITING

HISTORY A 3-day-old first born term male infant had an uneventful perinatal course and was discharged home at 12 hours of age. His mother notes that he initially fed well but has been vomiting for the past 24 hours. The vomiting initially consisted of formula but now is lightly green tinged. His mother feels his abdomen is "firm." He passed a small amount of meconium for the first time today. He has had no fever and has been alert and active.

EXAMINATION The baby appears systemically well. Vital signs are normal, and capillary refill time is 1.5 seconds. Heart and lung examination is normal. The abdomen is markedly distended without masses. It is not tender to deep palpation in all quadrants. Rectal examination reveals a normally located anus with normal sphincter location, size, and tone. Digital examination is normal and followed by passage of a large amount of meconium.

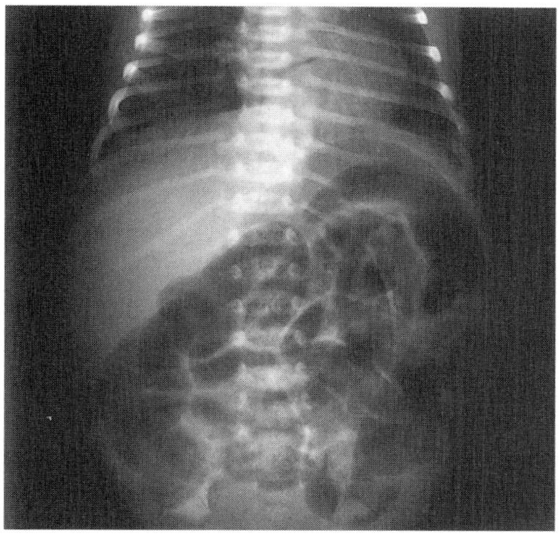

LABORATORY Complete blood count (CBC) and platelets are normal, and electrolytes are normal. Kidney, ureter, and bladder (KUB) and left lateral decubitus radiographs of the abdomen are shown in Figures 1–1 and 1–2.
Please answer all questions before proceeding to discussion section.

Figure 1–1. *Supine abdominal film.*

✓ QUESTIONS

1. The history, physical examination, and radiographs are most suggestive of:
   A. Malrotation with midgut volvulus causing bowel ischemia
   B. Ileal atresia
   C. Low intestinal obstruction
   D. Necrotizing enterocolitis
   E. Constipation due to milk intolerance

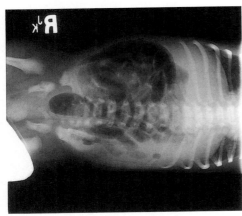

Figure 1–2. *Left lateral decubitus abdominal film.*

2. Proper management includes:
   A. Immediate exploratory laparotomy for relief of obstruction
   B. Exploratory laparotomy following fluid resuscitation and antibiotics
   C. Change to a soy-based formula with instructions to return if the baby develops fever or further vomiting
   D. Lower gastrointestinal contrast study
   E. Upper gastrointestinal contrast study

3. A barium enema is done and shown in Figure 1–3. This study shows:
   A. Pneumatosis intestinalis
   B. A transition zone in the sigmoid colon
   C. A rectal stricture
   D. A normal colon; the obstruction is apparently above this level
   E. A colon atresia

4. The next step in management is:
   A. Descending colostomy
   B. One stage pull-through procedure
   C. Rectal biopsy at the bedside
   D. Full thickness rectal biopsy in the operating room with frozen section examination
   E. A or B

5. When the diagnosis is confirmed, management may include:
   A. Ileostomy
   B. Descending colostomy
   C. Immediate one stage pull-through procedure
   D. Daily rectal irrigations followed by delayed surgical correction
   E. B, C, or D

6. The aganglionic bowel in this disease must be:
   A. Resected
   B. Bypassed
   C. Resected or bypassed
   D. Preserved for use in later reconstruction
   E. Stripped of its muscular layers

7. The definitive procedure that clearly has the lowest incidence of postoperative complications is:
   A. Duhamel
   B. Swenson
   C. Soave
   D. Any of the above via a laparoscopic approach
   E. None of the above

8. The patient undergoes definitive correction without complications. He is home and tolerating a normal diet with normal bowel habits. Four months later, he is seen in the emergency room with fever to 103°F, lethargy, watery diarrhea, and abdominal distention. Management includes:
   A. Immediate admission for rectal irrigation and antibiotics
   B. Immediate admission for nasogastric decompression, antibiotics, and bowel rest
   C. Stool cultures for *Salmonella, Shigella, Campylobacterium,*

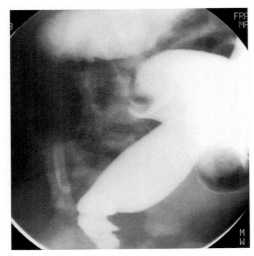

Figure 1–3. *Barium enema.*

rotaviruses, and *Clostridium difficile* followed by administration of oral metronidazole
   D. Acetaminophen, clear liquid diet, and instructions to return if fever persists or signs of dehydration develop
   E. Diagnostic barium enema to rule out a stricture

9. This disease is associated with:
   A. VATER syndrome
   B. Beckwith-Wiedemann syndrome
   C. Down syndrome
   D. Future development of malignant tumors
   E. An autosomal recessive mode of inheritance

10. The parents may be told that the risk of Hirschsprung disease in future children is:
   A. Less than 10%
   B. No greater than the general population
   C. Fifty percent since inheritance is autosomal dominant
   D. Fifty percent
   E. Twenty-five percent

ANSWERS AND DISCUSSION

1. **C** The plain films of the abdomen reveal multiple moderately dilated loops of intestine with air fluid levels on the left lateral decubitus view. This suggests an intestinal obstruction. Based on the number of loops, the obstruction appears to be fairly distal. Malrotation with volvulus and ischemia would produce signs of sepsis and shock as well as abdominal tenderness. The presence of a large amount of meconium on rectal examination suggests that the obstruction is unlikely to be complete (as with atresia). Necrotizing enterocolitis (NEC) presents with signs of sepsis and is usually seen in premature infants. Radiographs in NEC typically show pneumatosis intestinalis and may show portal venous gas or free intraperitoneal air. Milk intolerance is very rare in a newborn baby and does not present with obstipation and evidence of obstruction on x-ray.

2. **D** The differential diagnosis includes, Hirschsprung disease, meconium plug syndrome, and ileal or colonic stenosis (rare). A barium enema is the diagnostic study of choice. In addition to aiding in the diagnosis of Hirschsprung disease, the barium enema will localize the transition zone, which helps in planning operative correction. Laparotomy (**A** or **B**) is not indicated at this time since the diagnosis is not established and the patient is stable. A formula change (**C**) is not appropriate. Upper gastrointestinal contrast studies (**E**) in the setting of distal obstruction are seldom helpful. The multiple dilated loops fill with contrast and obscure the pathology.

3. **B** This barium study shows a "transition zone," which is diagnostic of Hirschsprung disease. As one examines a normal colon from the rectum proximally, the bowel caliber should remain constant or decrease. When there is a "transition" from "small" distal colon or rectum to more proximal colon, which is larger, Hirschsprung disease is very likely.

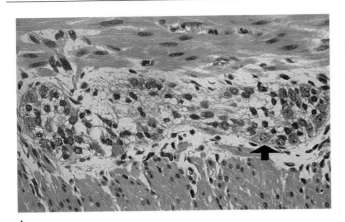

A

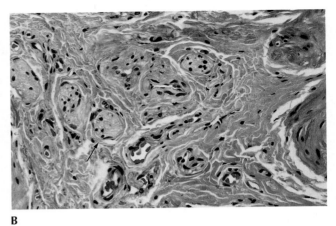

B

Figure 1–4. A. *This is a high power hematoxylin and eosin (H&E) stain of normal colon. Longitudinal smooth muscle is at the top of the image and circular smooth muscle at the bottom. The nerve plexus in between the muscle layers shows multiple ganglion cells (arrow points to one). These are large cells with complex nuclei.* **B.** *This is a neural plexus in a patient with Hirschsprung disease. Ganglion cells are absent and multiple areas of hypertrophied nerve fibers are seen (arrow). (See also color plates.)*

While barium enema is the most important radiograph in the diagnosis of Hirschsprung disease, the clinician must appreciate its limitations. Errors in interpretation of the barium enema may result from two factors: the age of the patient and the length of the aganglionic segment. In infants less than 1 month of age (such as this patient) the ganglionic segment may not yet have dilated. Thus, a transition zone is absent, and the study may be normal. In this situation, accuracy may be improved by obtaining an abdominal film 24 hours later. If barium is retained in the colon, Hirschsprung disease is likely. In long-segment Hirschsprung disease or total colon aganglianosis, the barium enema is often normal. In an older child with short segment disease, the aganglionic segment may be obscured by the large column of barium.

4. **C** Hirschsprung disease is caused by an absence of ganglion cells in the large intestine from the dentate line proximally to the transition zone. The diagnosis must be confirmed histologically. In a neonate, the diagnostic procedure of choice is a suction rectal biopsy. This is done at the bedside without anesthesia and allows excellent visualization of Meissner's submucosal plexus. The diagnosis of Hirschsprung disease requires an experienced pediatric pathologist. This is one of the few situations where the pathologist is asked to identify conclusively the absence of a structure rather than the presence of an abnormality. Figure 1–4 (see also color plate) illustrates the findings on hematoxylin and eosin stain. Acetylcholinesterase stain has been used, but fresh tissue is required.

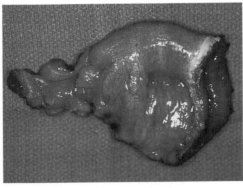

Figure 1–5. *This is a resected segment of sigmoid colon at the level of the transition zone. The collapsed bowel (on left) is aganglionic bowel distal to the transition zone. The dilated bowel (on right) has normal ganglion cells and is chronically distended due to the distal functional obstruction. (See also color plate.)*

5. **E** Definitive treatment of Hirschsprung disease includes resection of the aganglionic intestine with restoration of fecal continence by means of an anastomosis of ganglionic bowel to the anal verge (Figure 1–5; see also color plate). The standard of management against which all treatments are measured begins with a colostomy above the transition zone, in bowel with normal ganglion cells. The baby is then allowed to grow to 6 to 12 months of age at which time the ganglionic bowel is "pulled through" into the pelvis restoring fecal continence.

Some surgeons have advocated resection of aganglionic bowel and pull-through in one stage. When a family is reliable and motivated, they may elect to do daily rectal irrigations (fully decompressing the colon) until the child has reached an appropriate age for pull-through. The appropriate age is decreasing. Many surgeons now recommend pull-through at 3 to 6 months. A number of reports have advocated primary pull-through in the newborn. Short-term results have been impressive, but the long-term outcome is not yet known. The reader is referred to the Bibliography. A critical determinant of success in primary pull-through is the presence of a highly experienced pathologist. The surgeon must be absolutely certain about the presence of ganglion cells in the pulled through segment. This determination can be difficult on frozen section examination. If there is any degree of doubt, one should do a colostomy and await permanent sections. The consequences of pulling through aganglionic bowel are severe.

6. **C** There are several widely accepted and successful definitive operations to treat Hirschsprung disease. The original procedure was described by Swenson and bears his name. In this operation, all of the aganglionic bowel is resected, and the normal bowel is anastomosed at the dentate line. Critics of this procedure argue that it is technically difficult and that the incidence of postoperative enterocolitis may be higher than in other procedures. A multinational retrospective study disputes these arguments. The Soave procedure includes an intramural submucosal dissection of the distal rectum down to the dentate line. The normal bowel is then pulled through this muscular cuff, which is split longitudinally. Duhamel's operation is the simplest technical procedure to do. The distal aganglionic bowel is not resected. Rather, it forms the anterior wall of a neorectum while the ganglionic bowel forms the posterior wall.

   All three of these procedures have achieved good results reported in large series. The preponderance of evidence does not favor any of the three. The surgeon's choice depends on personal preference and experience. Overall results are good. Over 90% of patients may expect near normal bowel function over the long term. The most important early complication is anastomotic leak occurring in 4% to 7% of patients. This is usually treated with diverting colostomy. Stricture occurs in 4% to 8% of patients. Late complications are discussed in answer 8.

   Colostomy proximal to the transition zone will bypass the aganglionic bowel. The patient should remain symptom free until the definitive procedure.

7. **E** None of the procedures has proven superiority over the others (see answer 6). The laparoscopic approach has been successfully applied at all ages. It may shorten hospital stay and may result in smaller scars. No series has shown a decrease in the complication rate or a better long-term result.

8. **A** The most common late complication of Hirschsprung disease is enterocolitis. Enterocolitis may occur prior to colostomy or after a properly done pull-through. It presents with abdominal distention and pain, fever, and explosive watery diarrhea. The disease may be mild or may include fulminant gram-negative sepsis or intestinal perforation.

The hallmark of treatment for enterocolitis is rectal irrigations to decompress the colon. One should place a soft rubber tube in the rectum and stand back. There is usually high pressure gas and watery stool present. The colon is irrigated until clear. In severe enterocolitis, rectal irrigations should be done several times daily. Intravenous fluids, antibiotics, and bowel rest are important but will not be effective without properly done irrigations.

The etiology of enterocolitis is not clear. Some evidence has suggested that *Clostridium difficile* may play a role. If this organism is cultured from the stool, it should be treated.

Recurrent episodes of enterocolitis after pull-through may be caused by retained aganglionic distal bowel. Repeat biopsy is indicated after the enterocolitis has been successfully treated.

9. **C** Down syndrome is found in 4% to 5% of cases of Hirschsprung disease. Hirschsprung disease has few other associated anomalies. Congenital heart disease, Waardenburg syndrome, and Smith-Lemli-Opitz syndrome have been reported. Some authors have suggested an association with other neural crest disorders, such as neurofibromatosis and neuroblastoma.

10. **A** Specific gene mapping for Hirschsprung disease has not yet been successful. In rectosigmoid disease, such as this case, inheritance is thought to be a result of a sex-modified multifactorial trait or a recessive gene with low penetrance. Risk for future offspring is around 4%. Longer segment disease is associated with increased risk for future siblings. With total colonic Hirschsprung, inheritance is compatible with a dominant gene with incomplete penetrance. Sibling risk is around 30%.

BIBLIOGRAPHY

Andrassy RJ, Isaacs H, Weitzmann JJ. Rectal suction biopsy for the diagnosis of Hirschsprung's disease. *Ann Surg.* 1981;193:419.

Badner JA, Sieber WK, Garver KL, et al. A genetic study of Hirschsprung's disease. *Am J Hum Genet.* 1990;46:568.

Canty TG. Modified Duhamel procedure for treatment of Hirschsprung's disease in infancy and childhood: review of 41 consecutive cases. *J Pediatr Surg.* 1982;17:773.

Georgeson KE, Fuenfer MM, Hardin WD. Primary laparoscopic pull-through for Hirschsprung's disease in infants and children. *J Pediatr Surg.* 1995;30:1017–1022.

Hackam DJ, Superina RA, Pearl RH. Single-stage repair of Hirschsprung's disease: a comparison of 109 patients over 5 years. *J Pediatr Surg.* 1997;32:1028–1032.

Rothenberg SS, Chang JH. Laparoscopic pull-through procedures using the harmonic scalpel in infants and children with Hirschsprung's disease. *J Pediatr Surg.* 1997;32:894–896.

So HB, Schwartz DL, Becker JM, et al. Endorectal pullthrough without preliminary colostomy in neonates with Hirschsprung's disease. *J Pediatr Surg.* 1980;15:470.

Swenson O, Rheinlauder HF, Diamond I. Hirschsprung's disease: a new concept in etiology—operative results in 34 patients. *N Engl J Med.* 1949; 241:551.

Teitelbaum DH, Drongowski RA, Chamberlain JN, et al. Long-term stooling patterns in infants undergoing primary endorectal pull-through for Hirschsprung's disease. *J Pediatr Surg.* 1997;32:1049–1053.

Thomas DFM, Fernie DS, Becker JM, et al. Enterocolitis in Hirschsprung's disease: a controlled study of the etiologic role of *Clostridium difficile. J Pediatr Surg.* 1986;21:22.

A 1-WEEK-OLD BABY WITH VOMITING

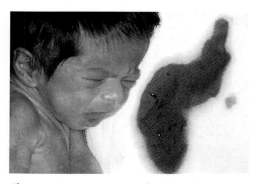

Figure 2–1. *Appearance of a 1-week-old baby who began vomiting yesterday. (See also color plate.)*

HISTORY   A healthy, 1-week-old, term infant presents with a 1-day history of vomiting, decreased stool and urine output, and lethargy. The last stool was streaked with blood. According to the baby's mother, he has fed well until yesterday.

EXAMINATION   The infant appears dehydrated and lethargic with delayed capillary refill. The heart and lungs are normal. The abdomen is scaphoid and soft without tenderness. Rectal examination is normal but confirms mucoid, blood-tinged stool. The baby is shown in Figure 2–1 (see also color plate).

LABORATORY   Blood work: Hematocrit is 33%, white blood cell count (WBC) is 16,000/mm³, and platelets are 350,000/mm³. Electrolytes: Na 135, Cl 98, K 3.8, CO_2 17. The infant's abdominal x-ray is shown in Figure 2–2.

Please answer all questions before proceeding to discussion section.

✓ QUESTIONS

1. The next most appropriate radiologic test would be:
   A. Doppler ultrasound of superior mesenteric vessels
   B. Barium enema
   C. Upper gastrointestinal series
   D. Abdominal computed tomography (CT) scan

2. Normal fetal intestinal rotation occurs:
   A. Between 4 and 10 weeks' gestational age
   B. Under the influence of maternal (transplacental) hormones
   C. Within the peritoneal cavity of the fetus
   D. Between 10 and 16 weeks' gestational age

3. Normal intestinal rotation involves:
   A. A 180-degree clockwise rotation of the cecocolic loop about the celiac axis
   B. A 270-degree counterclockwise rotation of the duodenojejunal loop about the superior mesenteric artery
   C. A 270-degree clockwise rotation of the duodenojejunal loop about the superior mesenteric artery
   D. A 360-degree counterclockwise rotation of the duodenojejunal loop about the superior mesenteric artery

4. Clinical presentations of malrotation include:
   A. Acute midgut volvulus
   B. Chronic duodenal obstruction
   C. Failure to thrive with chronic diarrhea
   D. All of the above

5. Thirty percent of patients with malrotation present within the first month of life:
   A. True
   B. False

6. Operation for malrotation:
   A. Is not indicated for asymptomatic patients
   B. Should not be undertaken until the diagnosis has been confirmed by contrast radiography
   C. Consists of laparotomy, reduction of volvulus, release of Ladd's bands, appendectomy, and cecopexy
   D. May require a second-look procedure

7. Complications following surgery for malrotation include:
   A. Recurrent volvulus
   B. Adhesive intestinal obstruction
   C. Short bowel syndrome
   D. All of the above

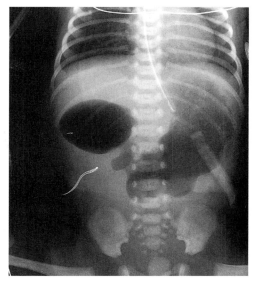

Figure 2–2. *Abdominal plain film demonstrating dilated proximal bowel loops and a paucity of distal intestinal gas, which is consistent with midgut volvulus.*

ANSWERS AND DISCUSSION

1. **C** The vomitus is green. Bilious vomiting indicates intestinal obstruction. The scaphoid abdomen suggests the obstruction is proximal. The onset of symptoms at 1 week of age argues against congenital causes of obstruction (ie, atresia). This baby has malrotation with midgut volvulus until proven otherwise. Upper gastrointestinal series with localization of the position of the duodenojejunal flexure remain the gold standard for diagnosis of malrotation (Figure 2–3). Barium enema localization of cecal position is unreliable in diagnosing malrotation since the cecum may be high or medially displaced based on its mobility (false positive), or it may reside in the right lower quadrant in cases of documented malrotation (false negative). Doppler sonographic interrogation of the position and relationship of the superior mesentric vessels is a recently described diagnostic technique. It is a specific but not a sensitive indicator of malrotation.

2. **A & 3. B** The result of normal intestinal rotation and fixation is stabilization of the midgut by broad-based attachment of its mesentery

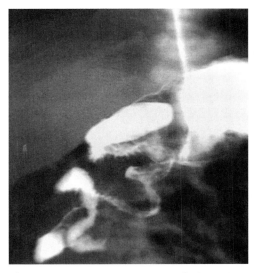

Figure 2–3. *Upper gastrointestinal (GI) series demonstrating malpositioned ligament of Treitz (below and to the left of the pedicle of the second lumbar vertebra). Note also the corkscrew appearance of the proximal jejunal loops suggesting volvulus.*

to the posterior abdominal wall. Between gestational weeks 4 and 10, the elongating midgut moves outside the abdomen into the base of the umbilical cord and the proximal and distal limits of the midgut (the duodenojejunal loop and the cecocolic loops, respectively) undergo a 270-degree counterclockwise rotation about the superior mesenteric vascular pedicle. As the intestines return into the peritoneal cavity, the duodenojejunal loop becomes fixed in the left upper abdomen, while cecocolic descent and attachment occurs gradually and often incompletely, accounting for the frequently observed high or mobile cecum seen in term or preterm infants. Disorders of intestinal rotation represent a spectrum of abnormality of midgut rotation and fixation with a propensity for midgut volvulus determined by the width and fixation of the superior mesenteric vascular pedicle.

4. **D** The presentation of malrotation is variable and is determined principally by the completeness of midgut volvulus and resulting intestinal luminal and vascular compromise, the presence of obstructing duodenal bands, called Ladd's bands, and the susceptibility to internal herniation because of a failure of intestinal fixation. When a midgut volvulus results in intestinal ischemia, the patient presents with dehydration, lethargy, bloody stool (and often vomitus), and a tender abdomen. If no vascular compromise is present, the presentation may be typical of intestinal obstruction either from luminal torsion caused by volvulus, from duodenal obstruction by Ladd's bands, or, rarely, by internal herniation associated with failures of fixation. If chronic volvulus exists that causes mesenteric venous and lymphatic obstruction only, the child may present with chronic diarrhea, fat malabsorption, and failure to thrive.

5. **B** Thirty percent of patients with malrotation present within the first week of life, 50% present within the first month, and 90% within the first year.

6. **D** Operation for malrotation is indicated for all symptomatic presentations. In instances where the diagnosis is suspected clinically and there is evidence of intestinal ischemia, it is appropriate to proceed to laparotomy without radiographic confirmation of the diagnosis. Asymptomatic malrotation may be discovered coincidentally in a patient who has a contrast study for unrelated symptoms. In these patients, operation is appropriate, because it is impossible to predict when (if ever) the malrotation might become symptomatic. The operation consists of reduction of volvulus, division of Ladd's bands, and broadening of the mesentery between the duodenojejunal junction and the cecum. Most surgeons remove the appendix, which would otherwise reside in the left lower abdomen, posing a confusing clinical picture in the event that the patient were to develop appendicitis in the future. Suture fixation of the duodenum or cecum is discouraged, because this may actually increase the risk of intestinal obstruction from adhesions or internal herniation, although it is recommended for patients who develop recurrent malrotation after an appropriate first operation. If an extensive portion of the intestine is necrotic or questionably viable, resection is delayed until a second-look procedure, which usually occurs within 48 hours (Figure 2–4; see also color plate).

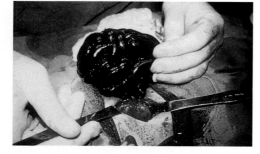

Figure 2–4. *Malrotation with midgut volvulus. The bowel in this case (different from the one discussed in Case 2) is clearly necrotic. In cases where intestinal viability is uncertain, the bowel is returned to the abdomen, and a second-look laparotomy is done in 24 to 48 hours. (See also color plate.)*

7. **D** Postoperative complications are similar to those associated with any abdominal operation, namely wound infection, intestinal obstruction from adhesions, and rarely, postoperative intussusception. If a significant length of small bowel has been lost, the short bowel syndrome may result. Recurrent malrotation with volvulus is an infrequent occurrence.

BIBLIOGRAPHY

Long FR, Kramer SS, Markowitz RI, et al. Radiographic patterns of intestinal malrotation in children. *Radiographics.* 1996;16:547.

Powell DM, Otherson HB, Smith CD. Malrotation of the intestine in children: the effect of age on presentation and therapy. *J Pediatr Surg.* 1989;24:777.

Spigland N, Brandt ML, Yazbeck S. Malrotation presenting beyond the neonatal period. *J Pediatr Surg.* 1990;25:1139.

Touloukian RJ, Smith EI. Disorders of rotation and fixation. In: O'Neill JA, Rowe MI, Grosfeld JL, et al. eds. *Pediatric Surgery,* 5th ed. St Louis: Mosby; 1998:1199–1214.

CASE

A CYANOTIC SPELL IN AN 8-HOUR-OLD INFANT

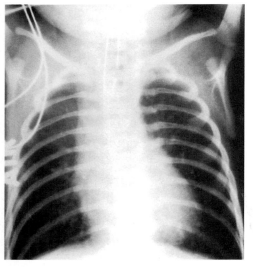

Figure 3–1. *Chest x-ray, frontal view, showing catheter curled up in proximal esophageal pouch.*

HISTORY   A 1900 g premature male infant develops deep cyanosis and bradycardia during the first (glucose water) feeding offered to him at 8 hours of age. He is the product of a pregnancy that was uncomplicated until his mother (19 years old, gravida 1, para 0) developed premature labor 5 weeks before her due date. Vaginal delivery was without difficulty. Apgar scores were 7 at 1 minute and 9 at 5 minutes. He was begun on intravenous fluids and placed in a 40% oxygen hood in the intensive care nursery. Initially, he appeared healthy, although he required hourly suctioning of secretions from the pharynx. The cyanosis and bradycardia improved after suctioning of the pharynx and administration of 100% O_2 via mask.

EXAMINATION   He is an irritable premature male infant. Gestational age is estimated at 34 weeks. Pulse is 160 per minute, blood pressure is 72/50, rectal temperature 37°C. Oxygen saturation is 95% with nasal cannula in place. There are no abnormalities of the head, face, palate, trunk, or extremities. The chest is symmetric, with the cardiac impulse palpable in the third intercostal space at the left sternal border. No cardiac murmur is audible. Breath sounds are equal and of normal quality bilaterally. The upper abdomen is mildly distended but soft, and there are no palpable masses or enlarged viscera. Genitalia are normal. The anus is patent and at the normal location. A drop of meconium is visible at the orifice. An orogastric tube is inserted.

LABORATORY   Hemoglobin is 14.5 gm%. Hematocrit is 55%. The white blood cell count (WBC) is 12,500/mm³, polymorphonuclear leukocytes are 65, bands are 3; lymphocytes are 28, and monocytes are 4. The blood glucose level is 80 mg/dL. The baby has not yet voided urine at 8 hours. The infant's chest x-rays are shown in Figures 3–1 and 3–2. Capillary blood gas levels (at 2 hours of age) are a pH of 7.32, Pco_2 of 39, a Po_2 of 50, and a Fio_2 of approximately 40%.

Please answer all questions before proceeding to discussion section.

✓ QUESTIONS

1. The most likely diagnosis is:
   A. Esophageal atresia with tracheoesophageal fistula (TEF)
   B. Esophageal atresia without fistula
   C. H-type TEF
   D. Double aortic arch
   E. Respiratory distress syndrome

2. The initial, *most* important maneuver to establish the diagnosis is:
   A. Barium esophagram
   B. Esophagram with water-soluble contrast
   C. An attempt to pass a catheter through esophagus to stomach
   D. Ultrasound examination of the esophagus
   E. Emergency bronchoscopy

3. The most common type of esophageal atresia is:
   A. Blind upper pouch, no fistula
   B. Fistula from upper pouch to trachea
   C. Blind upper pouch, fistula from trachea to lower pouch
   D. Double fistula (a fistula from each pouch to trachea)
   E. The H-type

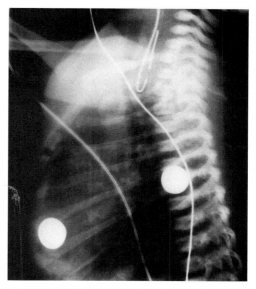

Figure 3–2. *Chest x-ray, lateral view, showing catheter in proximal esophagus. Metallic discs are monitor leads on side of chest.*

HOSPITAL COURSE The diagnosis is established, but the infant again becomes cyanotic and restless. His pulse drops to 90 beats per minute and systolic blood pressure to 40. Rhonchi are audible over both sides of the chest. After suctioning, administration of oxygen, and placement of a suction catheter in the upper esophagus, his vital signs return to normal. Echocardiogram shows a four-chambered heart, with right ventricular hypertrophy and pulmonic stenosis. During the echocardiogram, the infant experiences a third episode of cyanosis and bradycardia, which responds slowly to resuscitation. He becomes apneic; an endotracheal tube is inserted. His upper abdomen becomes increasingly distended as positive pressure ventilation is applied.

4. Which of the following is the *most* important emergency management of this infant?
   A. Antibiotics, O_2, and close monitoring of blood gases for 24 to 48 hours
   B. Gastrostomy
   C. Right thoracotomy with closure of the fistula and repair of the atresia
   D. Left thoracotomy with closure of the fistula and repair of the atresia
   E. Median sternotomy and open repair of the cardiac lesion

5. The pneumonitis/pneumonia associated with esophageal atresia/TEF may be the result of:
   A. Aspiration of saliva
   B. Aspiration of gastric acid
   C. Aspiration of formula, contrast material, or both
   D. Bacteria
   E. All of the above

6. Major anomalies associated with esophageal atresia are most common in which *one* of the following organ systems?
  A. Skeletal
  B. Gastrointestinal
  C. Cardiovascular
  D. Genitourinary
  E. Neurologic

7. Primary repair of esophageal atresia/TEF (without gastrostomy) is *most* appropriate for which of the following?
  A. Premature infant (birth weight 1900 g) with tetralogy of Fallot
  B. Term infant with trisomy 18 (Edward syndrome)
  C. Term infant with pectus excavatum
  D. Term infant with the CHARGE association
  E. Both C and D

8. A birth history often associated with esophageal atresia (although not noted in this case) is:
  A. Amnionitis caused by premature rupture of membranes
  B. Polyhydramnios
  C. Oligohydramnios
  D. Maternal cigarette smoking
  E. Maternal cocaine addiction

9. The extrapleural operative approach to the esophagus has the advantage of:
  A. Speed
  B. Lighter plane of anesthesia
  C. Better exposure
  D. Safety in case of an anastomotic leak
  E. Minimal trauma from retraction on the lung

10. All of the following statements regarding postoperative complications of esophageal atresia/TEF are true, *except:*
  A. Anastomotic complications are directly related to the gap between the proximal and distal pouches
  B. Most anastomotic leaks do not require operative treatment
  C. H-type TEF has the lowest complication rate
  D. Stricture at the anastomosis is often associated with gastro-esophageal reflux
  E. Recurrent TEF may be prevented by interposition of a patch of prosthetic mesh between the tracheal and esophageal suture lines

11. The technique of choice for esophageal anastomosis in the neonate is:
  A. One layer, interrupted, end-to-end, with fine, nonabsorbable suture (eg, silk)
  B. One layer, interrupted, end-to-end, with fine absorbable suture (eg, polyglycolic acid)
  C. One layer, running, end-to-end, with fine nonabsorbable suture (eg, polypropylene)
  D. Two layers, interrupted, end-to-end, with fine nonabsorbable suture (eg, silk)
  E. One layer, interrupted, end-to-side (with ligation of TEF), with fine silk

12. The current survival rate of babies with esophageal atresia treated in neonatal centers is:
    A. Ninety percent
    B. Seventy-five percent
    C. Fifty percent
    D. Thirty-five percent

ANSWERS AND DISCUSSION

1. **A** Esophageal atresia with tracheoesophageal fistula is the most likely diagnosis. Copious pharyngeal secretions are the result of the inability of the infant to swallow his own saliva. Attempted feeding causes overflow from the blind upper pouch, with aspiration and cyanosis. Chest x-rays show the radiopaque catheter advanced as far as it will go in the blind upper esophageal pouch. The presence of air in the stomach rules out esophageal atresia without fistula (**B**), because in the absence of a fistula, no pathway exists for air to enter the gastrointestinal tract. With H-type TEF (**C**), the esophagus is patent, and the tube passes into the stomach. H-fistulas are usually diagnosed after a few days or weeks of recurrent episodes of aspiration pneumonia rather than on the first day of life. Double aortic arch (**D**), a type of vascular ring that encircles the trachea and esophagus, is usually diagnosed after the first few days of life. The symptoms, stridor and cyanosis with feedings, typically worsen as the child grows and the ring tightens. Respiratory distress syndrome (**E**), which is common in premature infants, is characterized by reticulogranular infiltrates on chest x-ray, which are not noted in this patient.

2. **C** When the diagnosis of esophageal atresia is suspected, a well-lubricated 8 or 10 French catheter should be passed through the mouth or nostril to the stomach. If the catheter meets an obstruction 8 to 12 cm from the lip or nostril, the diagnosis of esophageal atresia is made. The catheter should be firm enough so that it will not curl up in the proximal pouch. A chest x-ray should be obtained with the catheter in place to document the level of the atresia and evaluate the heart, lungs, and skeletal structures. A few milliliters of air may be injected through the tube to outline the upper pouch. It is not necessary to confirm the diagnosis by radiographic contrast study. In fact, standard barium esophagram (**A**) is contraindicated, as is water-soluble contrast study (**B**) because of the danger of aspiration of the contrast material into the lungs. In some centers, a limited radiographic study is performed in order to confirm the diagnosis and rule out a proximal TEF. Caveats include having the infant in the upright position; injecting no more than 0.5 to 1.0 mL of dilute barium into the upper pouch; suctioning the barium immediately after a film is obtained; and having only experienced pediatric radiologists performing the study. (Such caveats usually mean that a procedure is more trouble than it is worth.) Many centers now use tracheobronchoscopy just prior to thoracotomy for repair of the esophageal anomaly. This procedure requires facility in neonatal endoscopy but yields crucial information (eg, the precise anatomic level of the fistula or the presence of rare variants, such as double fistula or right aortic arch). Bronchoscopy (**E**), however, is not the ini-

tial procedure of choice. The diagnosis should be made by the passage (or rather, nonpassage) of a catheter down the esophagus. Ultrasound of the esophagus (**D**) has not been used for diagnosis, as sonograms do not outline air-filled structures.

3. The anatomic spectrum of esophageal atresia/TEF, in several large series, is as follows:

   C Blind upper pouch with distal TEF: 86%
   A Isolated esophageal atresia (no fistula): 8%
   E H-type TEF (no atresia): 4%
   D Esophageal atresia with fistula to both pouches: 1%
   B Esophageal atresia with proximal TEF: <1%

4. **B** Although some pediatric surgeons might disagree, gastrostomy is the best choice for initial management of this infant, whose physiologic status is unstable. He has two risk factors for mortality: congenital heart disease and prematurity. High-risk infants tolerate a brief anesthetic for gastrostomy better than a longer anesthetic for thoracotomy and definitive repair. Venting the stomach protects against aspiration of gastric juice and prevents respiratory embarrassment from gastric distention. Thoracotomy and definitive repair of the anomaly (**C**) may be deferred until the infant is clinically stable. Left thoracotomy (**D**) is incorrect because the esophagus and fistula are ordinarily approached via the *right* chest, not the *left* (except in the rare instance of a right-sided aortic arch). Antibiotics and other supportive care (**A**) are helpful but will not halt the aspiration of gastric contents. They should be used in conjunction with gastrostomy. Median sternotomy and open heart surgery (**E**) may be necessary in the future but not on the first day of life. Stabilization of the infant takes priority, usually followed by repair of the esophageal anomaly, then cardiac repair. The use of gastrostomy, which formerly was the rule in many centers, has declined in the past two or three decades. At present, the majority of infants are managed by primary repair. Rarely, the gastrostomy creates a problem of its own: a vent so large that infants with severe respiratory distress syndrome and a large TEF may be difficult to ventilate. Urgent closure of the TEF is then required, either by operation or by endoscopic placement of a balloon to occlude the TEF.

5. **E** All of the factors—saliva, gastric acid, formula, contrast material, and bacteria—may contribute to the pneumonia. Gastric acid, the most important factor, incites a chemical pneumonitis that soon evolves into a bacterial pneumonia.

6. **C** The overall occurrence of associated anomalies is 50% to 70%. About two thirds of the anomalies are considered major (likely to complicate the early life of newborns with esophageal atresia with TEF), and one third are minor (not likely to be of significant consequence). The most important are cardiovascular anomalies (**C**), which are present in 29% to 35% of cases. The absence of a heart murmur at birth (as in this case) does not rule out the diagnosis of congenital heart disease. Imperforate anus is the most common of the gastrointestinal anomalies (**B**), which are associated with 24% of cases. Genitourinary anomalies are found in 20%, and neurologic defects in

10%. Skeletal anomalies (**A**), particularly of the thoracic vertebra and ribs, occur in 13% but usually are not of major significance at birth. The mnemonic VATER refers to the association of vertebral defects, anorectal atresia, tracheoesophageal fistula, esophageal atresia, and renal or radial limb anomalies. If one or two of these exist, the others should be looked for. The mnemonic has been revised to VACTERL, which includes all of the above, plus the most important association, congenital cardiac disease.

7. **C** Pectus excavatum is not a contraindication to primary repair. All the other choices include major risk factors. The two factors that have the greatest influence on survival are major cardiac anomalies and birth weight less than 1500 g. The infant with trisomy 18 (**B**) has a lethal condition; esophageal repair is contraindicated. The CHARGE association (coloboma, heart defects, atresia choanae, mental retardation, genital hypoplasia, and ear deformities) (**D**) carries a mortality of up to 70% from major cardiac anomalies.

8. **B** Polyhydramnios is noted in 32% of infants with esophageal atresia and distal TEF and in 85% of infants with isolated esophageal atresia. Oligohydramnios (**C**) is associated with congenital anomalies of the urinary tract. Other associations are amnionitis (**A**) and neonatal sepsis, maternal cigarette smoking (**D**) and prematurity, and maternal cocaine addiction (**E**) with neonatal necrotizing enterocolitis, plus, of course, withdrawal symptoms in the infant.

9. **D** The extrapleural approach to the esophagus may provide safety in case of anastomotic leak, a complication recognized in 10% to 20% of cases. An extrapleural leak is generally well tolerated, whereas a leak into the pleural space may lead to empyema. The importance of the extrapleural approach, however, has diminished as neonatal care has improved in the last two decades. A study from Detroit showed no difference in survival (transpleural vs extrapleural) since 1974, whereas before 1974, the transpleural approach had higher mortality. The transpleural approach is slightly faster (**A**) than the extrapleural. Plane of anesthesia (**B**), exposure (**C**), and trauma to the lung from retraction are comparable with the two approaches.

10. **E** Recurrent TEF, a complication that occurs in 2% to 5% of cases, most often follows an anastomotic leak and an inflammatory process in the mediastinum. Interposition of a flap of pleura, azygous vein, or other mediastinal tissue, may help to prevent recanalization of the fistula. A prosthetic patch is probably the *last* thing one would want to interpose between the suture lines. A foreign body might cause, rather than prevent, a recurrent TEF. Most anastomotic leaks (**B**) are minor and treated by nutritional support and antibiotics. Rarely is operative treatment required. The primary cause of anastomotic complications (eg, leak, stricture, recurrent TEF) is tension on the anastomosis, which is directly related to the distance between esophageal pouches (**A**). H-type TEF (**C**) has a low complication rate as there is no esophageal anastomosis to leak or stricture. H-fistulas are located in the proximal trachea and esophagus and can almost always be repaired through cervical incisions rather than thoracotomy. Gastroesophageal reflux (**D**), a postopera-

tive problem in nearly half of infants, is associated with recurrent anastomotic stricture. Control of reflux by medical or surgical treatment may correct the stricture problem.

11. There is no correct answer to this question. All of the techniques have been used successfully, except (**C**), which is a vascular technique and would probably work also. The original, two-layer telescoping anastomosis (**D**) of Cameron Haight was popular in the past. The end-to-side technique (**E**), developed to minimize mobilization of the distal esophagus, had various advocates. Most pediatric surgeons use a single layer of full thickness interrupted sutures. Both silk (**A**) and synthetic absorbable suture (**B**) have been selected. Given a gentle and meticulous technique, which is a *sine qua non* for esophageal atresia, it is the gap, not the suture material, that determines anastomotic complications.

12. **A** Approximately 90% of all infants with esophageal atresia will survive. Great progress has been made in the management of this anomaly, which carried a mortality of 100% until 1941, when the first successful repair was performed by Cameron Haight. Mortality steadily declined in the next five decades, associated with major improvements in neonatal care before, during, and after operation. Survival is now anticipated for all infants except those with the most complex cardiac anomalies, extreme prematurity, or trisomy 18. Because many such infants were not candidates for any type of corrective surgery, the current mortality of 8% to 10% may approach an irreducible minimum.

HOSPITAL COURSE AND FOLLOW-UP   After emergency gastrostomy, the infant has no further cyanotic spells. Forty-eight hours later he is taken to the operating room for definitive repair. Bronchoscopy demonstrates a large TEF located 1 cm above the carina. The dominant aortic pulsations are on the left anterior trachea. A right extrapleural thoracotomy is performed, the TEF is divided and closed, and end-to-end anastomosis of the esophagus is carried out without tension. The postoperative course is uncomplicated. Barium esophagram (Figure 3–3) shows no leak or stricture. At 6 weeks, cardiac catheterization confirms the diagnosis of tetralogy of Fallot. His cardiac status worsens, and a Blalock shunt (subclavian artery to pulmonary artery) is performed. The gastrostomy is used for supplementary feedings until he is 5 months old. It is then removed in the clinic. He subsequently does well and returns to the hospital at 1 year of age for total correction of tetralogy of Fallot.

Esophageal atresia is the anomaly which, by its urgency, its exacting requirements at the operating table, its demand for precise postoperative management, and the long-term follow-up essential in the growing child, becomes the ultimate congenital anomaly for which pediatric surgeons prepare. (Randolph, 1986)

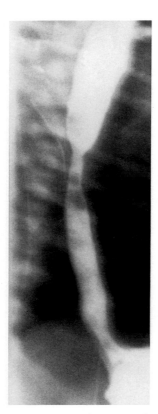

Figure 3–3. *Barium esophagram 7 days after repair showing patent esophagus.*

BIBLIOGRAPHY

Beasley SW. Esophageal atresia and tracheoesophageal fistula. In: Oldham KT, Colombani PM, Foglia RP, eds. *Surgery of Infants and Children: Scientific Principles and Practice.* Philadelphia: Lippincott-Raven; 1997: 1021–1034.

Bishop PJ, Klein MD, Philippart AI, et al. Transpleural repair of esophageal atresia without a primary gastrostomy: 240 patients treated between 1951 and 1983. *J Pediatr Surg.* 1985;20:823–828.

Guiney EJ. Oesophageal atresia and tracheo-esophageal fistula. In: Puri P, ed. *Neonatal Surgery.* Oxford, UK: Butterworth-Heinemann; 1996:227–236.

Haight C, Towsley HA. Congenital atresia of the esophagus with tracheo-esophageal fistula: extrapleural ligation of fistula and end-to-end anastomosis of esophageal segments. *Surg Gynecol Obstet.* 1943;76:672–688.

Harmon CM, Coran AG. Congenital anomalies of the esophagus. In: O'Neill JA Jr, Rowe MI, Grosfeld JL, et al. eds. *Pediatric Surgery,* 5th ed. St. Louis: Mosby; 1998:941–967.

Holder TM. Esophageal atresia and tracheoesophageal malformations. In: Ashcraft KW, Holder TM, eds. *Pediatric Surgery,* 2nd ed. Philadelphia: Saunders; 1993:249–269.

Kosloske AM, Jewell PJ, Cartwright KC. Crucial bronchoscopic findings in esophageal atresia and tracheoesophageal fistula. *J Pediatr Surg.* 1988; 23:466–470.

McKinnon LJ, Kosloske AM. Prediction and prevention of anastomotic complications of esophageal atresia and tracheoesophageal fistula. *J Pediatr Surg.* 1990;25:778–781.

Myers NA. Oesophageal atresia: the epitome of modern surgery. *Ann R Coll Surg Engl.* 1974;54:277–287.

Pietsch JB, Stokes KB, Beardmore HE. Esophageal atresia with tracheo-esophageal fistula: end-to-end versus end-to-side repair. *J Pediatr Surg.* 1978;13:677–681.

Randolph JG. In: Welch KJ, et al., eds. *Pediatric Surgery,* 4th ed, Chicago: Year Book Medical Publishers; 1986:682–694.

Randolph JG, Newman KD, Anderson KD. Current results in repair of esophageal atresia with tracheoesophageal fistula using physiologic status as a guide to therapy. *Ann Surg.* 1989;209:524–531.

Spitz L, Kiely EM, Morecroft JA, et al. Oesophageal atresia: at-risk groups for the 1990's. *J Pediatr Surg.* 1994;29:723–725.

4 CASE

A GIRL WITH A LUMP IN HER GROIN

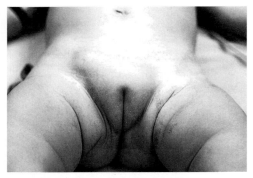

Figure 4–1. *Appearance of the groin in a 2-year-old girl with a lump in the right labia.*

HISTORY A relatively unconcerned mother brings in her 2-year-old daughter after a pediatrician notes a firm, pea-sized lump in her right labia that cannot be reduced. The mother says it has been there for months and has never caused a problem. She is only worried because the pediatrician said her daughter might need an operation. The patient's groin is shown in Figure 4–1.

Please answer all questions before proceeding to discussion section.

✓ QUESTIONS

1. Based on history alone, what is the most likely diagnosis?
   A. Indirect inguinal hernia containing bowel
   B. Femoral hernia
   C. Inguinal lymphadenopathy
   D. Direct inguinal hernia
   E. None of the above

2. If clinical findings are consistent with an incarcerated ovary, when should repair be effected?
   A. Emergently—put on the operating room add list
   B. Urgently—add to the next morning's list
   C. Soon—within a few days
   D. Electively—within a few weeks

3. Prior to repair of a known hernia, all parents must be taught the signs and symptoms of bowel strangulation or in this case, ovarian torsion. Which of the following could be used to distinguish between these diagnoses?
   A. Redness
   B. Swelling

    C. Tenderness

    D. Vomiting

    E. None of the above

4. This patient is taken to the operating room 48 hours later. Besides an ovary, which structure are you most likely to find in the sac?

    A. Bladder

    B. Salpinx

    C. Umbilical ligament

    D. Bowel

    E. Uterus

5. At operation, you find that the salpinx and a portion of the bladder comprise one wall of the hernia sac. Management options include:

    A. Placing a purse-string suture at the base of the sac and inverting it as you tie the suture

    B. Inverting the sac and closing the internal inguinal ring

    C. Closing the inguinal ring tightly around these structures to prevent bowel from passing through the defect

    D. A and B

    E. All of the above

6. Which of the following approaches are appropriate for the management of the left groin?

    A. If the parents note signs or symptoms of a hernia, exploration should be undertaken

    B. If on clinical examination a silk sign is present, exploration should be undertaken

    C. The risk of metachronous hernia is only 7% to 15%, so no exploration should be performed

    D. To prevent the risk of a second anesthesia the contralateral side should always be explored

    E. Nothing—anesthesia has so improved that there is less risk to a second operation or anesthesia

    F. All of the above

ANSWERS AND DISCUSSION

1. **E** These findings are typical of an inguinal hernia with an incarcerated ovary. An indirect inguinal hernia containing bowel is the most common cause (~1% of female children) of a bulge in this location, but it is usually soft and easily reducible. When a girl develops a nonreducible (incarcerated) hernia, the incarcerated structure is usually an ovary. A femoral hernia is very rare in children and accounts for about 1% of all hernias. Lymph nodes are common enough in the groin but quite unusual in the labia.

2. **C** It is true that when diagnosed, most incarcerated ovaries have been so for weeks or months, sometimes years. Strangulation is quite uncommon. The literature, however, contains rare anecdotal reports of strangulation. For this reason, no absolute right answer exists to this question except to say that sooner is better than later. Response **B** cannot be faulted, although the situation is not urgent enough to warrant intubation with a full stomach as in answer **A**.

3. **E** It can be very difficult to distinguish between these diagnoses, and the best policy is to operate early and prevent them. Vomiting, if bilious, may favor bowel incarceration but nonbilious vomiting can occur associated with the pain of torsion. An ultrasound of the mass might be successful in differentiating these diagnoses but would be an unwarranted delay when symptoms of strangulation or torsion are present. If the child is experiencing any of these symptoms, prompt operation is indicated.

4. **B** All of the listed structures are occasionally found in hernia sacs. In females, 21% of hernias will contain salpinx.

5. **D** The key to inguinal hernia repair is to ligate the hernia sac, thereby eliminating the communication of the peritoneal cavity from inside to outside the abdomen. When an intra-abdominal organ makes up part of the wall of the sac, the hernia is called a sliding hernia. In sliding hernias, ligation and excision of the sac is not possible as it would necessarily include resection of the involved viscera. In girls, the internal ring may be safely closed since no vital structures run through it. In boys, tight closure of the ring would compromise the vas deferens and spermatic vessels.

6. **F** There is no right answer to this question. There are, however, correct principles. In the risk–benefit analysis of contralateral groin exploration for hernias, it is certain that fewer complications are possible in girls when compared with boys. As such, any suggestion of a contralateral hernia should be operatively pursued. Statistically speaking, the incidence of metachronous hernias in children not premature is between 7% to 15%, diminishing with age. Therefore, those who advocate routine contralateral exploration must acknowledge an 85% to 93% rate of unnecessary operations. In the hands of anesthesiologists experienced with children, the mortality of a general anesthetic has been falling; formerly 1:10,000 it is now approaching 1:100,000—which is less than the risk of driving on many freeways. Many surgeons continue to perform routine contralateral explorations in girls.

BIBLIOGRAPHY

Marinkovic S, Kantardzic M, Bukarica S, Grebeldinger S, Pajic M. When to operate nonreducible ovary? *Med Pregl.* 1998;51:537–540.

Miltenburg DM, Nuchtern JG, Jaksic T, Kozinetz CA, Brandt ML. Meta-analysis of the risk of metachronous hernia in infants and children. *Am J Surg.* 1997;174:741–744.

Tackett LD, Breuer CK, Luks FI, et al. Incidence of contralateral inguinal hernia: a prospective analysis. *J Pediatr Surg.* 1999;34:684–688.

ABDOMINAL DISTENTION AND FAILURE TO PASS MECONIUM IN AN INFANT

HISTORY   A 36-hour-old infant has fed poorly and has now developed abdominal distention. He is a full-term male infant with no prenatal problems born to a healthy mother. He vomited his past two feedings and just vomited a small amount of bile. He has not passed meconium.

EXAMINATION   His weight is 2.9 kg. His respiratory rate is 50 with mild nasal flaring. Capillary refill time is 2.5 seconds, and other vital signs are normal. His abdomen is markedly distended with a few visible bowel loops but is soft and nontender to deep palpation. Rectal examination reveals some white mucous with no meconium.

LABORATORY   Hemoglobin is 17.5, WBC and platelets are normal. Abdominal x-rays (kidney, ureter, and bladder and left lateral decubitus) are shown in Figures 5–1 and 5–2.

Please answer all questions before proceeding to discussion section.

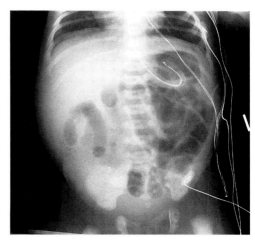

Figure 5–1. *Supine abdominal film.*

✓ QUESTIONS

1. The differential diagnosis includes all of the following *except:*
   A. Meconium plug syndrome
   B. Hirschsprung disease
   C. Ileal atresia
   D. Malrotation with midgut volvulus
   E. Meconium ileus

2. The most likely diagnosis is:
   A. Meconium plug syndrome
   B. Hirschsprung disease
   C. Ileal atresia
   D. Malrotation with midgut volvulus
   E. Meconium ileus

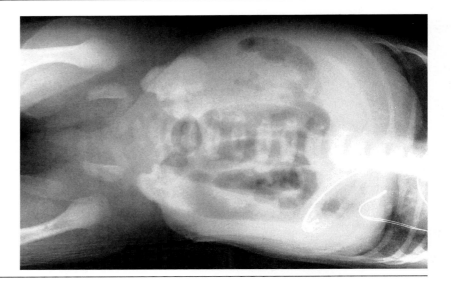

Figure 5–2. *Left lateral decubitus abdominal film.*

3. Following fluid resuscitation, the most appropriate initial therapy is:
   A. Immediate operation with ileostomy and appendectomy with examination for ganglion cells
   B. Rectal irrigation followed by suction rectal biopsy
   C. Lower gastrointestinal contrast study
   D. Immediate operation with T-tube irrigation of the intestine
   E. Immediate operation with bowel resection and primary anastomosis

4. The most common systemic disease associated with this condition is:
   A. Cystic fibrosis
   B. Hirschsprung disease
   C. Hypothyroidism
   D. VATER syndrome
   E. Crohn's disease

5. The prognosis regarding this infant's gastrointestinal function is:
   A. Normal following recovery
   B. Very poor, with a high likelihood that long-term parenteral nutrition will be necessary
   C. Good, if appropriate enteral supplements are given
   D. Poor, malabsorbtion should be expected
   E. Good except that he will be at continuing risk for bacterial overgrowth

6. Can this condition occur in the absence of severe systemic disease?
   A. Yes
   B. No

7. What can you tell the parents regarding the risk of recurrence for future pregnancies?
   A. This is a sporadic developmental anomaly, and future offspring are unlikely to be affected
   B. The condition is autosomal dominant, and the recurrence risk is 50%
   C. The condition is autosomal recessive, and the recurrence risk is 25%

   D. The condition is autosomal dominant, but only a small percentage of patients have gastrointestinal manifestations
   E. There is a very high likelihood of occurrence in future pregnancies and a high chance of late gestation fetal loss. Future pregnancies should be managed by a perinatologist

8. This type of intestinal obstruction has been resported to occur in the absence of systemic disease in the following ethnic group:
   A. Ashkenazi Jews
   B. Eastern Europeans
   C. Asians
   D. Japanese
   E. Native Americans

ANSWERS AND DISCUSSION

1. **D** This baby is vomiting green and, therefore, has an intestinal obstruction until proven otherwise. Physical examination reveals a distended abdomen suggesting a distal intestinal obstruction. This is confirmed by radiographic examination of the abdomen, which reveals multiple distended loops of intestine. The absence of meconium on rectal examination means that the obstruction is probably complete. All of the choices except **D** are causes of distal intestinal obstruction. Malrotation presents with green vomiting but the abdomen should be normal to scaphoid. Radiographs should reveal a normal gas pattern to a paucity of bowel gas. Midgut volvulus only causes bowel dilation in the setting of severe ischemia or necrosis. In this setting, the abdomen is tender, peritonitis is present, and there are systemic signs of sepsis.

2. **E** All of the conditions listed except malrotation and volvulus can have a clinical presentation identical to this case. Note that the decubitus film of the abdomen reveals multiple dilated loops in the absence of air fluid levels. This finding is highly suggestive of meconium ileus. In this condition, the same abnormally thick mucous that obstructs the ileum does not layer by gravity proximal to the obstruction. The "soap bubble" appearance in the right lower quadrant provides further support for this diagnosis. This appearance is caused by dispersion of air bubbles within the sticky gluelike meconium.

3. **C** The distinction between meconium ileus and ileal atresia prior to operation can be difficult. It is, however, extremely important, as up to 80% of cases of meconium ileus may be treated successfully without operation. In 1967, Noblett reported the use of hypertonic water soluble contrast media given via a fluoroscopically controlled enema. This contrast material fills the microcolon and obstructed terminal ileum and then passes into the dilated proximal loops (Figure 5–3). If the contrast does not reach the dilated bowel, the obstruction will not be relieved. The contrast "wets" the meconium and "loosens" it from the bowel wall. The addition of wetting agents such as Tween 80 or Mucomyst may improve results of contrast enema. Multiple contrast enemas separated by 12 to 24 hours may be necessary.

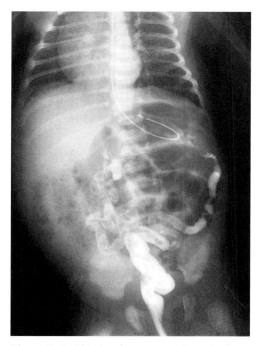

Figure 5–3. *This is a lower gastrointestinal study done with water soluble contrast. There is a "microcolon" or unused colon suggesting obstruction above this level. Multiple small "rabbit pellet" defects can be seen in the ileum and colon because of impacted meconium. The dilated bowel loops filled with air represent distended ileum behind the meconium impaction.*

This approach is only indicated in cases of uncomplicated meconium ileus, such as those without perforation, meconium peritonitis, localized volvulus, or intestinal atresia. In cases of complicated meconium ileus or whenever the obstruction cannot be relieved despite properly done contrast enemas, operation is indicated. The goal of operation in simple meconium ileus is complete evacuation of the meconium from the bowel with relief of the obstruction. Many different approaches have been advocated. These include ileostomy, ileotomy with catheter irrigation, placement of a T-tube for irrigation, and appendectomy with irrigation via the stump. For a complete discussion, refer to Andrassy and Nirgiotis, 1993.

4. **A** Meconium ileus is the earliest clinical manifestation of cystic fibrosis (CF) and is associated with CF in over 90% of cases. The severity of the bowel disease in infancy does not necessarily correlate with the severity of pulmonary complications later in life. Meconium ileus occurs in 10% to 20% of patients with CF. Cystic fibrosis is transmitted as an autosomal recessive trait, thus, both parents must be carriers. Among Caucasians, 5% to 6% are estimated to be carriers. The disease is rare in African-Americans and Asians.

5. **C** Pancreatic exocrine insufficiency is usually present at birth and pancreatic enzyme supplementation should be considered with the first feeding. With proper enzyme supplementation, gastrointestinal function is usually normal. The development of colonic strictures after high dose enzyme use has been reported. These high strength preparations have been withdrawn from the market, but many patients may still present with strictures.

6. **A** Meconium obstruction with all of the clinical and biochemical characteristics of classic meconium ileus (increased stool albumin) can occur in the absence of CF. A series of Chinese infants with meconium obstruction without CF was reported. In the absence of CF, the long-term prognosis appears to be good. All children with meconium ileus should undergo testing for CF.

7. **C** See answer to question 4.

8. **C** See answer to question 6.

BIBLIOGRAPHY

Andrassy RJ, Nirgiotis JG. Meconium disease of infancy. In: Ashcraft KW, ed. *Pediatric Surgery,* 2nd ed. Philadelphia: Saunders; 1993.

Chang PY, Huang FY, Yeh ML, et al. Meconium ileus like condition in Chinese neonates. *J Pediatr Surg.* 1992;27:1217–1219.

Kao SC, Franken EA Jr. Nonoperative treatment of simple meconium ileus: a survey of the Society for Pediatric Radiology. *Pediatr Radiol.* 1995;25(2):97–100.

Moss RL, Musemeche CA, Feddersen RM: Pan colonic fibrosis secondary to oral administration of pancreatic enzymes: a new surgical complication of cystic fibrosis. *Pediatr Surg Inter.* 1998;13:168–170.

Noblett HR. Treatment of uncomplicated meconium ileus by Gastrografin enema: a preliminary report. *J Pediatr Surg.* 1967;4:190.

A 5-YEAR-OLD BOY WITH MULTIPLE MEDICAL PROBLEMS AND ABDOMINAL PAIN

HISTORY A 5-year-old boy with trisomy 21 is transferred to your office because of recurrent vomiting episodes, this time bilious. He has severe vesicoureteral reflux and urinary incontinence treated with several abdominal operations. He now has a Mitroffanof valve—his appendix has been taken off the cecum and connects his bladder with his umbilicus—which is catheterized daily. He had a ventriculoperitoneal (VP) shunt placed at age 2 for hydrocephalus. He is reported to have frequent chest colds and his "intestines are up," but his mother was told that this problem was less important than his other ones. His bowel habit tends toward constipation (every 2 to 3 days) and is unchanged.

EXAMINATION He is able to talk and says his "tummy hurts," although no one knows when he last passed gas. Although his vital signs are normal, he vomits bilious material on your table after which he feels better. There is mild abdominal distention and some right lower quadrant tenderness to deep palpation but no guarding or rebound tenderness.

LABORATORY His white blood cell count (WBC) is 12,500 without left shift. His electrolytes, glucose, and creatinine are normal. His blood urea nitrogen (BUN) is elevated to twice normal, and his urinalysis shows ketones. Figure 6–1 shows his abdominal films and, upon reviewing these, it becomes apparent that he is known to have a congenital diaphragmatic hernia (CDH) through the foramen of Morgagni. One old report states: "Morgagni hernia containing bowel—unchanged."

Please answer all questions before proceeding to discussion section.

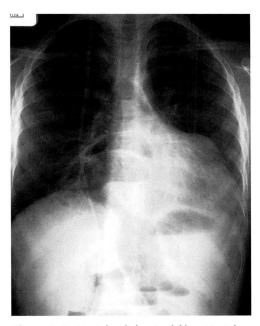

Figure 6–1. *Upright abdominal film. Upright view demonstrating ventriculoperitoneal shunt, bowel obstruction, and bowel in the chest.*

✔ QUESTIONS

1. Concerning hernias through the foramen of Morgagni (MH), which of the following is *false*?
   A. They represent 2% of all CDH

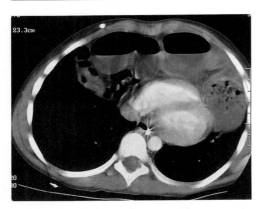

Figure 6–2. *Abdominal computed tomography scan demonstrates presence of dilated bowel loops in the mediastinum. The ventriculoperitoneal shunt is anterior.*

B. The right:left ratio is 5:1, and defects may be bilateral
C. This may explain the boy's coughing, interpreted as "chest colds"
D. They typically present at birth
E. There is an association with Down syndrome and the pentalogy of Cantrell

2. The mother asks you the following questions. To which do you answer "No."
A. Isn't MH usually asymptomatic?
B. Isn't bowel incarceration unusual?
C. Does her son need surgery for a MH if it is asymptomatic?
D. Is bowel obstruction from previous surgeries possible?
E. Is the bowel likely to be free in the chest (as opposed to being contained by a sac)?

3. You place a nasogastric (NG) tube and perform a thoracic and abdominal computed tomography (CT) scan with contrast that shows a very large MH involving the mediastinum and middle half of both hemidiaphragms (Figure 6–2). It also suggests partial small bowel obstruction in the right lower quadrant. The NG tube returns large volumes of bilious drainage associated with a rising WBC to 18,000. You decide on an operation. Concerning your selection of incision, which is *false?*
A. As a general principle acute CDHs should be approached through the abdomen, chronic CDHs through the chest
B. A McBurney incision is best
C. A thoracotomy would permit one to avoid the phrenic nerve(s) when excising the hernia sac
D. Most MHs can be fixed through a transverse supraumbilical incision
E. A midline abdominal incision is best for this patient

4. Entering the abdomen you note a loop of bowel, unappreciated on CT scan, traveling from the right lower quadrant up into a retrosternal hernia sac so large you can put your fist up into it. The proximal bowel is very distended and thick without signs of ischemia. The distal bowel is small and decompressed. There is no evidence of an obstructing lesion elsewhere in the abdomen. To your surprise, the bowel is incarcerated, and you cannot reduce it. You:
A. Extend the midline incision up to the xiphisternum to improve exposure
B. Close the abdomen and perform a right thoracotomy
C. Perform a median sternotomy
D. Place a self-retaining retractor then apply gentle traction to the bowel and attempt to dissect it from the inside of the hernia sac
E. A and D

5. You are pleased with your approach and are able to completely reduce the bowel without damage to it or the sac. Concerning repair of the defect, which answer is *false?*
A. Ideally, the sac should be excised
B. When a thoracotomy is chosen, the fifth interspace is preferred
C. Usually the posterior muscular rim can be sewn up to the xiphoid and costal margin
D. If the defect is huge, thin Goretex (1 mm) may be used

6. Anesthesia has gone well, and you have your hand up in the chest, prior to closure of the MH, when suddenly the patient's blood pressure drops, his pulse accelerates, and he becomes difficult to ventilate. The patient's arterial CO_2 is normal, and he does not feel warm. A stat chest x-ray shows no evidence of pneumothorax or hemothorax, and the endotracheal tube is correctly positioned. Rapidly, you conclude the following and make the appropriate suggestions:
   A. Latex allergy: give pressors, steroids, diphenhydramine (Benadryl)
   B. The chest x-ray is incorrect: perform bilateral needle thoracostomies: ICS2 in the mid-clavicular line
   C. Air embolism is likely: position the patient's head down in left lateral decubitus
   D. The chest x-ray is incorrect: place a left chest tube—and then a right one, if the left does not work
   E. Malignant hyperthermia: give dantrolene, avoid succinylcholine

7. Ultimately all goes well, until a precocious medical student corners you in the changing room and peppers you with difficult questions. Fortunately, the answer is "yes" to all *except:*
   A. Aren't there three sites through which MHs occur?
   B. Aren't MHs more likely to contain liver than bowel?
   C. Can I come to the next one?
   D. Aren't pericardial cysts, mediastinal teratomas, lung cysts, and paraesophageal hernias in the differential diagnosis?
   E. Aren't MHs formed when the costal and esophageal anlage of the diaphragm fail to join up with the sternal component?

ANSWERS AND DISCUSSION

1. **D** MHs probably occur more often on the right because the heart is on the left. In contrast to foramen of Bochdalek hernias that typically present with respiratory distress in the newborn, Morgagni hernias are usually asymptomatic. Often a MH is a fortuitous finding on a chest film done for other reasons. Cantrell's pentalogy includes defects of the abdominal wall, diaphragm, sternum, pericardium, and heart.

2. **E** First, her son is not asymptomatic. Probably his cough and possibly his bowel obstruction are related to his diaphragmatic hernia. Second, even an asymptomatic hernia should be fixed. Bowel incarceration is fairly uncommon but may be disastrous when it occurs. In MH, a sac is almost always present, except when associated with the pentalogy of Cantrell.

3. **B** The principle underlying **A** is that chronic hernias are more likely to be stuck to intrathoracic structures and require dissection from the interior of the intrathoracic sac. When the hernia is small and unilateral, any upper abdominal incision or a thoracic incision may be used. When it is bilateral, an abdominal incision is preferable. In this case, the patient has a bowel obstruction with dilated bowel in the lower abdomen. Since you are not certain whether bowel resection may be required, a midline incision is most versatile.

4. **E** It is early to embark on **C**, although this might be a fall-back position if the abdominal approach is unsuccessful. **B** would not permit dissection of the sac's component in the left hemithorax.

5. **B** The ninth interspace is preferred because one can extend it inferiorly through the costal margin for abdominal access if sac dissection from within the chest is difficult.

6. **A** This patient's history is quite typical for a patient with a latex allergy—a neurologically impaired child with multiple surgical procedures and daily bladder catheterizations. It would have been wise to observe latex precautions from the outset. Because patients with spinal dysraphisms and multiple exposures to latex are living longer and having more operations, latex allergy seems to be increasing. The operation should be terminated as soon as is safely possible, concomitant with the maneuvers described. If pneumothorax or hemothorax is suspected, the best solution is to look for abdominal protrusion of the diaphragm(s) and to open it if concerned. There is no reason to suspect air embolism unless a large vein has been opened or a large bolus of air inadvertently given through the IV line. Malignant hyperthermia will reliably cause CO_2 retention and increased patient temperature.

7. **C** Typically there are two slips of muscle that attach the diaphragm anteriorly to the sternum. MH can occur between these slips or to either side of them. If the student knows so much what more can you teach him?

BIBLIOGRAPHY

Kubiak R, Platen C, Schmid E, et al. Delayed appearance of bilateral Morgagni herniae in a child with Down's syndrome. *Pediatr Surg Intl.* 1998;13:600–601.

Stokes KB. Unusual varieties of diaphragmatic herniae. *Prog Pediatr. Surg.* 1991;27:127–147.

SUDDEN ABDOMINAL DISTENTION IN A 9-DAY-OLD PREMATURE INFANT

HISTORY This 34-week gestation, 1600 g female infant is born to a gravida 2, para 1, 23-year-old mother, whose pregnancy is uncomplicated until the onset of premature labor. Delivery is by repeat cesarean section. One minute Apgar score is 8. An attempt to insert an umbilical arterial catheter was unsuccessful. Respiratory distress develops shortly after delivery, manifested by tachypnea, grunting, and nasal flaring. At 2 hours of age arterial pH is 7.17. She is intubated, given oxygen and ventilatory assistance, and transported by air to a neonatal intensive care unit.

EXAMINATION She is an active female infant with endotracheal tube in place, receiving occasional breaths from the ventilator. The pulse is 140 beats per minute, rectal temperature is 36.2°C, blood pressure is 60 systolic, unassisted respirations 84 per minute. Gestational age is 34 weeks. There are no anomalies of the head, palate, trunk, or extremities. The chest expands symmetrically, with subcostal and intercostal retractions. No cardiac murmur is audible. The abdomen is soft, without masses. Peripheral pulses are full. During examination, meconium passes from the anus.

LABORATORY The hemoglobin is 16.2 gm%, and hematocrit is 48%. Arterial blood pH is 7.31, the P_{CO_2} is 47, the P_{O_2} is 32, and the F_{IO_2} is 50%. White blood cell count (WBC) is 16,200/mm^3, while segmented neutrophils are 60, lymphocytes are 36, and monocytes are 4. Platelets are 205,000 and the blood glucose level is 90 mg%. Total protein is 3.7 gm%. The x-rays or "babygrams" show diffuse alveolar infiltrates in both lungs with no abnormality of abdomen.

HOSPITAL COURSE Her respiratory status stabilizes and improves with oxygen and assisted ventilation. Phototherapy is given for hyperbilirubinemia. Gavage feedings are begun on the fifth hospital day, and she tolerates them well. She is weaned from the ventilator and is extubated on the seventh hospital day. A continuous cardiac murmur of

31

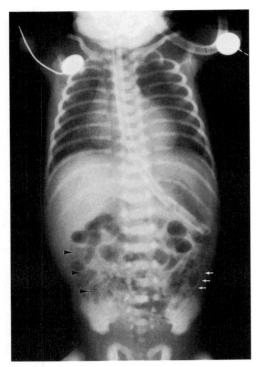

Figure 7–1. *Babygram, supine view, showing extensive pneumatosis intestinalis appearing as bubbles (black arrows) and streaks (white arrows) in the bowel.*

patent ductus arteriosus (PDA) is noted on the eighth hospital day, but there is no evidence of cardiac failure. The murmur disappears after she receives a course (three doses) of indomethacin. On the ninth hospital day, she suddenly develops abdominal distention and vomits. She becomes dusky and cyanotic and passes a bloody, foul-smelling stool. Cultures of blood and cerebrospinal fluid are obtained, and antibiotics are given. An orogastric tube is inserted and drains thick bilious material. A bolus of intravenous saline is given. Abdominal films are obtained (Figures 7–1 and 7–2). Abdominal paracentesis yields 3 mL of mahogany-colored fluid, whose Gram stain shows gram-positive rods.

Please answer all questions before proceeding to discussion section.

✓ QUESTIONS

1. Relative indications for operation in necrotizing enterocolitis (NEC) of the neonate include all of the following, *except:*
   A. Pneumatosis intestinalis
   B. Pneumoperitoneum
   C. Portal venous gas on x-ray
   D. A fixed loop on serial abdominal films
   E. Erythema of the abdominal wall

2. A positive paracentesis in NEC consists of:
   A. Brown fluid
   B. Bacteria on Gram stain of the peritoneal fluid
   C. Peritoneal WBC greater than 500/mm³
   D. A and B are correct
   E. A, B, and C are correct

HOSPITAL COURSE After resuscitation, including endotracheal intubation, the infant's vital signs stabilize, and she is taken to the operating room. At exploratory laparotomy, the findings are gangrene of the distal ileum with an ileal perforation. Most of the colon is also gangrenous, with the exception of a 3 cm "skip area" in the transverse colon. The distal sigmoid colon and rectum are viable.

3. The optimal operation is:
   A. Ileocolic resection and end-to-end anastomosis
   B. Right hemicolectomy (including distal ileum), left colectomy, four enterostomies

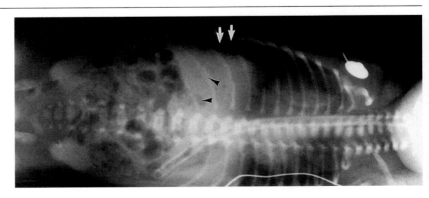

Figure 7–2. *Babygram, left lateral decubitus view, showing pneumatosis intestinalis, pneumoperitoneum (white arrows) and gas in the portal veins (black arrows).*

    C. Ileocolic resection, double enterostomy
    D. Proximal ileostomy, second-look laparotomy after 24 to 48 hours
    E. None of the above

4. A fulminant form of NEC is associated with:
    A. *Klebsiella pneumoniae*
    B. *Clostridium difficile*
    C. *Clostridium perfringens*
    D. *Candida albicans*
    E. Indomethacin administration

5. All of the following statements about the pathology of NEC are true, *except:*
    A. The necrosis may be patchy, with skip areas of normal bowel
    B. Thrombi in mesenteric arteries and veins are a frequent operative finding
    C. The ileocecal area is the site most commonly involved
    D. The bullae of pneumatosis intestinalis may be seen on gross inspection of the bowel
    E. Mucosal necrosis may occur without necrosis of the muscularis

6. Which of the following statements about the late complications of NEC is true?
    A. Intestinal stricture usually occurs in the ileum
    B. Perineal fistulas develop in 5% to 10% of cases
    C. Intra-abdominal abscess is the most frequent complication
    D. Malabsorption following NEC usually involves protein and fat but rarely carbohydrate
    E. None of the above

7. The following statements regarding enterostomy in NEC are true, *except:*
    A. The bowel ends should be brought out separately at any location where they reach the abdominal wall without tension
    B. The complication rate is similar for stomas brought through the abdominal incision and stomas brought through a separate stab wound
    C. A contrast study of the distal bowel should always be done prior to enterostomy closure
    D. Early enterostomy closure decreases the risk of complication from fluid and electrolyte losses
    E. Early enterostomy closure decreases the risk of stricture in the distal bowel

8. A 29-week, 1000 g premature infant survives after resection and ileostomy for NEC. Four weeks later, he has regained his birth weight but is unable to gain any further. He receives 120 calories per day of elemental formula by gavage feedings, which he tolerates well, without vomiting or abdominal distention. His ileostomy appears healthy and functions well. Laboratory studies are Hb 12.5 g; Hct 37%; WBC 10,000/mm³; differential: normal; Na 138; K 4.5; Cl 99; CO_2 25; BUN 8; glucose 70; pH 7.38. Which *one* of the following studies is most likely to identify a cause for his poor weight gain?
    A. Stool for reducing substances
    B. Serum levels of albumin and prealbumin

C. Liver function tests
D. Urinary sodium
E. Serum alpha-fetoprotein

9. Results of the additional laboratory studies in the above infant are as follows: Stool reducing substances: negative ×2; albumin 3.8 g; prealbumin pending (sent to a reference laboratory in California); bilirubin total 1.6 mg; direct bilirubin 0.9 mg; alkaline phosphatase, ALT, and AST: all normal; urinary sodium 4 mEq/L; AFP 138,700 ng/mL. Which *one* of the following is the best management of this problem?
   A. Insertion of central line for parenteral nutrition (in addition to oral intake)
   B. A change of formula to a soy preparation
   C. The addition of glutamine powder to the elemental formula
   D. An increase of dietary sodium to 5 to 7 mEq/day
   E. Resection of a liver tumor

ANSWERS AND DISCUSSION

1. **A** Pneumatosis intestinalis alone is not an indication for operation, since it is a reversible finding in about 50% to 60% of babies who receive vigorous and early medical treatment. Pneumoperitoneum (**B**) is recognized almost universally as an indication for operation in NEC. Portal venous gas (**C**) is an ominous sign usually seen in the sickest infants. Although some pediatric surgeons disagree, data from several centers support its inclusion among the indications. The fixed loop (**D**) and erythema of the abdominal wall (**E**) are signs that are predictive of intestinal gangrene and the need for operation, but they are not often present.

2. **D** Paracentesis findings of brown fluid or bacteria or both on Gram stain signify the presence of gangrenous gut and indicate the need for immediate operation. Most infants with ischemic bowel have ascitic fluid, which may be sampled by gentle aspiration with a 22- or 25-gauge needle inserted in the lateral abdomen or flank. The WBC count of the fluid (**C**) has not correlated with gangrene, although it is elevated in peritonitis.

3. **C** The principles of operation for NEC are (1) resection of gangrenous bowel; (2) exteriorization of the marginally viable ends; and (3) preservation of as much intestinal length as possible. Thus, the operation of choice is resection and double enterostomy (Figure 7–3; see also color plate). Primary anastomosis (**A**) is not performed in acute NEC by the majority of pediatric surgeons because the ischemia is progressive, risking subsequent anastomotic breakdown and peritonitis or anastomotic stricture. Further, the surgeon who does primary anastomosis may resect more bowel than necessary in order to ensure viability of the bowel ends. Resection and quadruple enterostomy (**B**) are not a good choice. The added risk of prolonging the operation to create four stomas outweighs any benefit of preserving 3 cm of transverse colon. Proximal enterostomy and a second-look operation (**D**) is an option for extensive NEC (pannecrosis), which is almost always fatal, but not for segmental involvement, which this infant appears to have.

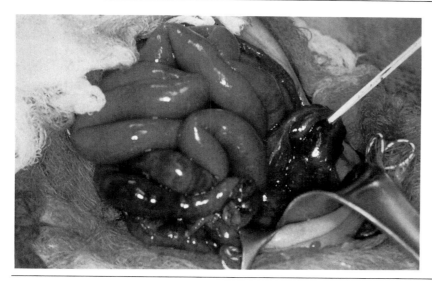

Figure 7–3. *Operative photograph of infant with necrotizing enterocolitis, showing gangrenous loops of ileum and colon in the foreground. There is a perforation of the ileum. The jejunum (in the background) is viable. (See also color plate.)*

4. **C** The most fulminant form of NEC, with a mortality as high as 87%, is associated with *C. perfringens*. This organism, which is the agent of gas gangrene, may be an innocuous member of the normal flora of the neonatal gut. In the presence of devitalized tissue, however, *C. perfringens* produces a deadly array of exotoxins, which cause hemolysis, rapidly advancing necrosis, and formation of large amounts of gas in the tissues. *Klebsiella pneumoniae* (**A**), also a member of the normal flora, is the organism most frequently found in the peritoneal fluid or blood of infants with severe NEC, but it is not as lethal as *C. perfringens*. *C. difficile* (**B**), the agent of antibiotic-associated (pseudomembranous) colitis, may colonize neonates, but it is rarely associated with NEC. *Candida albicans* (**D**) is a major pathogen of very low birth weight (VLBW) infants but does not produce the extreme toxicity of the bacterial pathogens. The role of indomethacin (**E**) in the pathogenesis of NEC is controversial. The drug, which is widely used for closure of patent ductus arteriosus in premature infants, is also a constrictor of the mesenteric vessels, and theoretically might induce ischemic damage to the gut. The vast majority of infants who receive the drug, however, never develop NEC. This issue is discussed further in Case 63 (patent ductus arteriosus).

5. **B** Thrombi in mesenteric arteries and veins are rarely found at operation, although they may be seen at autopsy. This pattern suggests that vascular thrombosis is a late event in NEC, following low flow in the mesenteric vessels, sepsis, and coagulopathy. The intestinal necrosis of NEC is typically patchy, with skip areas (**A**) of normal bowel between affected segments. The ileocecal region is the site most frequently involved (**C**). Pneumatosis intestinalis may sometimes be identified on gross inspection by the surgeon or pathologist. Mucosal necrosis (**E**) is an early event, followed by one of three outcomes: (1) extension of the necrotic process through the bowel wall, leading to gangrene and perforation; (2) extension into the muscularis, leading to stricture formation; or (3) mucosal healing with complete resolution of the process.

6. **E** None of the statements is true. Intestinal stricture (**A**) occurs in 15% to 25% of cases, usually in the colon. Fistulas (**B**) may develop between adjacent loops of bowel or between intestine and skin, but almost never in the perineum. Intra-abdominal abscess (**C**) from a walled-off perforation is surprisingly rare. Malabsorption (**D**), especially disaccharide malabsorption, is a frequent sequela. The baby may require feedings of an elemental formula for a prolonged period after recovery from NEC.

7. **A** Although "bring 'em out where they lie" was once advocated, evidence supports bringing out the two stomas close to one another in order to facilitate subsequent enterostomy closure. Mobilization of one of the stomas may be required at the initial operation but can be accomplished quickly. All of the other statements are true. Bringing the stomas through the laparotomy incision (**B**) does not increase the risk of wound complications. A contrast study of the distal bowel *must* be done before enterostomy closure (**C**), to rule out a stricture downstream. Evidence supports early enterostomy closure, which may decrease fluid and electrolyte imbalance (**D**) and may even decrease the risk of distal stricture (**E**).

8. **D** This infant with an ileostomy has excessive loss of sodium, which is diagnosed by an abnormally low urinary sodium level (less than 10 mEq/L). The serum sodium usually remains in the normal range, even in the face of a severe deficit of total body sodium. Bicarbonate losses from the ileostomy may result in metabolic acidosis as well. Reducing substances in the stool (**A**) are positive with disaccharide intolerance, which cannot occur when elemental (monosaccharide) formula is fed. Low serum albumin and especially prealbumin (**B**) reflect malnutrition, but the albumin in this infant is in the normal range. Liver function tests (**C**) in this infant show minimal abnormality, and serum alpha-fetoprotein (AFP) (**E**) is in the normal range. (Normal AFP at birth ranges from 10,000 to 180,000 ng/mL, falling to less than 1000 ng/mL by 60 days of age.)

9. **D** Sodium requirements are doubled in infants with enterostomies, from about 2.5 to 3.5 mEq/kg/day to 5 to 7 mEq/kg/day. Thus, the addition of sodium to the formula (or closure of the ileostomy) will correct the problem. Parenteral nutrition (**A**) is not needed in this infant since the sodium deficit can be corrected by oral means. (Axiom: enteral nutrition is safer than parenteral nutrition!) Soy formula (**B**) is preferred for infants with lactose intolerance, which is not the problem in this case. The amino acid glutamine (**C**) is the primary fuel of the enterocyte. It is present in elemental formulas and is not administered as a powder. The serum AFP level is in the normal range and is not indicative of a liver tumor (**E**).

HOSPITAL COURSE (*CONT.*)   The gangrenous bowel (ileum and colon) is resected, and double enterostomy is performed. In spite of vigorous supportive measures postoperatively, the enterostomy stomas become dusky, and urine output is minimal. At second-look laparotomy, performed 24 hours later, necrosis of virtually all of the remaining small and large bowel is found. No resection is performed. The baby dies 5 hours later. Pertinent autopsy findings are prematurity (34 weeks); extensive necrotizing enterocolitis; bilateral bronchopneumonia and atelectasis; and patent ductus arteriosus. Peritoneal fluid at operation had a heavy growth of *C. perfringens.* At autopsy, the fluid contained *C. perfringens, Klebsiella pneumoniae,* and *Streptococcus fecalis.*

BIBLIOGRAPHY

Albanese CT, Rowe MI. Necrotizing enterocolitis. In: O'Neill JA Jr, Rowe MI, Grosfeld JL, et al. eds. *Pediatric Surgery,* 5th ed. St. Louis: Mosby; 1998.

Ballance WA, Dahms BB, Shenker N, et al. Pathology of necrotizing enterocolitis. *J Pediatr.* 1990;199:S6–S13.

Bower TA, Pringle KC, Soper RT. Sodium deficit causing decreased weight gain and metabolic acidosis in infants with ileostomy. *J Pediatr Surg.* 1988;23:567–572.

Cooper A, Ross AJ III, O'Neill JA Jr, et al. Resection with primary anastomosis for necrotizing enterocolitis: a contrasting view. *J Pediatr Surg.* 1988;23:64–68.

Gertler JP, Seashore JH, Touloukain RJ. Early ileostomy closure in necrotizing enterocolitis. *J Pediatr Surg.* 1987;22:140–143.

Grosfeld JL, Chaet M, Molinari F, et al. Increased risk of necrotizing enterocolitis in premature infants with patent ductus arteriosus treated with indomethacin. *Ann Surg.* 1996;224:350–357.

Grosfeld JL, Cheu H, Schlatter M, et al. Changing trends in necrotizing enterocolitis: experience with 302 cases in two decades. *Ann Surg.* 1991;214:300–307.

Kosloske AM. Indications for operation in necrotizing enterocolitis revisited. *J Pediatr Surg.* 1994;29:663–666.

Kosloske AM. Necrotizing enterocolitis. In: Oldham KT, Colombani PM, Foglia RP, eds. *Surgery of Infants and Children: Scientific Principles and Practice.* Philadelphia: Lippincott-Raven; 1997:1201–1214.

Kosloske AM, Ball WS Jr, Umland E, et al. Clostridial necrotizing enterocolitis. *J Pediatr Surg.* 1985;20:155–159.

Musemeche CA, Kosloske AM, Ricketts RR. Enterostomy in necrotizing enterocolitis: an analysis of techniques and timing of closure. *J Pediatr Surg.* 1987;22:479–483.

Schwartz KB, Ternberg J, Bell MJ, et al. Sodium needs of infants and children with ileostomy. *J Pediatr.* 1983;102:509–513.

Tsuchida Y, Endo Y, Saito S, et al. Evaluation of alpha-fetoprotein in early infancy. *J Pediatr Surg.* 1978;13:155–156.

A 3.5-YEAR-OLD BOY WHO WALKS HOLDING HIS RIGHT SIDE

HISTORY   A 3.5-year-old boy develops abdominal pain 36 hours prior to admission. He cries and hold his epigastric area. Later he has three episodes of vomiting and a loose bowel movement. His mother gives him Pepto Bismol for the flu, and he goes to bed. The next morning, the pain is intense in the right side of the abdomen. He walks slowly, holding his right side. No one else in the family is ill. His parents drive him more than 100 miles to the emergency room.

EXAMINATION   He is a listless 3.5-year-old boy, lying still and crying softly. His pulse is 118 beats per minute, rectal temperature 38.4°C, respirations 40 per minute. His mucous membranes are dry, and his eyes are sunken. Tonsils are moderately enlarged. Lungs are clear to auscultation. No cardiac murmur is audible. The abdomen is moderately distended with hypoactive bowel sounds. There is generalized tenderness in all quadrants that is greatest in the right lower quadrant. Rebound tenderness is noted, referred to the right lower quadrant. Rectal examination elicits tenderness on both sides.

LABORATORY   Hematocrit is 38%, and WBC is 19,000/mm³ with segmented neutrophils at 83, bands at 7, lymphocytes at 7, eosinophils at 1, and monocytes at 2. Urinalysis reveals that the urine is gold, with a specific gravity of 1.032. The pH is 6.0, protein is 1+, acetone is 3+, glucose is negative, WBC is 5 to 10/hpf, RBC is 1 to 2/hpf, and casts are few granular. Chest x-ray is normal. Abdominal x-rays are not done.

HOSPITAL COURSE   He receives a bolus of intravenous fluid, antibiotics, nasogastric suction, and a Tylenol rectal suppository. He is given a dose of IV Demerol (0.5 mg/kg), which relieves his pain. After 3 hours, his condition is improved, and appendectomy is performed. Pus and loculations are found in the right lower quadrant, but no abscess cavity is present. The appendix is gangrenous, with a perforation from a fecalith near its midpoint. The omentum is nearby but is not adherent to the appendix. After appendectomy, the right lower quadrant and pelvis are irrigated with about 500 mL of saline. No drains are used. The McBurney incision is closed (after a change of gloves, using clean instruments), including the skin, which is closed loosely. Postoperatively, he is febrile for 48 hours, then becomes afebrile. Nasogastric suction is discontinued on the third postoperative day, and he tolerates oral feedings. Intravenous antibiotics are given for 1 week postoperatively. The wound heals primarily. He is discharged home on the evening of the seventh hospital day.

Please answer all questions before proceeding to discussion section.

✓ QUESTIONS

1. Acute appendicitis may present with a variety of signs and symptoms. The *most* important, single finding in establishing the diagnosis, however, is:
    A. Periumbilical pain that migrates to the right lower quadrant
    B. Persistent right lower quadrant abdominal tenderness
    C. Rebound tenderness
    D. Right-sided tenderness on rectal examination
    E. WBC greater than 12,000/mm³

2. Of the following diagnoses, which one is *most* difficult to differentiate from acute appendicitis?
    A. Right lower lobe pneumonia
    B. Pyelonephritis
    C. Pelvic inflammatory disease
    D. Primary peritonitis

3. Acute appendicitis in a 3-year-old child is a different disease from acute appendicitis in an adult. The following reasons for this difference all are true, *except:*
    A. The short, filmy omentum of the child is relatively ineffective in localizing infection
    B. Immunologic defense mechanisms, especially opsinization and phagocytosis of bacteria, are relatively ineffective in the child
    C. The delicate, thin-walled appendix of the child undergoes rapid necrosis and perforation
    D. The child is frequently unable to voice his complaints

4. The imaging study that is indicated in the *majority* of cases of perforated appendicitis in children is:
    A. Supine and upright views of the abdomen
    B. Barium enema
    C. Abdominal and pelvic ultrasound
    D. Abdominal and pelvic CT scan
    E. None of the above

5. In children under 2 years of age with appendicitis, the incidence of appendiceal perforation noted at appendectomy is:
    A. Greater than 80%
    B. Fifty percent
    C. Thirty percent
    D. Less than 20%

6. Which of the following statements is true regarding perforated appendicitis in children?
   A. Anaerobic bacteria, such as *Bacteroides,* are rarely present with gross perforation
   B. The presenting signs may be diarrhea, fever, and abdominal distention
   C. Wound infection occurs as a postoperative complication in 15% to 20% of cases
   D. Intra-abdominal or pelvic abscess occurs as a postoperative complication in 15% to 20% of cases
   E. Intestinal obstruction from adhesions occurs as a postoperative complication in 15% to 20% of cases

7. A combination of *therapeutic* antibiotics that is likely to be effective in a child with perforated appendicitis includes all of the following, *except:*
   A. A first-generation cephalosporin and metronidazole
   B. A second-generation cephalosporin and metronidazole
   C. Gentamicin and clindamycin
   D. Ampicillin, gentamicin, and clindamycin
   E. Ampicillin, gentamicin, and metronidazole

8. *Perioperative* antibiotics are recommended for *early* acute appendicitis. Which of the following is optimal timing for administration of perioperative antibiotics?
   A. Begin 12 to 24 hours prior to operation, continue for 24 hours postoperatively
   B. A single dose 2 hours prior to operation
   C. A dose with induction of anesthesia, continue for 24 hours postoperatively
   D. A dose at the end of operation, continue for 48 hours postoperatively
   E. None of the above

9. Which of the following statements is true regarding appendectomy in children?
   A. If perforation is suspected, a midline incision should be made to facilitate exposure
   B. Purse-string inversion of the appendiceal stump is not necessary
   C. Routine cultures of the peritoneal fluid should be done for aerobic and anaerobic bacteria
   D. When the skin is closed, the wound infection rate for acute appendicitis without perforation is 15% to 20%
   E. When the skin is closed, the wound infection rate for acute appendicitis with perforation is 15% to 20%

10. The insertion of transperitoneal drains following appendectomy in a child with perforated appendicitis provides which *one* of the following advantages (compared to not draining)?
    A. A decreased risk of intra-abdominal abscess
    B. A decreased risk of postoperative adhesions
    C. A decreased risk of all postoperative complications
    D. A shorter hospital stay
    E. None of the above

ANSWERS AND DISCUSSION

1. **B** Persistent right lower quadrant abdominal tenderness is the most important single finding in the diagnosis of acute appendicitis. Periumbilical pain that later migrates to the right lower quadrant (**A**) is the classic course often found in older children and adults. Children under the age of five, however, rarely follow classic courses, and the disease may progress to perforation without a clinical stage of localized pain and tenderness. Rebound tenderness (**C**), especially that referred to the right lower quadrant (Rovsing's sign) is a valuable sign when present, but occurs relatively late in the course of appendicitis, after inflammation of the parietal peritoneum has developed. It is not present in early appendicitis. Right-sided tenderness on rectal examination (**D**) is an excellent diagnostic sign for the inflamed pelvic appendix, but it is not present in intra-abdominal appendicitis or retrocecal appendicitis. A WBC greater than 12,000/mm^3 (**E**) is a nonspecific index of bacterial infection at any site.

2. **D** Primary peritonitis is virtually always diagnosed at operation for acute appendicitis and, thus, is the most difficult diagnosis among the choices given in this question. The most common organisms found in the peritoneal fluid in this condition are *Streptococcus pneumoniae,* other streptococci, and *Escherichia coli.* Primary peritonitis is often associated with renal or hepatic conditions in which ascites is present. Right lower lobe pneumonia (**A**) may present with right-sided abdominal pain, but generally physical examination and chest roentgenogram will identify it. Rarely, acute appendicitis and right lower lobe pneumonia occur simultaneously. Pyelonephritis (**B**) usually can be differentiated on the basis of pus cells and white cell casts in the urine and maximal tenderness in the flank. Appendicitis, however, occasionally produces pyuria if the appendix lies adjacent to the ureter or bladder. Pelvic inflammatory disease (**C**) is difficult to differentiate from appendicitis in the teenage girl. A history of sexual activity, exquisite cervical tenderness, or chronicity of the pain support the diagnosis of salpingitis. Imaging studies that may be helpful in this situation are ultrasound examination, barium enema or both. (More about imaging of appendicitis in question 4.)

3. **B** Immunologic defenses of a normal 3-year-old child are comparable to that of the normal adult. Although opsinization and phagocytosis of bacteria are diminished in the newborn infant, these functions reach adult levels of effectiveness at 1 month of age. The statements regarding the short filmy omentum, the thin-walled appendix, and the child's inability to voice his complaints are all correct.

4. **E** Routine imaging is not indicated. The majority of children with appendicitis, perforated or not, require no imaging study at all. In many centers, imaging is overused by primary care physicians who are unsure of the diagnosis. In this situation, the appropriate (and cost-effective) management is surgical consultation, not a trip to the radiology department. The studies should be used *selectively,* in cases in which the surgeon needs more data before making the decision

for (or against) appendectomy. Routine views of the abdomen (**A**) may show focal ileus in the right lower quadrant, which supports the diagnosis, or a calcified appendicolith, which is pathognomonic for appendicitis. Conversely, a colon packed with stool usually implicates constipation rather than appendicitis as the source of the abdominal pain. Barium enema (**B**) or abdominal-pelvic ultrasound (**C**) are particularly useful in the evaluation of teenaged girls with abdominal pain, in whom tubal or ovarian pathology may mimic appendicitis. Findings on barium enema that support the diagnosis of appendicitis include nonvisualization of the appendix, partial filling of the appendix, pressure defects on the cecum, and irritability of cecum or terminal ileum. The ultrasound is ideal for identification of abnormalities of the fallopian tubes or ovaries, or it may show a swollen, tubular mass (the inflamed appendix) in the right lower quadrant. The accuracy of ultrasound, like many radiographic studies, is operator-dependent. Computed tomography (CT) scans are generally useful later in the course of the disease, after perforation, abscess formation, and antibiotic treatment have obscured the clinical picture. The nonsurgical literature focuses on the sensitivity and specificity of these imaging studies, usually avoiding the fact that they are not necessary in the majority of cases of appendicitis in children.

5. **A** The incidence of appendiceal perforation in children under two is greater than 80%. Grosfeld reported a perforation rate of 94%, a morbidity of 50%, and a mortality of 9.3%. He advocated an "admit and observe" policy for any child under two with the suspicion of appendicitis. Perforated appendicitis in the newborn infant may be associated with necrotizing enterocolitis (NEC) or may be the presenting manifestation of Hirschsprung disease, when colonic distention leads to a "blow-out" of the appendix.

6. **B** A child under 2 or 3 years of age who presents with diarrhea, fever, and abdominal distention may have acute appendicitis with perforation without ever having localized tenderness in the right lower quadrant. Diarrhea or tenesmus may occur if an inflamed appendix lies adjacent to the rectum. Rectal exam is mandatory in this scenario. A tender mass may help to distinguish appendicitis from gastroenteritis. Abdominal distention is not a common finding in gastroenteritis, although it sometimes accompanies the severe enteritides (eg, *Salmonella* or *Shigella*). The child who is dehydrated and febrile should not go directly to the operating room because the administration of general anesthesia to such a child invites cardiac arrest and other complications. Preoperative preparation (as performed in this case) is mandatory, including hydration, nasogastric suction, reduction of fever, IV antibiotics, and relief of pain. The "resuscitation" may last 1 to 6 hours, after which appendectomy is carried out. Anaerobic bacteria, such as *Bacteroides* (**A**), are the most common inhabitants of the gastrointestinal tract and are invariably present with perforated appendicitis. A culture of the peritoneal fluid does not always identify them, however, because tissue antibiotic levels may suppress their growth, or improper handling of the specimen (eg, failure to transport the specimen in appropriate media, or failure to plate and incubate the specimen under proper anaerobic conditions) has occurred. The role of anaerobes in surgi-

cal infections was not appreciatd until the 1960s and 1970s when Altemeier and associates established their importance. The three most common complications of perforated appendicitis are wound infection (**C**), abdominal or pelvic abscess (**D**), and intestinal obstruction from adhesions (**E**). Pediatric series of the past two decades have reported *overall* complication rates from 7% to 20%; a rate of 15% to 20% for an individual complication is too high by current standards.

7. **A** The underlying principle in choosing antibiotics for peritonitis from bowel perforation is efficacy against both aerobic and anaerobic pathogens. The classic pathogens of experimental peritonitis are *E. coli* in the early phase and *Bacteroides fragilis* in the late, abscess phase. A first-generation cephalosporin and metronidazole (**A**) is the exception because it leaves a gap in the coverage of both the Enterobacteriaceae (eg, *E. coli, Klebsiella*) and enterococcus (ie, *S. fecalis*). A second-generation cephalosporin and metronidazole (**B**) is better against gram-negatives but still does not cover the enterococcus. Although the pathogenicity of enterococcus has been debated for adults, it is a recognized pediatric pathogen. Gentamicin and clindamycin (**C**) is a popular combination in adult colon surgery. Most pediatric surgeons add ampicillin (**D**) or (**E**) to the combination to cover the enterococcus. "Triple therapy" remains the standard for perforated appendicitis in children.

8. **C** Administration of perioperative antibiotics should be timed to achieve peak levels in the surgical wound when the (anticipated) contamination occurs. Thus, an IV dose with induction of anesthesia is recommended. Preoperative administration (**A**) usually misses the peak. Two hours prior to operation is too early (**B**), and the end of the operation (**D**) is too late. *Therapeutic* antibiotics should be continued as long as an inflammatory process persists. For early appendicitis, one to three doses suffice. For perforated appendicitis, most pediatric surgeons consider 7 days of IV antibiotic therapy appropriate. Gangrenous appendicitis, which has pathologic changes intermediate between the early and perforated stages, usually requires an intermediate duration of antibiotic treatment (eg, 3 or 4 days). The hospital stay is also commensurate with the pathologic stage of appendicitis. In the Montreal series of 420 children treated in the late 1980s, the average stay was 2.1 days after simple acute appendicitis, 3.7 days after gangrenous appendicitis, and 7.8 days after perforated appendicitis. Even with today's shorter hospital stays, this stratification of severity of illness and duration of necessary treatment holds true.

9. **B** Purse-string inversion of the appendiceal stump is not necessary. Many good surgeons simply ligate it. All of the other statements are false. A midline incision (**A**) affords better exposure than a muscle-splitting incision in the right lower quadrant but has a greater risk of poor healing. Routine cultures (**C**) rarely, if ever, change patient management and are not cost effective. Cultures should be reserved for complicated cases (eg, immunosuppressed patients, patients on prior antibiotic therapy, etc.) Wound infection rates in children are lower than those of adults. A wound infection rate of 15% to 20% is too high, both for nonperforated (**D**) and perforated (**E**) appendici-

tis. In two large studies of appendicitis from the Children's Hospitals of Buffalo and Montreal, the skin was closed in all cases, yet the wound infection rates reported were remarkably low: 3% and 1.7%, respectively. In a study of postoperative wound infection in children from New Mexico, the infection rate was 7.9% for contaminated wounds and 6.3% for clean wounds. One third of the most contaminated wounds were packed open and allowed to heal by granulation.

10. **E** Transperitoneal drainage of perforated appendicitis in children was a mainstay of therapy in the preantibiotic and early antibiotic eras, when perforated appendicitis carried a substantial mortality. The protocol of Robert E. Gross, a strong advocate of drainage, influenced generations of American pediatric surgeons. The excellent results of his Boston series occurred at a time when the only antibiotics were sulfadiazene, penicillin, and streptomycin, and limited information was available regarding the administration and pharmacokinetics of antibiotics. In the past two decades, the timely, appropriate use of antibiotic agents that are effective against both aerobic and anaerobic bacteria might obviate the need for drains. Two randomized series, one from Johns Hopkins, the other from New Mexico, compared drainage and antibiotics versus antibiotics alone in children with perforated appendicitis. The complication rate in both series was similar for drained and undrained children. The children with drains, however, had a significantly longer time in the hospital. Thus, the data do not support drainage of perforated appendicitis, unless a well-developed abscess is present. The authors of these studies have abandoned transperitoneal drainage for ruptured appendicitis in children.

BIBLIOGRAPHY

Altemeier WA. Bodily response to infectious agents. *JAMA.* 1967;202(12): 1085–1089.

Azizkhan RG. Appropriate use of antibiotics in infants and children with infections. In: Fonkalsrud EW, Krummel TM, eds. *Infections and Immunologic Disorders in Pediatric Surgery.* Philadelphia: Saunders; 1993; 153–168.

Bhattacharyya N, Kosloske AM. Postoperative wound infection in pediatric surgical patients: a study of 676 infants and children. *J Pediatr Surg.* 1990;25:125–129.

Bleacher JC, Krummel TM. Host resistance to infection. In: Fonkalsrud EW, Krummel TM, eds. *Infections and Immunologic Disorders in Pediatric Surgery.* Philadelphia: Saunders; 1993:63–75.

Grosfeld JL, Weinberger M, Clatworthy HW Jr. Acute appendicitis in the first two years of life. *J Pediatr Surg.* 1973;8:285–292.

Haller AJ, Shaker IJ, Donahoo JS, et al. Peritoneal drainage versus nondrainage for generalized peritonitis from ruptured appendicitis in children: a prospective study. *Ann Surg.* 1973;177:595–600.

Johnson DA, Kosloske AM, Macarthur CM. Perforated appendicitis in children: to drain or not to drain? *Pediatr Surg Int.* 1993;8:402–405.

Karp MP, Caldarola VA, Cooney DR, et al. The avoidable excesses in the management of perforated appendicitis in children. *J Pediatr Surg.* 1986;21:506–510.

Kosloske AM. Wound infections, drains, and irrigation in pediatric surgery. In: Fonkalsrud EW, Krummel TM, eds. *Infections and Immunologic Disorders in Pediatric Surgery.* Philadelphia: Saunders; 1993:177–182.

Neilson IR, Laberge J-M, Nguyen LT, et al. Appendicitis in children: current therapeutic recommendations. *J Pediatr Surg.* 1990;25:1113–1116.

Schwartz MZ, Tapper D, Solenberger RI. Management of perforated appendicitis in children. *Ann Surg.* 1983;197:407–411.

Stone HH. Bacterial flora of appendicitis in children. *J Pediatr Surg.* 1976; 11:37–42.

A 6-YEAR-OLD BOY WITH CRAMPY ABDOMINAL PAIN AND VOMITING

HISTORY You are called by the local emergency room to evaluate a 6-year-old boy with abdominal pain and vomiting. The boy was well until 8 hours ago when he was seized with midabdominal pain. The pain lasted for 5 minutes or so and then subsided. It has recurred several times per hour. The patient has been vomiting coffee ground material mixed with food. His last bowel movement was yesterday. His parents relate a history of similar episodes in the past that were less severe and resolved spontaneously.

EXAMINATION The child appears a bit pale and is in obvious discomfort. Temperature is 37.3°C; heart rate is 98; blood pressure is 110/70; respiratory rate is 20. He has distinctive pigmented melanotic spots of his lips, buccal mucosa, and palms of his hands (Figure 9–1; see also color plate). These lesions are 3 to 5 mm in size, and they are flat. The heart and lungs are normal. The abdomen is moderately distended. Rectal examination reveals maroon stool.

LABORATORY Hemoglobin 8.6; hematocrit 25; white blood cell count 8.5 with a normal differential. Urinalysis shows 2+ protein with no white or red blood cells.

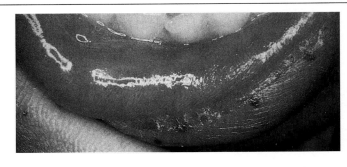

Figure 9–1. *Appearance of the lower lip in a 6-year-old boy with abdominal pain and vomiting. (From Misiewicz JJ et al. Atlas of Clinical Gastroenterology. 2nd ed. London, Wolfe-Mosby; 1994.) (See also color plate.)*

Please answer all questions before proceeding to discussion section.

✓ QUESTIONS

1. The most likely diagnosis is:
   A. Metastatic melanoma to the small intestine
   B. Ileocolic intussusception
   C. Midgut volvulus
   D. Peutz-Jeghers syndrome
   E. Henoch-Schoenlein purpura

2. Which of the following is true regarding this disease?
   A. It is inherited in an autosomal dominant fashion
   B. It is rarely associated with malignancy
   C. It most commonly affects the right colon
   D. Eighty percent of patients develop signs and symptoms in the first 10 years of life
   E. Operation is often required, but life expectancy is normal

3. The intestinal polyps in this syndrome are:
   A. Adenomatous
   B. Hamartomas
   C. Sometimes large enough to obstruct the lumen
   D. Hyperplastic mucosa
   E. Found only in the small intestine

4. You admit this patient to the hospital for observation, and he develops signs of a complete bowel obstruction. Which of the following would be included in the treatment plan?
   A. Barium enema
   B. Air enema
   C. Resection of multiple polyps with possible use of intraoperative endoscopy
   D. Short segment resection of the involved bowel via a small right lower quadrant incision
   E. Therapeutic upper gastrointestinal endoscopy

5. Which of the following tumors are associated with this syndrome?
   A. Testicular neoplasms
   B. Adenocarcinoma of the colon
   C. Ovarian tumors
   D. Adenocarcinoma of the cervix
   E. All of the above

6. The life expectancy of patients with this syndrome is:
   A. Normal
   B. Normal with aggressive surgical treatment
   C. Markedly reduced
   D. Dependent on whether the abnormality is inherited or spontaneous
   E. Greater in women than men

ANSWERS AND DISCUSSION

1. **D** This patient has findings suggestive of a small bowel intussusception. This finding associated with the typical mucocutaneous pigmentation are classic for Puetz-Jeghers syndrome. This syndrome, first reported in 1921, consists of polyposis of the intestinal tract and melanin spots on the face and hands.

   Melanoma is rare in children and even rarer presenting as a small bowel metastasis. The melanin spots on the patient's face and hands are caused by Peutz-Jeghers syndrome rather than neoplasm. Ileocolic intussusception typically occurs between age 3 months and 3 years. When intussusception occurs outside of this age range, it is usually because of a pathologic "lead point," and is most common in the small bowel. This patient probably has a small bowel intussusception caused by an intestinal polyp acting as a lead point.

   Midgut volvulus can present at any age. This disorder causes an acute and complete obstruction of the distal duodenum. It is associated with bilious vomiting and severe acute abdominal pain. In addition, x-rays in this case suggest a mid to distal bowel obstruction as opposed to the proximal obstruction seen in midgut volvulus. Henoch-Schoenlein purpura causes purpuric lesions within the submucosa of the small intestine. These lesions can act as lead points for small bowel intussusception. Henoch-Schoenlein purpura is associated with purpuric lesions on the dorsal surface of the distal legs and arms.

2. **A** While the specific genetic cause of Peutz-Jeghers syndrome has not yet been identified, its inheritance pattern is autosomal dominant. While many cases are observed within known cohorts of families afflicted with this syndrome, it is common to see spontaneous cases as well. While the multiple polyps in Peutz-Jeghers syndrome tend to be benign, the syndrome is strongly associated with malignancy both in the gastrointestinal tract and beyond. The polyps in Peutz-Jeghers syndrome most commonly occur in the small intestine (55%) but are also found in the stomach and duodenum (30%) and colon and rectum (15%). Roughly 30% of patients with Peutz-Jeghers syndrome present with signs and symptoms in the first 10 years of life, with 50% presenting by age 20 years. An operation may be required acutely if the patient develops a small bowel intussusception that does not reduce spontaneously. Many authorities also recommend elective laparotomy with intraoperative endoscopy for removal of all small intestinal polyps greater than 15 mm. Biannual esophagogastroduodenoscopy and colonoscopy with polyp removal is also recommended.

3. **B** The intestinal polyps in Peutz-Jeghers syndrome are classified histologically as hamartomas of the muscularis mucosa. It is possible for adenomatous polyps to occur concurrently with these hamartomas.

   These polyps rarely grow larger than 2 or 3 cm. While they may act as lead points for intussusception, it would be exceedingly unlikely for a polyp to obstruct the lumen of the intestine. As mentioned in answer 2, these polyps are most commonly found in the small intestine but can be found throughout the intestinal tract.

4. **C** Intermittent intussusception is a common feature associated with Peutz-Jeghers syndrome. In many cases, the signs and symptoms of intussusception resolve spontaneously. When operation is necessary for an intussusception, the surgeon should probably use this opportunity to examine the remainder of the gastrointestinal tract in order to excise any polyps larger than 5 mm. Intraoperative endoscopy at the time of laparotomy best facilitates this in the small intestine. The stomach and colon are accessible endoscopically without operation.

Barium enema and air enema are useful for diagnosis and reduction of ileocolic intussusception. Neither of these studies is helpful in the patient with small bowel intussusception. Short segment resection of the involved intestine may be necessary, however, the intussusception can usually be reduced manually. Even if short segment resection is required, this should be combined with endoscopy and examination of the remaining small bowel. Upper gastrointestinal endoscopy is an important adjunct in the management of patients of Peutz-Jeghers syndrome but will be of little value in the management of this acute situation.

5. **E** There are many reports in the literature of intestinal tumors developing in patients with Peutz-Jeghers syndrome. Malignant changes have been reported to occur in the hamartomatous polyps of this syndrome. Adenomas and adenocarcinomas have been found in the small and large intestines of these patients in far greater frequency than in the general population. Compared with an age-matched general population, patients with Peutz-Jeghers syndrome have a relative risk of death from gastrointestinal cancer that is 13 times greater than that of the general population.

Patients with Peutz-Jeghers syndrome have a much higher risk of extraintestinal tumors as well. These tumors include testicular and ovarian neoplasms, cervical cancer, bile duct cancer, pancreatic cancer, gallbladder cancer, thyroid cancer, and breast cancer. Phillips and Spigelman (1994) have proposed the following annual evaluation for patients with this syndrome:

1. History for symptoms related to polyps
2. Complete blood count to detect anemia
3. Breast and pelvic examination with cervical smear and pelvic ultrasound in female patients
4. Testicular examination with ultrasound in male patients
5. Pancreatic ultrasonography
6. Biannual esophagogastroduodenoscopy and colonoscopy with polyp removal
7. Frequent mammography

It is unclear whether this aggressive management will actually reduce the risk of death from cancer in patients with this syndrome. Retrospective data suggests that patients with Peutz-Jeghers syndrome have a 60% chance of dying by age 60.

6. **C** The incidence of malignancy in patients with Peutz-Jeghers syndrome is not dependent on whether the abnormality is inherited or spontaneous. There is no known difference in outcome between the sexes.

BIBLIOGRAPHY

Dormandy TL. Gastrointestinal polyps with mucocutaneous pigmentation (Peutz-Jeghers syndrome). *N Engl J Med.* 1957;236:1093–1141.

Ishida H, Murata N, Tada M, et al. A new simple technique for performing intraoperative endoscopic resection of small-bowel polyps in patients with Peutz-Jeghers syndrome. *Surg Today.* 1999;29:581–583.

Phillips RKS, Spigelman AD, Thompson JPS, et al. Peutz-Jeghers syndrome. In: Phillips RKS, et al. eds. *Familial Adenomatous Polyposis and Other Polyposis Syndromes.* Boston: Little-Brown; 1994.

Shibata S, Seam RK, Kapoor HL. Malignant Sertoli cell tumor of the testis in a child. *J Surg Oncol.* 1990;44:129.

Tovar JA, Eizaguirre AA, Jimenez J. Peutz-Jeghers syndrome in children: report of two cases and review of the literature. *J Pediatr Surg.* 1983;18:1.

Westerman AM, Entius MM, de Baar E, et al. Peutz-Jeghers syndrome: 78-year follow-up of the original family. *Lancet.* 1999;353(9160):1211–1215.

A 5-WEEK-OLD BABY
WITH VOMITING

You are working in the emergency room. A mother calls you on the phone and says that her 5-week-old baby is vomiting. He was born at term without perinatal problems. He is breast fed. The vomiting began 2 days ago and is now occurring after every feeding. There is no blood or mucous in the vomitus, and the baby has not had diarrhea. The baby is not febrile but seems a bit lethargic.

Please answer all questions before proceeding to discussion section.

✓ QUESTIONS

1. What is the most important question you should ask the mother to narrow the differential diagnosis?
   A. Is the vomiting projectile?
   B. Is the abdomen tender?
   C. What color is the vomitus?
   D. Are there any other family members ill with similar symptoms?

This baby's vomiting consists of milk and is not projectile. You ask the mother to bring the baby to see you. On physical examination his weight is identical to his birth weight. Temperature is 36.8°C; pulse is 148; blood pressure is 87/45; and respiratory rate is 20. His lungs are clear with equal breath sounds. Heart tones are normal without murmur. His abdomen is soft and mildly distended with voluntary guarding. There is no hepatosplenomegaly, and you are not able to palpate a mass. Skin turgor is somewhat depressed. Capillary refill time is 3.5 seconds in his toes.

2. Which of the following are true?
   A. He is mildly dehydrated (about 10% decrease in plasma volume)
   B. The presence of a normal heart rate confirms he is no more than 15% dehydrated

C. He is significantly dehydrated (greater than 20% of plasma volume)

D. It is normal for a 5-week-old baby to weigh a bit less than his birth weight

E. Accurate assessment of hydration status requires placement of a urinary catheter

3. The differential diagnosis of nonbilious vomiting at this age includes:
   A. Overfeeding
   B. Gastroesophageal reflux
   C. Pyloric stenosis
   D. Congenital adrenal hyperplasia
   E. All of the above

4. Electrolytes are as follows: sodium 137, potassium 2.9, chloride 80, bicarbonate 38, BUN 9, and creatinine 0.6. This abnormality can potentially be explained by:
   A. Ingestion of an exogenous acid, such as aspirin poisoning
   B. Gastric outlet obstruction with loss of hydrochloric acid
   C. A "contraction alkalosis" secondary to severe dehydration
   D. Early renal failure
   E. All of the above

5. Fluid resuscitation should include:
   A. Lactated Ringer's by bolus until capillary refill time is normal
   B. D5 ½ normal saline (NS) with 40 mEq/L of potassium chloride by bolus until capillary refill is normal followed by maintenance infusion of the same solution
   C. Five percent albumin by bolus until capillary refill is normal
   D. Normal saline by bolus until capillary refill is normal followed by D5 ½ NS with 40 mEq/L of potassium chloride at maintenance rate
   E. Normal saline by bolus until capillary refill is normal followed by the same fluid at maintenance rate

6. Most of the potassium loss has occurred in the:
   A. Vomitus
   B. Stool
   C. Urine
   D. Potassium has not been lost; it is intracellular

7. A supine abdominal film is ordered by the referring physician and is shown in Figure 10–1. Which of the following is true?
   A. The findings are consistent with duodenal atresia
   B. The findings are consistent with a complete obstruction, which could be in the duodenum or proximal jejunum.
   C. The film shows free intraperitoneal air consistent with bowel perforation
   D. The film shows evidence of gastric outlet obstruction
   E. The findings are consistent with severe gastroesophageal reflux

8. Palpation of a hypertrophied pylorus:
   A. Obviates the need for any further radiologic investigations prior to surgery

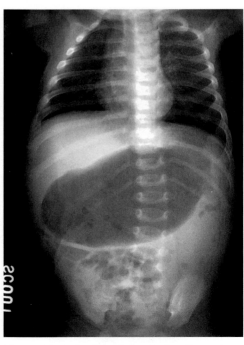

Figure 10–1. *Supine abdominal radiograph.*

B. Requires diagnostic confirmation with an abdominal ultrasound prior to surgery

C. Requires diagnostic confirmation with an upper gastrointestinal (GI) series prior to surgery

D. Is possible in only 10% of patients with pyloric stenosis

9. The diagnostic study of choice is:
   A. Abdominal ultrasound
   B. Upper gastrointestinal series with barium
   C. Upper gastrointestinal series with water soluble contrast
   D. Plain film of the abdomen
   E. A or B

ANSWERS AND DISCUSSION

1. **C** It is critical to determine whether or not this baby has evidence of intestinal obstruction. Intestinal obstruction causes green vomiting. The differential diagnosis of green vomiting includes malrotation with midgut volvulus, which is an acute surgical emergency. This is discussed elsewhere. The differential diagnosis of clear or milk vomitus is entirely different and is discussed here. Projectile vomiting suggests a mechanical cause. This is not, however, a particularly reliable sign. Abdominal tenderness is difficult for a parent to ascertain at this age. The presence of other ill family members is important but a secondary consideration.

2. **C** Infants and children have an excellent autonomic nervous system and do not have peripheral vascular disease. They are able to compensate effectively for large losses of intravascular volume with little hemodynamic compromise. Tachycardia and hypotension are very late signs of hypovolemia in the infant, occurring with plasma losses of around 25% and 35%, respectively. The most sensitive indicator of volume status in the infant is capillary refill time. Normal is 1 to 1.5 seconds. This patient's capillary refill time (>3.5 seconds) is markedly abnormal and indicates significant dehydration. A 5-week-old baby should not weigh less than his birth weight. If this weight loss is acute, it is due to dehydration. If it is chronic, it is due to poor nutrition.

3. **E** The differential diagnosis also includes increased intracranial pressure because of hydrocephalus or a mass. Overfeeding is diagnosed by history. These babies have excellent weight gain and are not dehydrated. Gastroesophageal reflux tends to cause vomiting since birth, but it may present in a manner such as this patient's course. Congenital adrenal hyperplasia is the only cause of vomiting associated with hyperkalemia.

4. **B** This patient has a hypochloremic, hypokalemic, metabolic alkalosis. This is caused by a gastric outlet obstruction, which uniquely causes loss of hydrogen ions and loss of chloride far in excess of loss of sodium. Overdose of aspirin would cause a metabolic acidosis not an alkalosis. Acute dehydration causes an acidosis as well because of lactate production. Contraction alkalosis may be due to overuse of diuretics and is not consistent with this clinical situation. Renal fail-

ure does not cause this type of electrolyte abnormality. The potassium level should be elevated and bicarbonate level depressed.

5. **D** This patient has lost chloride in excess of sodium and is hypokalemic. Ideally, the fluid replacement would include hydrochloric acid. This is impractical and sclerosing to veins. Hydrochloric acid is only given in cases of extreme alkalosis and only by central venous line. Normal saline is the appropriate choice for bolus fluid to restore intravascular volume acutely to normal. Ringer's lactate is not appropriate in the setting of hypochloremic alkalosis since it contains only 109 mEq of chloride, and it contains lactate, which will be metabolized to bicarbonate. Potassium is not included in the initial bolus fluid for two reasons: Rapid infusion of potassium can be dangerous, and potassium should not be given until urine output is seen confirming the absence of acute renal failure. Once urine output is established, potassium should be given liberally in the maintenance fluid since serum levels tend to underestimate the total body deficit.

6. **C** Gastric juice contains only about 10 to 20 mEq/L of potassium. The majority of this patient's losses have occurred in the urine. Dehydration leads to maximal reabsorbtion of sodium in the distal tubule of the kidney. This is done by means of an adenosine triphosphate (ATP) driven ion exchange pump. For every molecule of sodium reabsorbed, a molecule of either a hydrogen ion or a potassium ion must be excreted. In the alkalotic patient, the hydrogen ions are preferentially preserved leading to a very large excretion of potassium in the urine. When potassium levels are dangerously low, the kidney again begins to excrete hydrogen ions despite the presence of a serum alkalosis. This is called paradoxic aciduria. It is a sign of severe hypokalemia.

7. **D** This supine abdominal radiograph shows a markedly dilated stomach bubble that fills the upper abdomen. This finding is often diagnostic of gastric outlet obstruction, but it may be seen with air swallowing after a crying episode. Duodenal and jejunal atresia are

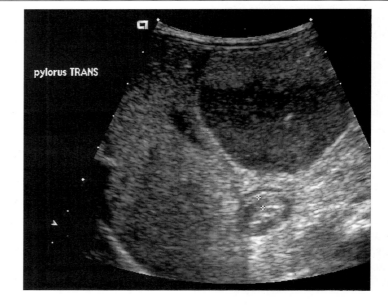

Figure 10–2. *This is a transverse scan of the hypertrophied pylorus. The structure appears as a "target" as the highly echogenic mucosa and serosa offset the thickened muscle, which appears dark. The cursors are positioned at the inner and outer edges of this muscle layer. There are a variety of sonographic measurement criteria for diagnosis. In general, a muscle layer that is greater than 4 mm thick or a pyloric channel greater than 2 cm in length is diagnostic.*

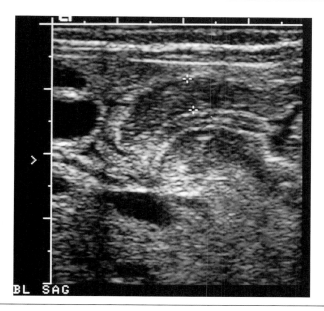

Figure 10–3. *In this image, the hypertrophied pylorus is seen longitudinally. The "bright" echogenic mucosa can be seen lining the long narrow pyloric channel. Again the cursors are measuring the muscle thickness.*

completely obstructive processes, and no distal gas should be seen on the radiographs. Further, one should see a dilated duodenum or jejunum or both that are not present here. Free intraperitoneal air can appear in the midabdomen on a supine film (ie, the "football" sign with necrotizing enterocolitis), but the air generally projects over the liver and other loops of intestine. In addition, the contrast of gas both inside and outside the bowel wall causes the characteristic "double wall" sign seen with free air.

8. **A** If the hypertrophied pylorus can be palpated by the responsible surgeon, there is no need for any complementary study. Physical examination of the infant with pyloric stenosis can often be facilitated by gastric tube decompression and sham feeding with warm sugar water in a peaceful and warm environment. This usually results in rectus muscle relaxation, which makes rolling of the "olive" beneath the fingertips possible.

9. **A** Abdominal ultrasound is the diagnostic study of choice when pyloric stenosis is suspected. It has excellent sensitivity and specificity, is noninvasive, and requires no radiation exposure. Upper gastrointestinal series can achieve similar accuracy. This study can also identify gastroesophageal reflux and abnormalities of rotation. Plain films often reveal gastric distention with little distal gas, but this is a nonspecific finding. A representative study is shown in Figures 10–2 and 10–3.

BIBLIOGRAPHY

Benson CD, Alpern EB. Preoperative and postoperative care of congenital pyloric stenosis. *Arch Surg.* 1957;75:877.

Greason KL, Thompson WR, Downey EC, et al. Laparoscopic pyloromyotomy for infantile hypertrophic pyloric stenosis: report of 11 cases. *J Pediatr Surg.* 1995;30:1571–1574.

Hulka F, Campbell TJ, Campbell JR, et al. Evolution in the recognition of infantile hypertrophic pyloric stenosis. *Pediatrics.* 1997;100(2):E9.

Olson AD, Hernandez R, Hirschl RB. The role of ultrasonography in the diagnosis of pyloric stenosis: a decision analysis. *J Pediatr Surg.* 1998; 33:676–681.

Rice HE, Caty MG, Glick PL. Fluid therapy for the pediatric surgical patient. *Pediatr Clin North Am.* 1998;45:719–727.

Schechter R, Torfs CP, Bateson TF. The epidemiology of infantile hypertrophic pyloric stenosis. *Paediatr Perinat Epidemiol.* 1997;11:407–427.

Schwartz MZ. Hypertrophic pyloric stenosis. In: O'Neill JA, Rowe MI, Grosfeld JL, et al. eds. *Pediatric Surgery.* St Louis: Mosby Year Book; 1998.

A 2.5-YEAR-OLD GIRL WITH A 24-HOUR HISTORY OF VOMITING AND INTERMITTENT ABDOMINAL PAIN

HISTORY She was well until yesterday morning when, after stealing a piece of chicken from her brother's plate, she developed crampy abdominal pain and later vomiting with diarrhea. The vomit is yellow but not frankly bilious, the pain lasts for 10 to 15 minutes during which time she is difficult to console. By "diarrhea" the parents mean: "she usually goes once every two days but in the last day she's gone three times, and it's dark red sometimes." No one else in the home is ill.

EXAMINATION Her vital signs are normal, her lips dry; she smiles and says her abdomen does not hurt. Suddenly, in the midst of the exam, she doubles up and starts to cry, asking for her parents. In the brief examination before this occurs her abdomen feels a little distended, but there is no significant tenderness, guarding, or rebound. You have specifically looked for a right upper quadrant abdominal mass and do not feel one. You are surprised and initially relieved when your rectal inspection discloses what looks like a rectal prolapse with some blood in the lumen.

RADIOLOGY The parents bring you a plain film taken the night before at their local clinic where they were told their daughter probably has gastroenteritis (Figure 11–1).

Please answer all questions before proceeding to discussion section.

✓ QUESTIONS

1. The findings suggest:
   A. Malrotation with or without volvulus
   B. Intussusception
   C. Gastroenteritis
   D. *Salmonella* food poisoning
   E. Rectal prolapse

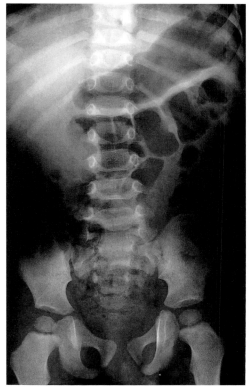

Figure 11–1. *Abdominal flat plate of 2.5-year-old girl with abdominal pain.*

2. What is the best *screening* study to confirm your suspicions, assuming skilled radiology is available?
   A. Abdominal ultrasound
   B. Water soluble contrast enema
   C. Water enema
   D. Air enema
   E. Barium enema

3. If an enema is chosen, which of the following points is *incorrect?*
   A. The study is worthless without skilled buttock taping ± balloon inflation of the catheter
   B. Water soluble contrast is probably a better idea than barium
   C. One should proceed cautiously in the presence of peritoneal signs from translocation
   D. Air enema, used at pressures up to 120 torr, may succeed in reduction more often than liquid
   E. It should be preceded by antibiotic administration and intravenous access

4. Which of the following are true concerning intussusception and rectal prolapse?
   A. The latter complicates the former from time to time
   B. Computed tomography (CT) scan is used for differentiation
   C. Endoscopy is used for differentiation
   D. Clinical examination is used for differentiation
   E. Silver nitrate coagulation is usually successful in solving the local bleeding

5. What feature is uncommon in this disease?
   A. Absence of a palpable, sausage-shaped mass in the right upper quadrant
   B. Vomiting
   C. Her age
   D. The rectal findings
   E. Stool color and consistency

6. Following the use of pressures of 80 torr, 100 torr, and then 120 torr (each for 5 minutes without much sedation), air enema successfully solves the problem. About this conclusion, which of the following is *false?*
   A. Reduction is not "successful" unless contrast refluxes well up into the ileum
   B. It is common to have fevers for the first 24 to 48 hours—antibiotic coverage is prudent
   C. Recurrent symptoms probably herald recurrent intussusception
   D. The chance of successful reduction may be 85%
   E. Recurrent symptoms should be treated with operation

7. When an operation is required for reduction, which is *false?*
   A. There is a greater chance of necrotic bowel. When this requires resection, the distal incision should be made on the outside of the recipient bowel at the level of the intraluminal bulge
   B. It is important to squeeze the distal bowel toward the proximal
   C. The "intussusci*piens*" is the reci*pient* bowel

    D. Laparoscopic reduction is possible; otherwise a right transverse abdominal incision is appropriate

    E. The appendix should be removed

8. Lead points occur in 2% to 6% of children with intussusception, more commonly after age 3 years. Of the following, which could not cause a lead point?

    A. Henoch-Schoenlein purpura

    B. Urachal remnant

    C. Vitelline duct remnant

    D. Carcinoid tumor

    E. Ileal duplication

    F. Peyer's patch

    G. Appendix

    H. Lymphoma

    I. Cystic fibrosis

    J. Polyp

9. Intussusception usually begins at the ileoceccal region. What can be said of ileal–ileal intussusception?

    A. It is best detected with a contrast enema

    B. It often occurs following retroperitoneal surgery

    C. It occurs almost exclusively in age group: 3 months to 3 years

    D. Nasogastric tube (NG) suction is usually sufficient therapy

    E. It is best treated with a contrast enema

ANSWERS AND DISCUSSION

1. B The intussusception can be seen on the plain film from last night, already at the hepatic flexure. The proximal mass with a central depression is protruding into the early transverse colon, and there are signs of bowel obstruction. She is too well for 24 hours of volvulus (**A**), and the intermittent obstruction of Ladd's bands in malrotation is not so periodic. The latter is true for the pain of rectal prolapse. *Salmonella enteritidis* is a famous contaminant of chicken causing bloody diarrhea. It is a possible but less likely cause of the rectal findings and might be expected to involve other consumers of the contaminated food.

2. A The *pseudokidney sign* (Figure 11–2), a *target lesion* (Figure 11–3), or both are found on ultrasound, which in the hands of an experienced radiologist or technician connote intussusception. That said, in many centers this expertise is unavailable; in this circumstance options **B, D,** and **E** are useful for both diagnosis and therapy. **C** requires ultrasound skill to monitor reduction.

3. C Seldom is an odious task (like buttock taping) more important to the success of a procedure than in intussusception. Failure to provide a hermetic seal is responsible for many failed enema reductions. As the findings are obvious no matter what the contrast, water soluble ones are safer if a perforation occurs (Figure 11–4). Air may be safer still and cause smaller perforations. The presence of peritoneal signs suggests perforation not translocation, although this is possible. If there is frank peritonitis, the patient should be resuscitated

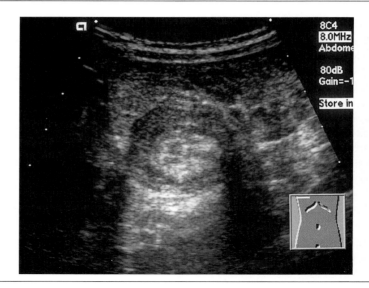

Figure 11–2. *Target sign found on abdominal ultrasound in a patient with intussusception. The intussusceptum appears as a ring within the intussuscipiens.*

and taken to the operating room. A second-generation cephalosporin with anaerobic coverage is one choice of antibiotic.

It is essential that children with suspected intussusception receive adequate fluid resuscitation and antibiotics prior to an attempt at radiologic reduction. A dehydrated patient may become cold and unstable in the x-ray department. The administration of a column of air or contrast on top of an ischemic intussusception can cause bacterial translocation.

4. **D** The coexistence of these disease entities defies Occam's razor and is reportable. This patient has an intussusception traversing the entire colon and exiting the rectum. In this location it may be distinguished from rectal prolapse in two ways. The most obvious way is to insert a finger up between the perianal skin and the prolapse. This is impossible in rectal prolapse. A second, less obvious than it sounds method, is to examine the mucosal pattern. Ileum or colon

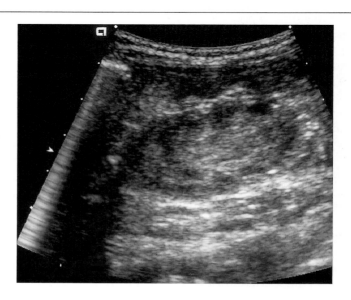

Figure 11–3. *Pseudokidney sign with an echogenic center is seen when the intussusception is viewed in the long axis.*

will demonstrate transverse markings (valvulae conniventes, plicae semilunares) suggesting intussusception; the rectum will demonstrate longitudinal folds (crypts above the dentate line) suggesting prolapse.

5. **D** The finding in **A**—caused by intussusception of the ileum up the cecum toward the proximal transverse colon—is more often described than found, especially when the intussusception is this extensive, which is a rare event. Vomiting is so constant that in its absence one must be hesitant about the diagnosis of intussusception. The vomiting is often—but not necessarily—bilious. The peak incidence occurs between the ages of 3 months and 3 years. The stool, when classical, is compared with "currant jelly." The described posture is very typical.

6. **E** The point made in **A** cannot be made strongly enough. While **B** is true, in uncomplicated cases admission is often just 24 to 36 hours, depending on one's postreduction feeding regimen. Recurrence is usually within the first 48 hours and happens in approximately 10% of patients, increasing the chances of a pathologic lead point. Success with nonoperative therapy is widely variable from 50% to 95% depending on the skill of the radiologist, persistence, the techniques used (air and water advocates claim higher rates of reduction), and the time delay from onset to therapy. In children ages 3 months to 3 years, recurrence should be treated several times before an operation is undertaken. This is not true for older patients in whom pathologic lead points are more likely.

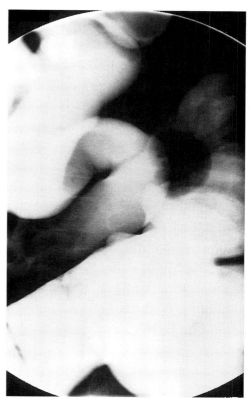

Figure 11–4. *Water soluble contrast enema of nearly complete reduction.*

7. **A** Manual reduction is most successful when gentle proximal traction is aided by squeezing the distal bowel like a tube of toothpaste. The intussusceptum is the proximal bowel. While early reports of laparoscopic reduction are emerging, this therapy is most likely to be successful when attempts at reduction in the radiology suite have not been energetic. The final point cannot be stressed enough. When intestine necroses, it is usually the intussusceptum's blood supply that is compromised. The sheath of intussuscipiens is typically viable, even though it contains the lump of intussusceptum. Therefore, when operative reduction is unsuccessful, the intussuscipiens should be initially preserved and resected only if nonviable. Because the scar usually resembles a McBurney incision (confusing future practitioners) and because the appendix may serve as a lead point, it is routinely removed.

8. **B** The urachus is nowhere near the bowel. A Meckel's diverticulum is one example of **C**.

9. **B** This is a separate disease entity that occurs at any age, typically during the postoperative period following retroperitoneal surgery (kidneys, pancreas, adrenals, other). An abdominal CT scan with contrast is the best diagnostic tool, and therapy is always surgical. A nasogastric (NG) tube temporizes. Because the obstruction occurs high above the ileocecal valve, enemas introduce insufficient retrograde pressure to be diagnostic or therapeutic.

BIBLIOGRAPHY

Anderson DR. The psuedokidney sign. *Radiology.* 1999;211:395–397.

Ein SH, Alton D, Palder SB, Shandling B, Stringer D. Intussusception in the 1990s: has 25 years made a difference? *Pediatr Surg Intl.* 1997; 12:374–376.

Eshel G, Barr J, Heyman E, et al. Intussusception: a 9-year survey (1986–1995). *J Pediatr Gastroenterol Nutr.* 1997;24:253–256.

Littlewood Teele R, Vogel SA. Intussusception: the paediatric radiologist's perspective. *Pediatr Surg Intl.* 1998;14:158–162.

Rohrschneider WK, Troger J, Nutzenadel W. Childhood intussusception: management perspectives in 1995 (letter; comment). *J Pediatr Gastroenterol Nutr.* 1997;25:118–120.

A 7-YEAR-OLD BOY STRUCK BY A CAR

HISTORY   A 7-year-old boy was struck by a car that was traveling an estimated 30 miles per hour. He was thrown 15 feet and landed against a tree. After a brief, initial period of unconsciousness, he was awake and verbal. He was transported with a cervical collar on a spine board with supplemental mask O_2. A peripheral IV was placed in the field, and he received 250 mL of Ringer's lactate en route to hospital. His vital signs in the field were heart rate (HR) 110, blood pressure (BP) 110/65, respiration rate 24.

EXAMINATION   Physical examination reveals an alert and verbal 7 year old in moderate distress, complaining of left chest and shoulder discomfort. His estimated weight is 25 kg. Head and neck examination is negative. He has palpable left chest wall crepitus and diminished breath sounds on the left side. He has a large left flank abrasion, and some upper abdominal pain and tenderness. As you complete your examination, he suddenly begins to complain of severe left chest pain and shortness of breath. He becomes pale and sweaty, and his vital signs now are HR 160, BP 90/50, respiration rate 40 and shallow.

Please answer all questions before proceeding to discussion section.

✓ QUESTIONS

1. Your next step would be:
    A. Administer 20 mL/kg crystalloid, and proceed with rapid sequence induction and endotracheal intubation
    B. Administer 20 mL/kg O-negative blood; obtain a chest x-ray and abdominal computed tomography (CT) scan
    C. Administer 20 mL/kg crystalloid; prepare for left chest tube placement
    D. Administer 20 mL/kg crystalloid, and proceed with left-sided needle thoracentesis

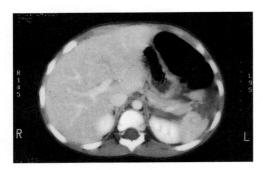

Figure 12–1. *Computed tomography scan through upper abdomen demonstrates a perfusion defect at the inferior pole of the spleen. The capsule appears disrupted, and there is perisplenic free fluid.*

2. Following the appropriate intervention, his vital signs stabilize, with the heart rate decreasing to 120, BP 110/70, respiratory rate 28. After obtaining blood work and placing a Foley catheter and nasogastric tube, the following tests are performed:
   A. C-spine, chest, pelvis x-rays, head CT, abdomen/pelvis CT scan with IV and oral contrast
   B. C-spine, chest, pelvis, skull x-rays, and diagnostic peritoneal lavage (DPL)
   C. C-spine, chest, pelvis x-rays, head CT scan, abdominal ultrasound
   D. C-spine, chest x-ray, head CT scan followed by exploratory laparotomy

3. An abdominal CT scan is shown in Figure 12–1. After an additional 20 mL/kg of Ringer's lactate and 1 mg of morphine IV, his heart rate is 100 and blood pressure 110/72. He still complains of some left chest and shoulder pain and has localized epigastric tenderness with an otherwise soft abdomen. His laboratory work returns: hematocrit 31, hemoglobin 10.5, sodium 137, potassium 3.8, chloride 102, carbon dioxide 22, amylase 50. At this point you would:
   A. Proceed with peritoneal lavage to rule out a possible small bowel injury
   B. Obtain shoulder x-rays and an orthopedic consult
   C. Admit to the pediatric intensive care unit for monitoring, serial physical exams, and hematocrit checks
   D. Proceed with exploratory laparotomy and splenectomy

4. Eight hours after pediatric intensive care unit (PICU) admission, he complains of increased upper abdominal pain. His heart rate has climbed slowly to 140, but blood pressure remains stable at 110/60. His urine output for the last hour is 20 mL. His stat hematocrit comes back at 23. His nasogastric (NG) tube is draining clear, coffee-grounds stained fluid, and his abdomen is soft but for some epigastric and left upper quadrant tenderness. Now, you would:
   A. Administer 20 mL/kg of Ringer's lactate, and observe hemodynamic response
   B. Administer 20 mL/kg of cross-matched blood, and observe hemodynamic response
   C. Administer blood, and repeat the abdominal CT scan
   D. Administer blood, and proceed to the operating room for laparotomy

5. After a blood transfusion, his heart rate decreases to 105, and his hematocrit increases to 32. Thereafter he remains hemodynamically stable, and the following evening his hematocrit is 30. At this point, the PICU director requests that you transfer the patient out of the unit to make room for a postoperative liver transplant patient. You should:
   A. Tell the PICU director to call in more nurses because your patient is not ready for PICU discharge
   B. Transfer the patient to the ward, only if a repeat CT scan shows no additional free fluid and no anatomic progression of the splenic injury
   C. Transfer the patient to the ward, for reasons other than those of the PICU director
   D. Discharge the patient from hospital

6. The patient's continuing care should consist of:
   A. Five days (total) hospitalization on bedrest, with unlimited physical activity after discharge
   B. Seven days (total) hospitalization on bedrest, with limited activities for 3 months postinjury
   C. Two weeks (total) hospitalization without activity restriction, with limited physical activities for 6 months postinjury
   D. None of the above

7. Regarding overwhelming postsplenectomy infection (OPSI), all of the following are true *except:*
   A. The risk is highest in children under age 5, within the first 2 years after splenectomy
   B. The risk is highest in children undergoing splenectomy for non-traumatic causes
   C. The most commonly associated causative organism is *Haemophilus influenzae*
   D. The incidence can be reduced by both immunization and antibiotic prophylaxis

ANSWERS AND DISCUSSION

1. **C** In the context of a blunt chest and abdominal injury with rib fractures, the sudden onset of severe respiratory distress, diminished breath sounds, and hypotension is diagnostic of a tension pneumothorax. Although needle thoracentesis will temporarily decompress the pleural space and improve ventilation and venous return, all trauma patients require chest tubes to prevent reaccumulation of air (or blood, if this represents a hemopneumothorax). Therefore, a preliminary needle thoracentesis is unnecessary unless there will be some delay in obtaining or placing a chest tube. The diagnosis of tension pneumothorax is clinical rather than radiologic, therefore a chest x-ray should not be obtained until *after* a thoracostomy tube has been placed.

2. **A** All significantly injured trauma patients require radiographic C-spine clearance, a chest x-ray, and pelvic x-ray. This child's period of unconsciousness at the scene mandates that he have a head CT scan as well. His injury mechanism, the presence of lower rib fractures, and his abdominal and shoulder pain make a splenic injury likely, and some additional abdominal investigation is required, with the choices being diagnostic peritoneal lavage, abdominal sonogram, and CT scan. Diagnostic peritoneal lavage for suspected liver or spleen injury is of limited use in children, since the presence of gross or microscopic hemoperitoneum has no impact on therapeutic decision making. Abdominal sonography is emerging as an inexpensive, accurate, and immediately available diagnostic tool in some emergency departments, but its use depends on the expertise of those available to interpret the scan. In most centers, abdominal/pelvic CT scanning with intravenous and oral contrast will be the imaging modality of choice, since it provides quality images (not only of intraperitoneal organs but of the retroperitoneum as well), which are more easily interpreted by surgeons, who are often the "first line" of radiologic interpretation in the emergency department.

3. **C** The CT scan demonstrates a splenic fracture extending to the hilum (grade III) with a moderate amount of perisplenic fluid and some free fluid in the pelvis. Nonoperative management of a child with a splenic injury is justified if the patient: (1) maintains stable vital signs, (2) has no evidence of an associated abdominal injury requiring laparotomy, and (3) requires initial or ongoing blood replacement, or both, of less than one-half the blood volume (= 40 mL/kg). Children managed without surgery require admission to an intensive care area where they have frequent, but generally noninvasive, hemodynamic monitoring, urine output recording, serial hematocrit measurement, and physical examination. The diagnosis of an associated injury (usually a small bowel perforation) may be difficult to make at the outset, particularly if localized tenderness is attributed to the splenic injury. Computed tomography findings of free air or contrast extravasation are seen rarely. The presence of free fluid from a small bowel injury will mean little if there is significant hemoperitoneum from the splenic injury. Peritoneal lavage and microscopic examination of the bloody lavage fluid may be helpful in this situation; however, in most instances, the decision to operate to exclude an associated small bowel injury will be based on physical findings at presentation or those evolving after hospital admission. The shoulder pain is most likely the result of diaphragmatic irritation from perisplenic blood rather than a mechanical injury.

4. **B** The initial resuscitative fluid used to treat hypovolemia after traumatic hemorrhage is crystalloid. Advanced trauma life support (ATLS) protocols recommend giving two 20 mL/kg boluses of crystalloid, and thereafter blood, until stable hemodynamic criteria are met. In the absence of peritonitis mandating abdominal exploration or exsanguinating hemorrhage, the decision to take a child with a ruptured spleen to laparotomy is based on ongoing resuscitative requirements (one half of the blood volume or more). There is little correlation between splenic injury grade and need for operation, meaning that CT scans have little predictive value in the success or failure of nonoperative management and, therefore, add little to ongoing care once the diagnosis of a splenic injury has been made.

5. **C** The criteria for transfer of a nonoperatively managed patient with a splenic injury out of the PICU are clinical and laboratory evidence of cessation of bleeding over a defined period of time, usually 24 hours. In other words, the patient should have stable vital signs, evidence of adequate end organ perfusion (urine output), and a stable hematocrit.

6. **B** Because the phenomenon of delayed, post-traumatic splenic hemorrhage is rare, little data exist on which to base a recommendation for duration of hospitalization. Most pediatric surgeons arbitrarily choose 5 to 7 days of postinjury hospitalization, usually with mandatory bedrest, and then discharge to home with instructions to avoid contact sports for 3 to 6 months.

7. **C** Overwhelming postsplenectomy infection (OPSI) is a virulent septic syndrome with a mortality rate that approaches 50%. The infection is usually caused by one of three encapsulated bacteria: pneumococcus (most common), *Haemophilus,* and meningococcus.

It affects 1% to 2% of asplenic individuals and can occur decades after splenectomy. The risk of developing OPSI is highest in children less than 5 years, usually within the first 2 years after splenectomy, and in children who undergo elective splenectomy for hematologic disease, mainly sickle cell anemia and thalassemia. Although fatal pneumococcal sepsis has occurred in vaccinated children receiving antibiotic prophylaxis, there is good evidence that vaccination and antibiotics significantly decrease the risk of postsplenectomy infection. The issue of whether antibiotic prophylaxis should be lifelong or not remains controversial.

BIBLIOGRAPHY

Eichelberger MR, Moront M. Abdominal trauma. In: O'Neill JA, Rowe MI, Grosfeld JL, et al. eds. *Pediatric Surgery.* St Louis: Mosby Year-Book; 1998.

Jugenburg M, Haddock G, Freedman MH, et al. The morbidity and mortality of pediatric splenectomy: does prophylaxis make a difference? *J Pediatr Surg.* 1999;34:1064–1067.

Taylor GA, Sivit CJ. Computed tomography imaging of abdominal trauma in children. *Semin Pediatr Surg.* 1992;1:253–259.

Wesson DE, Filler RM, Ein SH, et al. Ruptured spleen—when to operate. *J Pediatr Surg.* 1981;16:324–326.

A 2-YEAR-OLD BOY
WITH A SCROTAL MASS

HISTORY   While operating on a 2-year-old boy with a large left-sided scrotal hydrocele, you note a 2-cm, firm, intratesticular mass that was nonpalpable preoperatively due to the tension of the hydrocele sac. The testicle is delivered through your inguinal incision and you are able to visualize the mass.

Please answer all questions before proceeding to discussion section.

✓ QUESTIONS

1. The most appropriate treatment at this point would be:
   A. Radical orchiectomy and retroperitoneal lymph node dissection
   B. With vascular occlusion of the spermatic cord, testicular biopsy with frozen section, and radical orchiectomy if malignant histology
   C. Wedge biopsy and closure with subsequent therapy based on permanent sections and serum tumor markers
   D. Wedge biopsy and closure with contralateral blind needle biopsies of contralateral testis

2. Testicular tumors in children are more often benign than malignant.
   A. True
   B. False

3. The most common malignant testicular tumor of childhood is:
   A. Rhabdomyosarcoma
   B. Yolk sac (endodermal sinus) tumor
   C. Seminoma
   D. Lymphoma

4. Testicular yolk sac carcinoma may metastasize to all of the following *except:*
   A. Bone marrow
   B. Bone cortex
   C. Liver
   D. Lung
   E. Retroperitoneal lymph nodes

5. Which of the following are risk factors for the development of testicular neoplasms?
   A. Duplication of the short arm of chromosome 12
   B. Gonadal dysgenesis
   C. Cryptorchidism
   D. Acute lymphoblastic leukemia
   E. All of the above

6. The preoperative work-up for a patient with a palpable intratesticular mass consists of all of the following *except:*
   A. Chest x-ray
   B. Abdominal computed tomography (CT) scan
   C. Serum levels of alpha fetoprotein and beta-human chorionic gonadotropin
   D. Fine-needle aspiration cytology of testicular mass

ANSWERS AND DISCUSSION

1. B Approximately 20% of all prepubertal testicular tumors present unexpectedly as a mass at the time of hydrocele or hernia repair. Such a finding should prompt an immediate determination of histology and, if a malignant testicular primary neoplasm is diagnosed, radical orchiectomy (Figure 13–1). It is important to occlude the testicular vessels during manipulation and biopsy of the testicle to minimize the risk of hematogenous dissemination of tumor cells. For malignant germ cell tumors, the role of retroperitoneal lymph node dissection is somewhat controversial. Most authors recommend selective lymph node dissection for those patients with a CT scan suggesting lymph node metastases or for patients with persistently elevated alphafetoprotein levels after orchiectomy for yolk sac carcinoma. The 15% to 20% false-negative rate of CT scanning for retroperitoneal nodal disease, however, has prompted the recommendation by some that all patients undergo modified ipsilateral lymph node sampling since current therapy for stage 1 disease (confined to the testicle) does not include adjuvant chemotherapy or radiation. If a patient has normal or unknown tumor markers at diagnosis (and normal markers after orchiectomy), then a negative ipsilateral retroperitoneal node sampling is required to confirm stage 1 disease.

2. B False

3. B Yolk sac tumors (endodermal sinus tumors) are the most common prepubertal tumor, accounting for 60% of all tumors in this age group. More than 75% of childhood yolk sac tumors are encountered during the first 2 years of life. Teratomas (Figure 13–2; see also color plate) are the second most common testicular tumor in

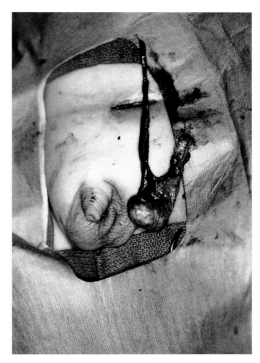

Figure 13–1. *Radical orchiectomy specimen of patient with solid testicular neoplasm. A high ligation of the vessels at the level of the internal ring is performed prior to testicular manipulation.*

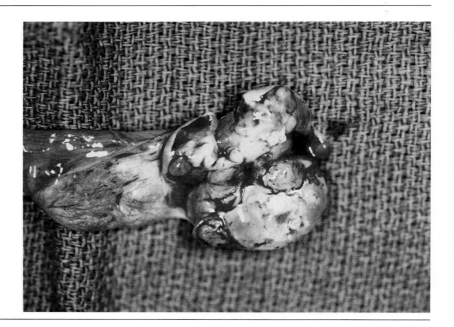

Figure 13–2. *Tumor on cut section demonstrates fat and cartilage consistent with mature teratoma. (See also color plate.)*

children. These tumors are composed of tissues derived from more than one germ cell layer (endoderm, mesoderm, and ectoderm) and may have solid and cystic components. Teratomas are classified as mature, if they are composed of well-differentiated tissues without mitotic activity, or immature (grades I to III), if they contain poorly differentiated tissues with mitotic activity as well as neuroepithelial elements. Gonadal stromal tumors represent approximately 8% of prepubertal testicular tumors, and the most common is the Leydig cell tumor. These tumors have a peak age incidence of 4 to 5 years, and usually produce testosterone, so that many of these young boys often present with precocious puberty. Gonadoblastomas are rare tumors that occur in children with mixed gonadal dysgenesis (45X, 46XY karyotype). These children typically have gonadal asymmetry and an ambiguous gender phenotype and, because of the risk of malignant transformation, should undergo gonadectomy at diagnosis. Secondary tumors of the testis include leukemia and lymphoma. Occult testicular involvement has been found in up to 20% of patients with acute lymphoblastic leukemia and may be an early indication of relapse or persistent disease. It has been postulated that the blood-testis barrier prevents chemotherapeutic agents from reaching malignant cells. Rhabdomyosarcoma is the most common paratesticular neoplasm, arising from the tunica of the testis and the spermatic cord. It has a peak age incidence of 2 to 5 years and accounts for 10% of all cases of rhabdomyosarcoma.

4. **A** The sites of metastases in decreasing order of frequency are: lungs, retroperitoneal lymph nodes, liver, and bones. Approximately 15% of patients will have metastases at presentation.

5. **E** A duplication of the short arm of chromosome 12 (also known as isochromosome 12p) and abnormalities of chromosome 1 have been reported in association with germ cell tumors. The relationship between gonadal dysgenesis and gonadoblastoma has already been discussed. Leukemic deposits in the testis may signify persistent or re-

current disease and may be related to defects in host tumor surveillance associated with the blood-testis barrier. Studies of patients with testicular tumors have characterized relative risks of cancer development to vary widely between 3- and 50-fold. The relative risk is highest for patients with bilateral, or intra-abdominal cryptorchidism, or both versus those without. The germ cell and tubular degeneration associated with cryptorchid testes is thought to be causally related to the increased risk of malignancy, and the testicular tumor most commonly associated with cryptorchidism is seminoma, which occurs at the same time as tumors in normally descended testes (ie, 20 to 40 years).

6. **D** A prepubertal patient presenting with an intratesticular mass should have serum levels of alpha-fetoprotein (AFP) and beta-human chorionic gonadotrophin (beta-hCG) drawn prior to surgery. Alpha fetoprotein is produced by fetal yolk sac, liver, and intestine, and by gonadal and extragonadal germ cell tumors. It has a half-life of 5 days, and if a tumor producing AFP is removed completely, levels should return to baseline within five half-lives. Beta-hCG is produced by embryonal carcinoma, choriocarcinoma, and mixed teratomas and has a half-life of 24 hours. Testicular ultrasound may be helpful in predicting benign lesions, particularly if a cystic component (either epidermoid cyst or cystic teratoma) is present, which may facilitate testis-sparing surgery. Patients with a solid testicular mass should undergo preoperative imaging with abdominal CT scanning and chest x-ray or CT scan to look for nodal and hematogenous metastatic disease, respectively. Except in the instance of a suspected leukemic testicular relapse, there is *no* indication for transscrotal needle biopsy of the testis. Scrotal violation by malignant cells occurs during needle biopsy and mandates that hemiscrotectomy be part of the subsequent surgical treatment of the testis tumor.

BIBLIOGRAPHY

Andrassy RJ, Corpron C, Ritchey M. Testicular tumors. In: O'Neill JA, Rowe MI, Grosfeld JL, et al., eds. *Pediatric Surgery.* St Louis: Mosby Year Book, 1998.

Skoog SJ. Benign and malignant pediatric scrotal masses. *Pediatr Clin North Am.* 1997;44:1229–1250.

14 CASE

A 4-YEAR-OLD BOY WITH FATIGUE AND AN ABDOMINAL MASS

HISTORY You see a 4-year-old boy regarding an abdominal mass. His parents have noted that he has been increasingly lethargic over the past several months. They think he is pale, and he has recently started to take long afternoon naps. He stopped napping when he was 2 years. His appetite has been poor, and he has lost 4 pounds in the last 2 months.

EXAMINATION The child is thin and pale. Temperature 37.4°C; heart rate 102; blood pressure 145/85; respiration rate 22. He is very cooperative with your examination. His lungs are clear with equal breath sounds. His heart tones are normal. His abdomen is quite full. You feel a large mass under the left costal margin that is firm and immobile. His extremities are thin and without edema or clubbing.

LABORATORY Hemoglobin 8.6; hematocrit 25; white blood cell count 8.5 with a normal differential. Urinalysis shows 2+ protein with no white or red blood cells.

Please answer all questions before proceeding to discussion section.

✓ QUESTIONS

1. The most likely diagnosis is:
   A. Wilms tumor
   B. Hodgkin disease
   C. Non-Hodgkin's lymphoma
   D. Neuroblastoma
   E. Rhabdomyosarcoma

2. A computed tomography (CT) scan of the abdomen is shown in Figure 14–1. Which of the following is true?
   A. This tumor is very unlikely to invade surrounding structures

72

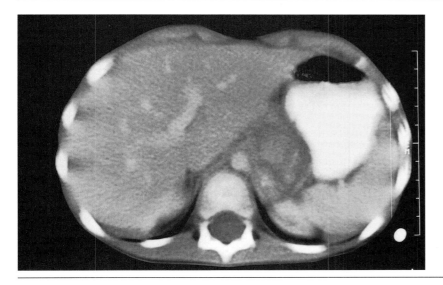

Figure 14–1. *Abdominal CT scan of a 4 year old with an abdominal mass.*

    B. Prompt excision via an abdominal approach is the treatment of choice

    C. You should proceed with percutaneous drainage and culture of the fluid

    D. The calcifications within the tumor suggest it is long-standing and likely to be benign

    E. The prognosis is very poor

3. Which of the following factors influence this patient's prognosis?
    A. Age
    B. Stage of the tumor
    C. Histologic appearance
    D. Cytogenetic analysis
    E. All of the above

4. Mass screening programs for the early detection of these tumors:
    A. Have not influenced patient survival
    B. May decrease the mortality rate by as much as 50%
    C. Have been found to decrease mortality by about 10% but with a very large increase in financial cost
    D. Have not changed the rate of detection
    E. None of the above

5. You are asked about a 1-week-old baby with a massive abdominal neuroblastoma metastatic to the liver and bone marrow. The baby also has multiple subcutaneous nodules found to be tumorous. Which of the following techniques have been successfully used for such patients?
    A. Placement of a silastic abdominal sheath after laparotomy
    B. Radiation to the liver
    C. Daily administration of cyclophosphamide (5 mg/kg/d)
    D. No intervention
    E. All of the above

6. Which of the following are associated with an increased incidence of neuroblastoma?
   A. Hirschsprung disease
   B. Beckwith-Weidemann syndrome
   C. Fetal alcohol syndrome
   D. Maternal phenytoin use
   E. All of the above

7. A bone marrow biopsy reveals small round blue cells consistent with heuroblastoma. Which of the following is the most appropriate initial treatment for this 4-year-old boy?
   A. Fine-needle aspiration cytology under local anesthesia
   B. Wide resection of the mass with resection of all contiguous structures
   C. Laparotomy and tumor biopsy followed by chemotherapy
   D. Limited resection with preservation of all vital structures followed by chemotherapy
   E. Chemotherapy without biopsy

8. Which of the following should be included in the initial evaluation of patients with neuroblastoma?
   A. A CT scan of the head
   B. Bone marrow biopsy
   C. Lumbar puncture
   D. MIBG scan
   E. All of the above

ANSWERS AND DISCUSSION

1. **D** The most common solid, abdominal tumors of childhood are Wilms tumor and neuroblastoma. Patients with Wilms tumor are typically asymptomatic and present when they are found to have a large abdominal mass on routine examination. Children with neuroblastoma, on the other hand, typically present with a variety of constitutional symptoms. Weight loss, fatigue, failure to thrive, abdominal pain and distention, anemia, and fever are common. The abdominal mass is usually tender. Hypertension is found in 25% of cases and appears to be related to catecholamine production by the tumor. Another common clinical finding is biliateral orbital ecchymoses, termed "panda eyes," which is caused by orbital metastases.

   When the tumor involves the stellate ganglion, the patient may present with Horner syndrome (ptosis and meiosis of the affected eye). Hodgkin disease typically presents as a cervical node or mediastinal mass. When non-Hodgkin's lymphoma occurs in the abdomen, it typically occurs in the mesenteric lymph nodes. Rhabdomyosarcoma most commonly occurs in the prostate, bladder, or pelvic retroperitoneum.

2. **E** The CT scan of the abdomen shows a large, left, suprarenal mass with multiple areas of internal calcification. The mass surrounds the celiac axis. These findings are diagnostic of neuroblastoma.

   A large, unresectable neuroblastoma in a child of this age carries a very poor prognosis. The most appropriate treatment includes administration of chemotherapy in an effort to control the systemic disease and shrink the tumor. The goal of therapy is to reduce the tumor size to a level where it can be safely resected. Recommendations include intensive multiagent chemotherapy using combinations of cyclophosphamide, doxorubicin, cis-platinum, etoposide, and vincristine. Because of consistently poor survival with advanced stage neuroblastoma, myoablative therapy followed by bone marrow transplantation has been tried. This has resulted in some modest improvement in survival for stage III disease; results for stage IV disease are less clear.

3. **E** The age of the patient at the time of diagnosis has a profound influence in outcome for neuroblastoma. Survival rates for children with neuroblastoma under 1 year of age are between 70% and 90%, while survival rates for children older than 1 year are on the order of 20% and 30%. Much of this discrepancy is explained by the unusual maturation seen in neuroblastoma in infancy (see the following answers). The size of the tumor is loosely related to survival, but the anatomic stage is a more important predictor. The Shimada classification system of the tumor's histologic appearance has been able to divide tumors into favorable versus unfavorable histology. The Shimada system is based primarily on the stromal characteristics of the cells, as well as on neuroblastic differentiation. This information combined with the patient's age helps predict prognosis.

   The N-*myc* oncogene is a valuable predictive marker in neuroblastoma. Cytogenetic analysis can determine the number of copies of this gene present in the cell. When the gene is amplified (more than ten copies present), prognosis is poor. It is thought that overexpression of the N-*myc* oncogene may impair neuroblastic differentiation and promote proliferation of immature neural crest cells. The presence of N-*myc* amplification is far more ominous in children greater than 1 year of age than in infants. Elevated serum ferritin levles are associated with a poor prognosis. Table 14–1 shows the factors commonly affecting prognosis in neuroblastoma.

4. **A** Because age has such a profound effect on outcome for neuroblastoma, experts have hypothesized that earlier detection of these tumors may lead to better outcome. In Japan, a mass screening program was initiated based on detection of catecholamine metabolites in the urine. This screening program resulted in a marked increase in the detection of cases in infants younger than 1 year of age. The percentage of cases of neuroblastoma among all pediatric cancers nearly doubled from 10% to 19%. Early detection of neuroblastoma, however, did not reduce the number of cases seen in older children. Experience with neuroblastoma in children under 1 year of age suggests that many of these tumors mature and may never cause clinical disease. One could infer that most of the tumors seen in older children that carry a poor prognosis are those with biologic characteristics that cause them to behave aggressively. The answer to effective treatment of these tumors probably lies in better forms of therapy rather than in earlier detection.

5. **E** This question describes the most unusual group of patients with neuroblastomas, infants with stage IV-S disease. These patients have hepatomegaly, subcutaneous tumor nodules, and tumor in the bone marrow, but they do not have other metastatic disease. They have

TABLE 14–1 NEUROBLASTOMA: FACTORS AFFECTING PROGNOSIS[a]

Factor	Good Prognosis	Poor Prognosis
Age	<1 year	>1 year
Stage	I, II, IV-S	III, IV
Shimada histology	Stroma rich	Stroma poor
Site	Mediastinum, pelvis, neck	Adrenal, celiac axis
>10 Copies N-*myc*	No	Yes
DNA-flow cytometry	Hyperdiploid	Diploid
Elevated trk-A	Yes	No
Elevated serum		
Ferritin	No	Yes
Neuron-specific enolase	No	Yes
Lactate dehydrogenase	No	Yes
Loss of heterozygosity chromosome 1p	No	Yes
Multidrug resistant-gene	No	Yes
Multidrug resistent protein-gene	No	Yes
Somatostatin receptors	Yes	No
Vasoactive intestinal peptide secretion	Yes	No
MHC class I antigen	Yes	No
Detection by screening	Yes	No

[a] This table shows a wide spectrum of biologic, histologic, and clinical prognostic factors that have either a positive or negative impact on survival in infants and children with neuroblastoma.
Reproduced, with permission, from Grosfeld JL. Neuroblastoma. In: O'Neill JA, Rowe MI, Grosfeld JL, et al., eds. *Pediatric Surgery,* 5th ed., Vol. 2. St. Louis: Mosby; 1998.

primary tumors that would be classified as stage I or II, except for the features already mentioned. Stage IV-S neuroblastoma accounts for roughly 30% of the disease seen during the first year of life. Treatment for this disease is quite controversial. The natural history for most of these tumors is one of maturation and resolution. There are numerous reports in the literature of patients similar to the one described in this question who have done well with no intervention.

When these patients succumb to their disease, it is often because of local complications of the tumor mass rather than progression of disease. The hepatomegaly in these patients can result in increased abdominal pressure with respiratory difficulty, gastroesophageal reflux and vomiting, and protein and calorie malnutrition due to poor feeding. Some authors have successfully used a decompressive silastic sheath following laparotomy in order to reduce intra-abdominal pressure. Septic complications have been reported with this technique. Other authors have reported that liver irradiation reduces hepatic size and, therefore, symptoms of the disease. Some oncologists recommend daily administration of low-dose cyclophosphamide. This regimen, however, has not been clearly shown to be superior to no intervention.

There is some evidence to suggest that patients with stage IV-S disease and significant N-*myc* amplification do poorly. Most oncologists believe that these patients should be treated with aggressive therapy.

6. **E** Hirschsprung disease is a disorder of ganglion cell migration in the large intestine. These ganglion cells are thought to be neural crest in origin. Beckwith-Weidemann syndrome results in an increased incidence of a number of abdominal tumors, including

TABLE 14–2   EVANS STAGING SYSTEM

Stage	Description
I	Tumor confined to organ of orgin
II	Tumor extends beyond organ of orgin but does not cross the midline; umilateral lymph nodes may be involved
III	Tumor extends beyond midline; bilateral lymph nodes may be involved
IV	Distant metastases (skeletal, other organs, soft tissues, distant lymph nodes)
IV-S	Would be stage I or II; remote disease confined to liver, subcutaneous tissues, and bone marrow, but without evidence of bone cortex involvement

Wilms tumor, neuroblastoma, hepatoblastoma, and adrenocortical carcinoma. Fetal alcohol syndrome and maternal Dilantin use have been found to correlate with neuroblastoma by unknown mechanisms.

7. **C** This patient has a large stage IV tumor. It encases the aorta as well as the celiac access in the superior mesenteric artery. Complete resection is neither possible nor indicated. The best procedure would be small laparotomy with tumor biopsy for histologic and cytogenetic analysis. This information can be used to guide the most appropriate course of chemotherapy.

   Resection is appropriate for stage I or II neuroblastomas. As a general rule, the tumor should be separated from contiguous structures. Wide *en bloc* excision does not appear to confer an increased survival rate. Table 14–2 shows the Evans staging system for neuroblastoma.

8. **B** Neuroblastoma is commonly metastatic to the bone marrow. In fact, the diagnosis can often be made by means of bone marrow examination without biopsy of the primary tumor. Brain mestastases are rare, and a CT scan of the head is not considered part of the routine preoperative evaluation of the patient with neuroblastoma. The same is true of lumbar puncture. MIBG (I-123-metaiodobenzylguanidine) is an analog taken up by a variety of neuroendocrine tumors including neuroblastoma. It is sometimes useful in identifying hidden metastatic disease. Its role in the intitial evaluation of the patient with neuroblastoma remains unclear.

BIBLIOGRAPHY

Askin FB, Perlman EJ. Neuroblastoma and peripheral neuroectodermal tumors. *Am J Clin Pathol.* 1998;109:S23–S30.

Bessho F, Hashizume K, Nakajo T, et al. Mass screening in Japan increased the detection of infants with neuroblastoma without a decrease in cases in older children. *J Pediatr.* 1991;119:237–241.

Evans AE, D'Angio GJ, Randolph JG. A proposed staging for children with neuroblastoma. *Cancer.* 1971;27:374–378.

Grosfeld JL. Neuroblastoma. In: O'Neill JA, Rowe MI, Grosfeld JL, et al. eds. *Pediatric Surgery,* Vol. 2. St. Louis: Mosby; 1998.

Grosfeld JL, Rescorla FJ, West KW, et al. Neuroblastoma in the first year of life: clinical and biologic factors influencing outcome. *Semin Pediatr Surg.* 1993;2:37–46.

Haase GM, Perez C, Atkinson JB. Current aspects of biology, risk assessment, and treatment of neuroblastoma. *Semin Surg Oncol.* 1999; 16:91–104.

Look AT, Hayes FA, Shuster JJ, et al. Clinical relevance of a tumor cell ploidy and N-*myc* gene amplification in childhood neuroblastoma: a POG study. *J Clin Oncol.* 1991;9:581–591.

Meitar D, Crawford SE, Rademaker AW, et al. Tumor angiogenesis correlates with metastatic disease, N-*myc* amplification and poor outcome in neuroblastoma. *J Clin Oncol.* 1996;14:405–414.

Shimada H, Stram DO, Chatten J, et al. Identification of subsets of neuroblastomas by combined histopathologic and N-*myc* analysis. *J Natl Cancer Inst.* 1995;87:1470–1476.

A 9-YEAR-OLD GIRL WITH RIGHT LOWER QUADRANT PAIN

HISTORY A 9-year-old female child was admitted through the emergency department with a 12-hour history of abdominal pain and is referred for surgical opinion. The pain, which was initially diffuse and crampy, is now constant and localized to the right lower quadrant. She has no fever, no history of vomiting or diarrhea, and no urinary symptoms. She feels mildly nauseated. The girl is premenarchal and in excellent physical health.

EXAMINATION A quiet 9-year-old girl is resting comfortably on a gurney. Temperature 36.5°C, heart rate 88. Her abdomen is soft and nontender. There is a suprapubic fullness, and a ballotable, mildly tender mass arising from the pelvis. Rectal exam is normal. She has prepubertal breast development and no pubic hair. The remainder of her general physical examination is within normal limits.

LABORATORY Hematocrit 36; white blood cell count 11,000 without left shift; platelets 265,000; urinalysis normal.

Because of diagnostic uncertainty, an abdominal ultrasound is done, which demonstrates a 9-cm cystic mass thought to be arising from the right ovary. A computed tomography (CT) scan of the abdomen and pelvis is shown in Figure 15–1.

Please answer all questions before proceeding to discussion section.

✓ QUESTIONS

1. The most likely diagnosis, based on the CT findings is:
   A. Mature cystic ovarian teratoma (dermoid cyst)
   B. Follicular cyst
   C. Hemorrhagic corpus luteal cyst
   D. Ovarian granulosa-theca cell neoplasm

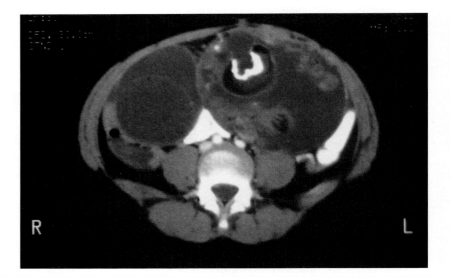

Figure 15–1. *Abdominal computed tomography (CT) scan showing large bilateral cystic ovarian masses. The left ovarian mass is heterogeneous, containing both a calcified mass resembling a tooth and fat, pathognomonic of a mature cystic teratoma.*

2. Prior to definitive therapy, which of the following tests should be done?
   A. Serum levels of estradiol and progesterone
   B. Follicle stimulating hormone/luteinizing hormone (FSH/LH) suppression test
   C. Percutaneous cyst aspiration cytology
   D. Serum levels of alpha-fetoprotein and beta-human chorionic gonadotropin (beta-hCG)

3. The most appropriate therapy for this patient is:
   A. Percutaneous cyst aspiration and close sonographic follow-up
   B. Laparoscopic ovarian cyst fenestration and close sonographic follow-up
   C. Laparoscopic ovarian cystectomy
   D. Laparotomy and oophorectomy

4. Fetal ovarian cysts are now frequently diagnosed by antenatal ultrasound. Which of the following statements regarding fetal ovarian cysts is *false?*
   A. Most fetal cysts will resolve spontaneously and, thus, should be observed without intervention
   B. Because of a significant risk of dystocia, it is recommended that term fetuses within ovarian cysts larger than 7 cm be delivered by cesarean section
   C. Fetal follicular cysts are formed in response to ovarian stimulation by maternal and placental hormones
   D. Large fetal cysts should be aspirated in utero if the mass effect of the cyst is likely to result in either pulmonary hypoplasia or fetal hydronephrosis

5. A baby is born with a 6-cm simple, anechoic ovarian cyst. All of the following statements are true *except:*
   A. Appropriate therapy includes cyst aspiration and sonographic follow-up
   B. Laparotomy and cystectomy may reduce the risk of torsion and ovarian loss

C. The risk of cyst malignancy is approximately 25%
D. The majority of small (< 4 cm) cysts will spontaneously involute because of withdrawal of maternal and placental hormone stimulation

6. Complications of ovarian cysts include:
   A. Mass effect
   B. Torsion
   C. Hemorrhage or rupture
   D. Precocious puberty
   E. All of the above

7. Which of the following correctly lists pediatric ovarian neoplasms in decreasing order of frequency?
   A. Teratoma, dysgerminoma, epithelial tumors, sex-cord/stromal cell tumors
   B. Epithelial tumors, teratoma, dysgerminoma, sex-cord/stromal cell tumors
   C. Teratoma, sex-cord/stromal cell tumors, epithelial tumor, dysgerminoma
   D. Teratoma, epithelial tumors, sex-cord/stromal cell tumors, dysgerminoma

8. Is the following statement regarding *pediatric* ovarian neoplasms true or false? Although the incidence of benign and malignant ovarian neoplasms increases with advancing age, the risk that an ovarian mass is malignant is inversely related to patient age.
   A. True
   B. False

ANSWERS AND DISCUSSION

1. **A** The absence of gastrointestinal symptoms and the presence of a mass makes the diagnosis of appendicitis less likely and warrants further study. The CT scan shows a 9-cm predominantly cystic, pelvic mass containing fat and areas of calcification with some associated pelvic free fluid. The presence of fat and calcification in association with a predominant cystic component is virtually diagnostic of a mature cystic teratoma or dermoid cyst.

2. **D** Although the radiographic features of this cyst point to a diagnosis of mature cystic teratoma, consideration must be given to the possibility that this cyst is malignant, particularly if the cystic component is complex or there is a large solid component. Serum should be obtained preoperatively for quantitative beta-hCG and alpha fetoprotein. There is usually no reason to measure ovarian hormones or gonadotropins unless precocious pseudopuberty is present. Cyst aspiration of a potentially malignant ovarian neoplasm is contraindicated for two reasons. First, cytologic examination of aspirated cyst fluid cannot reliably distinguish between benign and malignant ovarian cysts, and second, there is a risk peritoneal seeding if the cyst fluid contains malignant cells.

3. **D** The appropriate therapy for this presumed benign neoplasm is oophorectomy. Although partial ipsilateral ovarian preservation may be technically possible, the fact remains that until the entire tumor has been studied histologically (in particular the solid component), one cannot preclude the possibility that there might be immature or even malignant tumor elements present. For ovarian masses more likely to be malignant (complex cystic elements or large solid components) operative staging should also be performed. This includes peritoneal washings or ascites fluid for cytology, ipsilateral pelvic and paraortic sampling, contralateral ovarian evalutation with biopsies of suspicious lesions, omentectomy, and peritoneal biopsies. Minimally invasive approaches to these ovarian lesions and, in particular, the large cystic ones, are becoming increasingly popular. Operative cyst decompression greatly facilitates tumor removal but increases the risk of intraoperative spillage, which is significant if the tumor proves to be malignant. Although laparoscopy may play an important role in diagnosis of ovarian lesions, its appropriate role in surgical treatment remains incompletely defined.

4. **B** With increased availability of antenatal ultrasound, ovarian cysts in the fetus are increasingly recognized. Most are follicular cysts and result from maternal, placental, and fetal gonadotropin stimulation. The natural history of most fetal ovarian cysts is to resolve, particularly after birth when maternal and placental stimulation is removed. Fetal ovarian cyst aspiration is recommended only for extremely large cysts, whose mass effect on developing structures is likely to result in irreversible organ injury, for example, with pulmonary hypoplasia or fetal hydronephrosis. Large fetal ovarian cysts (> 4 to 5 cm) may have a higher rate of spontaneous torsion and ovarian loss. Unless or until this risk is known, however, it is hard to justify the potential fetal and maternal risks of prophylactic in utero cyst aspiration. The route of delivery should be dictated by obstetric indications, because dystocia is so unlikely.

5. **C** After birth, most asymptomatic ovarian cysts will regress because of the withdrawal of gonadotropin stimulation. Small cysts (< 4 to 5 cm) can be safely followed with ultrasound; however, large cysts (> 5 cm) have an increased risk for complications, usually torsion, that may result in ovarian loss. The treatment options for large neonatal ovarian cysts include needle aspiration and sonographic follow-up or laparotomy and cystectomy (with ovarian preservation). The probability that a simple, anechoic cyst is malignant is extremely low. Laparotomy should be performed when cysts recur after aspiration and, in cases of torsion, bleeding and rupture, or in the presence of a complex cyst pattern when neoplasia cannot be excluded.

6. **E** Patients with true precocious puberty usually have multiple small cysts from increased secretion of gonadotropin. Precocious pseudopuberty results in some patients with large, autonomously functioning follicular cysts, which elaborate estrogen independent of gonadotropin secretion. Mass effect, torsion, hemorrhage, and rupture are all well-characterized complications of ovarian cysts.

7. **A** Germ cell tumors account for approximately two thirds of all pediatric ovarian neoplasms, and the vast majority of these are mature

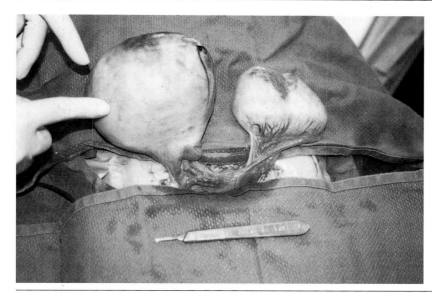

Figure 15–2. *Findings at laparotomy revealed bilateral ovarian teratomas. (See also color plate.)*

teratomas (Figure 15–2; see also color plate). Dysgerminoma is the most primitive of germ cell tumors, the commonest malignant neoplasm of children, and may be bilateral. It is histologically equivalent to seminoma of the testis, and is, hence, extremely chemo- and radiosensitive. The other malignant germ cell tumors are the endodermal sinus or yolk sac tumors (which elaborates alpha-fetoprotein), embyonal carcinoma, choriocarcinoma (which elaborates beta-hCG), and malignant teratoma. Non-germ cell tumors account for about one third of all malignant ovarian neoplasms and include the usually well-differentiated epithelial tumors and the sex-cord/stromal cell tumors (granulosa-theca cell tumors), which usually present with isosexual precocious puberty.

8. A True.

BIBLIOGRAPHY

Haase GM, Vinocur CD. Ovarian tumors. In: O'Neill JA, Rowe MI, Grosfeld JL, et al. eds. *Pediatric Surgery.* St Louis: Mosby Yearbook; 1998.

Helmrath MA, Shin CA, Warner BW. Ovarian cysts in the pediatric population. *Sem Pediatr Surg.* 1998;7:19–28.

CHOKING IN AN 18-MONTH-OLD BOY

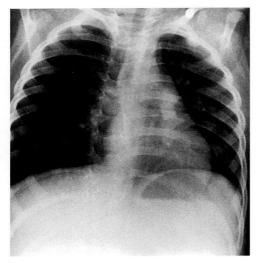

Figure 16–1. *Inspiratory chest x-ray showing abnormal lucency of right lung. Mediastinum is in the midline.*

HISTORY This 18-month-old boy had a choking spell and turned blue while playing outside after his older sibling shared a bag of peanuts with him. His mother rushed out, slapped him on the back, and noted prompt improvement of his cyanosis. He cried but did not vomit. A wheeze was audible. His mother brought him immediately to the emergency room. The episode happened 30 minutes after he ate a big lunch.

EXAMINATION He is a well-developed boy in no respiratory distress who alternately coughed and cried during examination. Pulse is 110 beats per minute, blood pressure is 88 systolic, temperature is 37.8°C, respirations are 28 with crying. There is a watery nasal discharge. The pharynx is slightly edematous with no exudates. Several small cervical nodes are palpable bilaterally. The chest expands symmetrically. There is no dullness or hyperresonance to percussion. On auscultation, there are inspiratory and expiratory wheezes over both sides of the chest, which are more prominent on the right. No cardiac murmur is audible. There are no abdominal masses. The remainder of the physical examination is within normal limits.

LABORATORY Hemoglobin 12 gm%, hemocrit 38%, white blood cell count 11,200/mm³, polymorphonuclear leukocytes 62, bands 2, eosinophils 3, lymphocytes 28, and monocytes 5. Patient refuses to void, so no urine data is available. Chest x-ray obtained on inspiration (Figure 16–1) and expiration (Figure 16–2).

Please answer all questions before proceeding to discussion section.

✓ QUESTIONS

1. The diagnosis is:
   A. Foreign body in the right mainstem bronchus

B. Foreign body in the left mainstem bronchus
C. Foreign body in the trachea
D. Foreign body in the bronchus intermedius

2. The objects most commonly aspirated by children are:
   A. Peanuts
   B. Popcorn
   C. Coins
   D. Small plastic toys
   E. Other

3. Chest roentgenogram after aspiration of a foreign body may show:
   A. Atelectasis of the affected lobe(s)
   B. Emphysema of the affected lobe(s) on expiration
   C. Mediastinal shift away from the affected lobe(s) on expiration
   D. Normal chest on inspiration
   E. All of the above

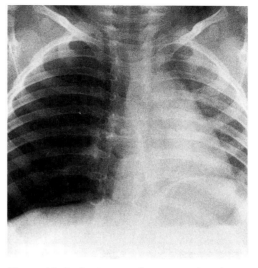

Figure 16–2. *Expiratory chest x-ray showing marked increase in lucency of right lung. Mediastinum is shifted to the left.*

4. Of the following modes of treatment, which one is the *most* appropriate for this child?
   A. Immediate bronchoscopy
   B. Bronchoscopy after a few hours' preparation for general anesthesia
   C. Inhalation of a bronchodilator, such as albuterol, followed by postural drainage and percussion
   D. Intravenous fluids and antibiotics

CLINICAL COURSE   The child was made NPO and begun on intravenous fluids. Bronchoscopy was carried out 2.5 hours later. Figure 16–3 shows what was removed from his right mainstem bronchus.

5. A toddler has choked on a peanut. After a spasm of coughing, he cries for his mother. His color is good, although he has an audible wheeze. Emergency management is:

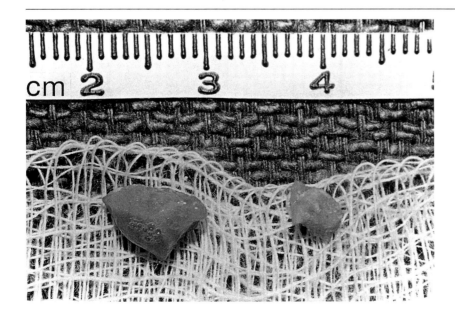

Figure 16–3. *Two peanut fragments removed from right mainstem bronchus.*

    A. Finger sweep of the pharynx
    B. Back blows and chest thrusts
    C. Heimlich maneuver
    D. Standard cardiopulmonary resuscitation (CPR)
    E. None of the above

6. Aspirated peanuts and other nuts are associated with an increased incidence of a specific complication:
    A. Atelectasis
    B. Pneumonia
    C. Arrhythmias
    D. Bronchial stricture

7. All of the following bronchoscopic techniques are appropriate for removal of an aspirated peanut from an 18-month-old child *except:*
    A. Extraction with the optical telescopic forceps via the rigid bronchoscope
    B. Extraction with a Fogarty catheter via the rigid bronchoscope
    C. Extraction with grasping forceps via the flexible bronchoscope
    D. A "second look" into the affected bronchus following extraction

8. Bronchoscopy is begun for extraction of a foreign body in an infant. Shortly after the bronchoscope (4.0 mm inside diameter) is inserted into the trachea, the oxygen saturation falls from 100% to 88%. The optimal management now is:
    A. Removal of the bronchoscope, insertion of an endotracheal tube
    B. Removal of the bronchoscope, insertion of a 3.5-mm bronchoscope
    C. Removal of the bronchoscope, mask ventilation
    D. Removal of the central telescope, continued ventilation
    E. Call code blue

9. During bronchoscopy for removal of a peanut from the right mainstem bronchus, the peanut falls back into the trachea just as the bronchoscope is brought out. Mask ventilation fails to inflate the chest. The oxygen saturation falls precipitously. Emergency management is:
    A. Immediate insertion of an endotracheal tube
    B. Immediate tracheostomy
    C. Immediate reinsertion of the bronchoscope for a therapeutic maneuver
    D. Heimlich maneuver

ANSWERS AND DISCUSSION

1. **A** An aspirated foreign body in the right mainstem bronchus is the most likely diagnosis. The history is typical. The patient is most likely to be an adventurous boy 1 to 2 years of age. Chest x-rays localize the foreign body to the right, rather than the left (**B**), mainstem bronchus. The foreign body produces high-grade partial occlusion of the bronchus, with a one-way valve that allows air to enter the lung but not to exit freely. Thus, the inspiratory view may be normal, but the expiratory view shows air-trapping in the affected lung or lobe. During expiration, the mediastinum shifts away from

the side of the pathology, thus exaggerating the normal loss of volume in the unaffected lung. It was once taught that most foreign bodies lodge in the right mainstem bronchus because of an anatomically "straight shot" down the trachea, whereas the left bronchus has a more acute angulation. Some series, however, in which children under 2 years of age predominate, have shown nearly equal numbers of lodgements in right and left mainstem bronchi (Figure 16–4), although, overall, right-sided lodgement is greater. Tracheobronchial angulation may be more nearly equal in the elastic medistinum of the small infant and probably evolves to the adult-type as the child grows older.

2. **A** Peanuts and other nuts are by far the most common aspirated foreign body. Popcorn, carrots, and an extraordinary variety of other objects may be found. Because only about 10% of aspirated foreign bodies are radiopaque, x-ray diagnosis relies on changes produced by unilateral blockage of airways.

3. **E** All of the findings listed may be seen after foreign body aspiration. An individual patient, however, has either obstructive emphysema (**B**) or atelectasis (**A**) of the affected lobe(s), but not both findings. If there is obstructive emphysema on expiration, the mediastinum shifts away from the side of the emphysema (**C**). The inspiratory film may be normal (**D**), and occasionally both inspiratory and expiratory films are normal (eg, bilateral foreign bodies, tracheal foreign bodies). A good history of foreign body aspiration is an indication to proceed with bronchoscopy in such cases.

4. **B** Bronchoscopy should be performed after appropriate preparation for general anesthesia. It would be unwise to administer general anesthesia 30 to 45 minutes after the child has eaten a big meal. Immediate "crash" bronchoscopy (**A**) is indicated only for the rare case of acute respiratory embarrassment. A nonendoscopic method of removal of foreign bodies consisting of an inhalation treatment, followed by postural drainage and percussion (**C**), was developed at the University of Colorado in the 1970s, but it is not recommended because of instances of cardiorespiratory arrest because of laryngospasm from migration of the foreign body. Intravenous fluids and antibiotics (**D**) are valuable adjuncts to therapy, particularly if the child is dehydrated or has pneumonia, but they do not address the primary problem.

5. **E** None of the measures is appropriate because the child is able to breathe and even speak. He should be taken without further ado to the emergency room. (If the mother calls 911, she should receive this advice.) First aid for the choking child (who cannot breathe or speak) consists of back blows and chest thrusts (**B**) for the child under 1 year of age, and the Heimlich maneuver (**C**) for the child 1 year or older. Finger sweeps (**A**) of the pharynx are not recommended, and standard CPR (**D**) will not work if the airway is completely blocked.

6. **B** Aspirated nuts are associated with an increased incidence of pneumonia when compared to other aspirated objects. Peanut oil may be especially irritating to the bronchial mucosa, producing excessive edema and pooling of secretions distal to the foreign body.

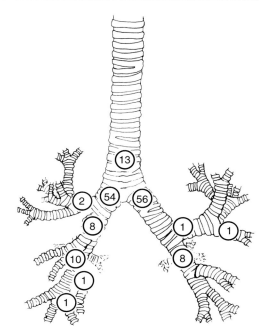

Figure 16–4. *Anatomic location of 155 aspirated foreign bodies removed from 145 children (New Mexico series).*

Atelectasis (**A**) may occur with any type of foreign body. Arrhythmias (**C**) may occur during bronchoscopic extraction under general anesthesia but are not related to the type of foreign body. Bronchial stricture (**D**) has not been reported as a late complication of aspiration, and it must be exceedingly rare, if it occurs.

7. **C** The flexible bronchoscope is unsuitable for foreign body extraction in small children because it lacks a channel for ventilation. This question (and the next two) cover important technical points for the endoscopist. The standard instrument for extraction of foreign bodies is the Storz pediatric ventilating bronchoscope with the Hopkins rod-lens system, which has been in use throughout the world since the 1970s. Either the optical forceps (**A**) or the Fogarty catheter technique (**B**) are the preferred methods of extraction of a peanut with the Storz bronchoscope. Occasionally, the Dormia basket may be useful as well. After the peanut is grasped or drawn into the tip of the bronchoscope, the entire assembly (bronchoscope, instrument, and foreign body) is removed. A "second look" (**D**) into the affected bronchus should be made to rule out retained fragments of foreign body and to suction secretions out of the affected lobe.

8. **D** This scenario is a common one, easily remedied by removal of the telescope, which occupies a large proportion of the lumen, to allow better ventilation via the 4.0-mm bronchoscopic tube. It is not a code blue situation. The bronchoscope need not be removed to restore oxygenation.

9. **C** This scenario is a desperate emergency, requiring an understanding of the pathoanatomy and pathophysiology of foreign body aspiration. The peanut is in one of two places, either at the vocal cords/subglottic area or, less likely, in the left mainstem bronchus, occluding it in combination with edematous obstruction of the right mainstem bronchus ("the degassing phenomenon"). Either scenario produces total obstruction of the airway. Laryngospasm may be an additional factor. Neither endotracheal tube (**A**) nor tracheostomy (**B**) is certain to reestablish the airway. The optimal way to oxygenate this patient is to reinsert the bronchoscope (**C**), and either remove the peanut quickly from the larynx or push it back into the right mainstem bronchus to establish one-lung ventilation. Every second counts. A muscle relaxant, given intravenously, will facilitate the procedure. The Heimlich maneuver (**D**) has not been reported in this situation.

BIBLIOGRAPHY

Azizkhan RG, Caty MG. Subglottic airway. In: Oldham KT, Colombani PM, Foglia RP, eds. *Surgery of Infants and Children: Scientific Principles and Practice.* Philadelphia: Lippincott-Raven; 1997:897–913.

Kosloske AM. Foreign bodies in children. In: Buntain WL, ed. *Management of Pediatric Trauma.* Philadelphia: Saunders; 1995:459–477.

Kosloske AM. Foreign bodies in the pediatric airway. In: Otherson HB, ed. *The Pediatric Airway.* Philadelphia: Saunders; 1991:168–180.

Kosloske AM. Respiratory foreign body. In: Hilman BL, ed. *Pediatric Respiratory Disease: Diagnosis and Treatment.* Philadelphia: Saunders; 1993:513–520.

A 5-YEAR-OLD BOY STRUCK BY A CAR

HISTORY A five-year-old boy was walking across the street when he was struck in the midabdomen by a car traveling about 25 miles per hour. He was thrown to the pavement but did not strike his head. He was alert and oriented at the scene and complained only of left ankle pain. He is brought to the emergency department with a cervical collar and a back board.

EXAMINATION He is alert and responsive. Temperature 37.0°C, heart rate 110, blood pressure 110/75, respiratory rate 22. There is no evidence of head or facial trauma, neck is nontender, lungs are clear with equal breath sounds. Heart tones are normal. Abdomen is nondistended with no guarding or rigidity. There is mild diffuse tenderness over the epigastrium. The left ankle is tender but not unstable. Neurologic examination is normal.

LABORATORY Hemoglobin 13.2, hematocrit 39, white blood cell count 14.2. Urinalysis is normal with no hematuria, amylase is normal. Chest, cervical spine, and pelvis x-rays are normal. Arterial bood gas: pH 7.37, P_{CO_2} 36, P_{O_2} 120 on 2 L nasal cannula.

Please answer all questions before proceeding to discussion section.

✓ QUESTIONS

1. The most common visceral injury after blunt abdominal trauma in this age group is:
   A. Small bowel rupture
   B. Colon perforation
   C. Kidney fracture
   D. Liver laceration
   E. Gastric perforation

2. This patient has a mechanism of injury suggesting abdominal trauma and some tenderness on physical examination. The next diagnostic maneuver should be:
   A. Kidney, ureter, and bladder (KUB) and upright films of the abdomen to look for free intraperitoneal air
   B. Ultrasound of the abdomen
   C. Diagnostic peritoneal lavage
   D. Liver spleen scan to look for the most common injuries
   E. Computed tomography (CT) scan of the abdomen

3. A CT scan of the abdomen is obtained, and the findings are shown in Figure 17–1, which shows:
   A. Splenic fracture
   B. Liver laceration
   C. Subcapsular hematoma of the liver
   D. Pancreatic contusion
   E. Pancreatic transection

4. What fraction of patients with severe pancreatic injuries will have an elevated serum amylase level at initial evaluation?
   A. One hundred percent
   B. Ninety percent
   C. Fifty percent
   D. Twenty percent

5. Proper management should include:
   A. Bowel rest, nasogastric suction, NPO status
   B. Distal pancreatectomy
   C. Whipple procedure
   D. Operative drainage of the lesser sac
   E. Percutaneous drainage of the injury

6. If you decide to operate on the patient, which of the following are true?
   A. Preservation of the spleen is much more likely when operation is done early rather than late

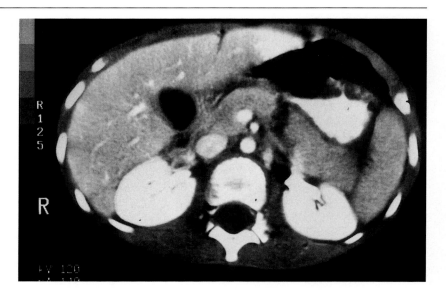

Figure 17–1. *Abdominal computed tomography (CT) scan.*

   B. Preservation of the spleen is more likely when operation is delayed as long as possible following the acute injury

   C. Blood loss should be expected to be very high

   D. Associated injury to the retroperitoneal great vessels is common

   E. The spleen should be removed

7. A different patient is seen 3 weeks after she suffered a blunt injury to the pancreas without transection or major duct disruption. After initially improving, she has developed bilious vomiting, abdominal distention, and a persistent elevation of her serum amylase. What is the most likely diagnosis?

   A. Persistent pancreatitis

   B. A missed jejunal perforation

   C. Intramural duodenum hematoma

   D. Duodenal fistula

   E. Pancreatic pseudocyst

ANSWERS AND DISCUSSION

1. **D** The most commonly injured organ in this setting is the liver followed closely by the spleen. Intestinal perforation certainly occurs in this setting. Bowel rupture can be difficult to diagnose since the initial physical examination can be normal. A CT scan and peritoneal lavage will identify only a minority of these injuries. Serial physical examination will reveal the development of peritonitis. Kidney injuries occur and usually present with hematuria. Gastric perforation occurs uncommonly.

2. **E** The diagnostic study of choice is a CT scan of the abdomen. This is the best way to evaluate the patient for the presence of solid organ injury (liver, spleen, kidney, pancreas). Plain films of the abdomen are of little value unless free air is seen. Even in the presence of traumatic bowel rupture, free air is a fairly uncommon finding. Ultrasound is showing some promise in the setting of abdominal trauma, but its role has yet to be defined. Peritoneal lavage is very sensitive for identifying the presence of intraperitoneal blood. Since most organ injuries are treated nonoperatively, simply finding blood is not helpful. A liver spleen scan has no role in this setting. A CT scan will provide the greatest anatomic detail, but it is not particularly sensitive for identifying hollow organ (bowel and bladder) injury.

3. **E** This image reveals a transection of the pancreas at its midportion just over the vertebral column. The pancreas is particularly vulnerable in this area to a blow to the epigastrium. The soft pancreas is crushed between the striking object (the car bumper in this case) and the spine. When diagnosed early, the only finding is this subtle lucency in the substance of the pancreas. If untreated, marked edema and large lesser sac fluid collections will develop. Unless an adequate bolus of IV contrast has resulted in enhancement of the pancreas, this injury may be missed.

4. **D** Serum amylase shortly following trauma will usually be normal despite the presence of severe pancreatic injury. Even if the CT scan is normal, amylase should be repeated around 24 hours after injury.

At this point it is a very sensitive marker for pancreatic injury. Cases of traumatic pancreatitis due to contusions may present with normal initial serum amylase and CT scan, but the amylase will rise markedly by the second hospital day. Trauma to the salivary glands can cause a marked elevation in the serum amylase level in the absence of pancreatic injury. If this is suspected, the amylase in the serum may be "fractionated" to determine the relative proportions of salivary and pancreatic amylase.

5. **B** Traumatic transection of the pancreas should be treated with distal pancreatectomy. When the pancreas is completely disrupted, pancreatic duct disruption can be assumed. This is best treated with resection of the distal pancreas (Figure 17–2). Drainage alone is likely to lead to the development of a pancreatic fistula. As long as the pancreas to the right of the spine is preserved, exocrine and endocrine insufficiency should not occur. If a large portion of proximal pancreas is destroyed, the surgeon can consider Roux-en-Y drainage of the distal pancreas. This procedure is associated with a significantly higher risk of septic complications than distal pancreatectomy. Whipple resection is reserved for severe injuries of the pancreatic head, duodenum, or both.

   In general, the spleen may be preserved during this resection. Dissection of the posterior pancreas from the splenic vein, however, can be tedious and time consuming. This decision must be made in the context of the patient's other injuries.

6. **A** If this injury is not diagnosed early, a large leak of pancreatic juice into the peritoneal cavity occurs. This results in an intense inflammatory reaction and the development of pancreatic fluid collections. When this occurs, pancreatic resection is much more difficult. The splenic vein becomes densely adherent to the inflamed pancreas

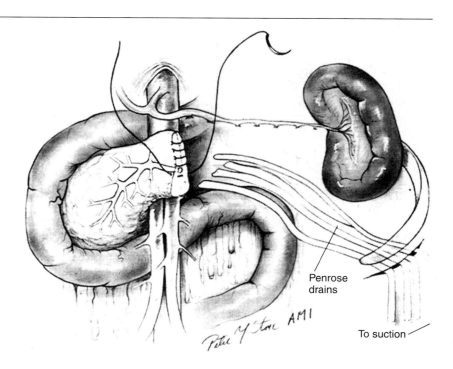

Figure 17–2. *Distal pancreatectomy with preservation of the spleen. (Reproduced with permission from Moront M, Eichelberger MR. Abdominal trauma. In: O'Neill JA Jr, Rowe MI, Grosfeld JL, et al., eds. Pediatric Surgery, 5th ed. St. Louis: Mosby-Yearbook; 1998, p. 279.)*

Penrose drains

To suction

and preservation is difficult. When the operation is done early, blood loss should not be great. Associated injury to the retroperitoneal vessels from blunt trauma is very uncommon.

7. **E** Pancreatic pseudocysts generally present about 3 to 4 weeks after pancreatic injury. They typically occur in the lesser sac and are readily identified by CT scan or ultrasonography (Figure 17–3). In the absence of evidence of infection, pseudocysts are usually treated conservatively for around 4 to 6 weeks. Many will resolve without intervention. When those that have not resolved develop a mature wall, they can be treated in a variety of ways. Options include cystgastrostomy, Roux-en-Y jejunal drainage, and percutaneous catheter drainage. Details of management are beyond the scope of this case.

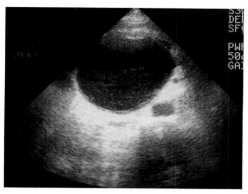

Figure 17–3. *Ultrasound image of pseudocyst.*

BIBLIOGRAPHY

Arkovitz MS, Johnson N, Garcia VF. Pancreatic trauma in children: mechanisms of injury. *J Trauma.* 1997;42:49–53.

Eichelberger MR, Hoelzer DJ, Koop CE. Acute pancreatitis: the difficulties of diagnosis and therapy. *J Pediatr Surg.* 1982;17:244.

McGahren ED, Magnuson D, Schaller RT, et al. Management of transected pancreas in children. *Aust N Z J Surg.* 1995;65:242–246.

Moretz JA, Campbell DP, Parker DE, et al. Significance of pancreatic amylase level in evaluating pancreatic trauma. *Am J Surg.* 1975;130:739.

Moss RL, Musemeche CA. Clinical judgment is superior to diagnostic tests in the treatment of pediatric small bowel injury. *J Pediatr Surg.* 1996;31:1178–1182.

Simon HK, Muehlberg A, Linakis JG. Serum amylase determinations in pediatric patients presenting to the ED with acute abdominal pain or trauma. *Am J Emerg Med.* 1994;12:292–295.

Sivit CJ, Eichelberger MR, Taylor GA, et al. Blunt pancreatic trauma in children: CT diagnosis. *AJR Am J Roentgenol.* 1992;158:1097–1100.

Takishima T, Sugimoto K, Asari Y, et al. Characteristics of pancreatic injury in children: a comparison with such injury in adults. *J Pediatr Surg.* 1996;31:896–900.

AN 8-MONTH-OLD GIRL WITH A "PROLAPSE" AT THE INTROITUS

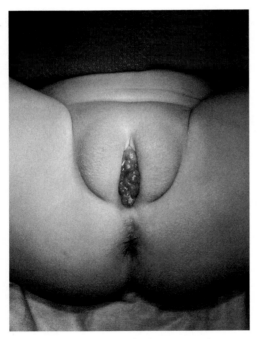

Figure 18–1. *Photograph showing prolapsing tissue at the introitus. (See also color plate.)*

HISTORY   You are asked to evaluate an 8-month-old girl with a history of blood-tinged spotting of her diaper. Her parents first noticed this 1 week ago and have found a red spot in her diaper at every diaper change. She has not been observed to pass grossly bloody urine, and her stools have been normal. She has not had easy bruising or evidence of bleeding elsewhere in her body.

EXAMINATION   She is a very healthy appearing active baby in no apparent distress. Her height and weight are in the 50th percentile. Vital signs are normal. Her lungs are clear; heart is regular without a murmur. Her abdomen is soft and not distended. There is no tenderness to deep palpation in all quadrants and no palpable masses. Perineal exam reveals prolapsing tissue at the introitus (Figure 18–1; see also color plate). This tissue obscures both the vaginal and urethral openings but does not appear to obstruct these orifices.

LABORATORY   Hemoglobin 12.5, hematocrit 35, white blood cell count (WBC) and differential normal. Electrolytes; blood, urea, and nitrogen (BUN); and creatinine are normal. Urinalysis shows trace blood with 1 to 2 red blood cells per high power field, with no white blood cells per high power field, and leukocyte esterase negative.

Please answer all questions before proceeding to discussion section.

✓ QUESTIONS

1. The lesion is most likely:
   A. Prolapsing vaginal mucosa
   B. Malignant neoplasm
   C. Benign multiloculated vaginal cyst
   D. *Candida albicans* infection
   E. Sacrococcygeal teratoma

2. Diagnostic evaluation should include:
   A. Computed tomography (CT) scan of the abdomen
   B. Computed tomography (CT) scan of the chest
   C. Cystoscopy
   D. Vaginoscopy
   E. All of the above

3. This lesion is most often successfully treated with:
   A. Combined chemotherapy
   B. Radiation therapy
   C. Radiation therapy followed by chemotherapy
   D. Simple excision
   E. Radical excision with vaginectomy, hysterectomy, and possible cystectomy

4. The most important factor determining prognosis for this patient is:
   A. Age
   B. Size of the mass
   C. Histology
   D. Involvement of the upper third of the vagina
   E. Serum level of alpha-fetoprotein

5. The goal of operation for this lesion is:
   A. Complete excision with wide margins
   B. Complete excision
   C. Submucosal resection with preservation of tissue
   D. Excision with lymph node dissection
   E. Biopsy

6. Assuming that metastatic disease is not present, the expected 5-year survival for this lesion is:
   A. Greater than 85%
   B. Fifty percent
   C. Less than 20%
   D. Near zero

7. Significant improvements in this lesion's response to chemotherapy have been made over the past several years. The addition of which agent has been primarily responsible for these gains?
   A. Actinomycin D
   B. Adjuvant external beam radiation
   C. Intravaginal brachytherapy
   D. Doxorubicin
   E. Interferon

8. Preliminary cytogenetic studies with this lesion suggest:
   A. A hyperdiploid state portends an improved prognosis
   B. Tumors with a normal content of DNA are less aggressive
   C. A single 10/23 translocation is found in 90% of cases
   D. Gene therapy has resulted in improved survival

9. The lesion is successfully treated with chemotherapy and a complete response is obtained. The oncologist asks you to do a "blind biopsy" in the treated tumor bed to rule out recurrence per study protocol. You do this, and the pathologist reports finding a mixture of vaginal

mucosa with mature rhabdomyoblasts. Which of the following is true?

A. This is a premalignant condition, and immediate resection is warranted
B. Cytogenetic analysis is necessary to determine recommended therapy
C. If rhabdomyoblasts are present at the margins of resection then re-excision is recommended. If the margins are clear, no further therapy is needed
D. No intervention is necessary; biopsy should be repeated in 4 to 6 months
E. Vimentin immunoreactivity is likely to be present

ANSWERS AND DISCUSSION

1. **B** A mass with this appearance is essentially diagnostic of rhabdomyosarcoma, a malignant tumor. Referred to in older literature as sarcoma botryoides, rhabdomyosarcoma of the vagina usually presents in infancy and early childhood as a painless prolapsing vaginal mass. In a review by Hays and coworkers of 28 girls with vaginal rhabdomyosarcoma, the mean age was 23 months with a range from birth to 4 years. The lesion may also present as vaginal bleeding. Vaginal bleeding in a child (except when traumatic resulting from sexual abuse) should always be assumed to be secondary to a neoplasm until proven otherwise.

   Prolapsing vaginal mucosa (**A**) is exceedingly rare in the pediatric population. A benign multiloculated vaginal cyst (**C**) does not exist. *Candida albicans* infection (**D**) is very common in this location but does not present as a mass. Sacrococcygeal teratoma (**E**) occurs in this age group but originates from the coccyx and rarely involves the anterior perineum.

2. **E** Initial evaluation should include a comprehensive search for metastatic disease as well as a complete examination of the local disease. A CT scan of the chest and abdomen are essential. Most experts recommend a radioisotopic bone scan as well. Bone marrow examination is also important. Assessment of local disease requires an examination in the operating room under general anesthesia. Vaginoscopy will reveal the extent of the tumor and whether or not the cervix is involved. Bimanual palpation of the uterus will supplement CT scan results. Cystoscopy is essential to rule out bladder extension.

3. **A** Traditionally, this tumor was treated by means of radical resection. At best, this included vaginectomy and hysterectomy. At worst, it included pelvic exenteration. Cure rates were high with this aggressive therapy. Over the past 15 years, efforts of cooperative study groups have focused on maintaining the high cure rates while significantly decreasing the morbidity of therapy. Refinement of multiagent chemotherapy and, most importantly, the addition of doxorubicin, dramatically improved the response of this tumor. Andrassy and associates reported that virtually all patients can be successfully treated without radical resection.

Review of specimens from seven patients who underwent radical resection after chemotherapy showed no tumor in six patients and maturing rhabdomyoblasts (a benign finding) in the seventh. A report by Andrassy and coworkers confirms that on long-term follow-up, no patients treated with modern chemotherapy have relapsed.

4. **C** Histology is, without question, the most important factor determining survival. Tumors with embryonal histology are far less aggressive and more responsive to therapy than tumors with alveolar or undifferentiated histology. Almost all vaginal tumors have embryonal histology. Age does not necessarily correlate with survival. The size and location of the mass are of some importance, but histology is paramount. Alpha-fetoprotein is an important marker for sacrococcygeal teratoma but is not elevated in these tumors.

5. **E** Since treatment with chemotherapy is virtually always successful, the surgeon's goal should be to stage the local disease accurately and provide adequate tissue for diagnosis without compromising function. Complete excision is not necessary and does not improve outcome. Lymph node dissection has no role in the treatment of this disease.

6. **A** See answer 5.

7. **D** See answer 3.

8. **A** Cytogenetic analysis of rhabdomyosarcoma is in its infancy. In a study by Shapiro and colleagues, a hyperdiploid state was associated with favorable histology and improved survival. The identification of t(2;13)(q35;q14) is a useful aid in the accurate diagnosis of rhabdomyosarcoma, distinguishing it from other small round cell tumors and supporting the distinction between alveolar and embryonal forms. Using fluorescence in situ hybridization, accurate diagnosis is now possible from very small amounts of tissue.

9. **D** The phenomenon of maturation on chemotherapy has been reported with this tumor. Evidence suggests that mature rhabdomyoblasts represent maturation of the tumor to a nonmalignant state. When this is found after therapy, no additional treatment is recommended. Repeat biopsies over a yet to be determined time frame are essential to make sure that the tumor does not recur. Cytogenetic analysis is not necessary to differentiate rhabdomyoblasts from tumor cells. Since rhabdomyoblasts are thought to be benign, their presence at the margin is not relevant. Vimentin immunoreactivity is usually lost by mature cells.

BIBLIOGRAPHY

Andrassy RJ, Wiener ES, Raney RB, et al. Progress in the surgical management of vaginal rhabdomyosarcoma: a 25 year review from the Intergroup Rhabdomyosarcoma Study Group. *J Pediatr Surg.* 1999;34:731–734.

Andrassy RJ, Hays DM, Raney RB, et al. Conservative surgical management of vaginal and vulvar pediatric rhabdomyosarcoma: a report from the intergroup rhabdomyosarcoma study—III. *J Pediatr Surg.* 1995;30:1034–1037.

d'Amore ES, Tollot M, Stracca-Pansa V, et al. Therapy associated differentiation in rhabdomyosarcomas. *Mod Pathol.* 1994;7:69–75.

Hays DM, Shimada H, Raney RB, et al. Sarcomas of the vagina and uterus: the intergroup rhabdomyosarcoma study. *J Pediatr Surg.* 1985;20:718–724.

Hays DM, Shimada H, Raney RB, et al. Clinical staging and treatment results in rhabdomyosarcoma of the female genital tract among children and adolescents. *Cancer.* 1988;61:1893–1903.

Heij HA, Vos A, de Kraker J, et al. Urogenital rhabdomyosarcoma in children: is a conservative surgical approach justified? *J Urol.* 1993;150:165–168.

Kamii Y, Taguchi N, Tsunematsu Y, et al. Primary chemotherapy for children with rhabdomyosarcoma of the "special pelvic" sites: is preservation of the bladder possible? *J Pediatr Surg.* 1994;29:461–464.

Kilpatrick SE, Teot LA, Geisinger KR, et al. Relationship of DNA ploidy to histology and prognosis in rhabdomyosarcoma. *Cancer.* 1994;74:3227–3233.

McManus AP, O'Reilly MA, Jones KP, et al. Interphase fluorescence in situ hybridization detection of t(2;13)(q35;q14) alveolar rhabdomyosarcoma—a diagnostic tool in minimally invasive biopsies. *J Pathol.* 1996;178:410–414.

Raney RB, Gehan EA, Hays DM, et al. Primary chemotherapy with or without radiation therapy and/or surgery for children with localized sarcoma of the bladder, prostate, vagina, uterus, and cervix: a comparison of the results in intergroup rhabdomyosarcoma studies I and II. *Cancer.* 1990;66:2072–2081.

Shapiro DN, Parham DM, Douglass EC, et al. Relationship of tumor-cell ploidy to histologic subtype and treatment outcome in children and adolescents with unresectable rhabdomyosarcoma. *J Clin Oncol.* 1991;9:159–166.

HEAD AND NECK
SHOW AND TELL

Please answer all questions before proceeding to discussion section.

✓ QUESTIONS

1. The 3-month-old infant in Figure 19–1 (see also color plate) comes to your office with a lump beneath the lateral aspect of his left eyebrow. It is 1.1-cm, firm, and nontender, and it appears to be fixed on its deep aspect. The diagnosis is:
   A. Lipoma
   B. Osteoma
   C. Dermoid
   D. Calcifying epithelioma of Malherbe
   E. Nonaccidental trauma

2. Prior to excision, appropriate management includes:
   A. Skull films
   B. Computed tomography (CT) scan of the head
   C. Neurosurgical consultation
   D. Ophthalmologic consultation
   E. None of the above

3. A 4-year-old girl comes to your office with a painless cyst (Figure 19–2; see also color plate) beneath her tongue. She has no other masses of the head or neck, and she has been healthy until 1 week ago, when the cyst appeared. The diagnosis is:
   A. Cystic hygroma
   B. Cystic lymphangioma
   C. Cystic teratoma
   D. Thyroglossal duct cyst
   E. Ranula

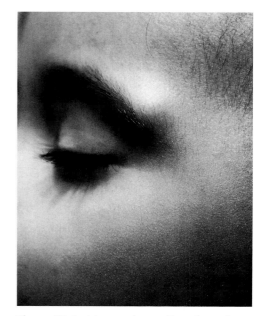

Figure 19–1. *Mass on brow. (See also color plate.)*

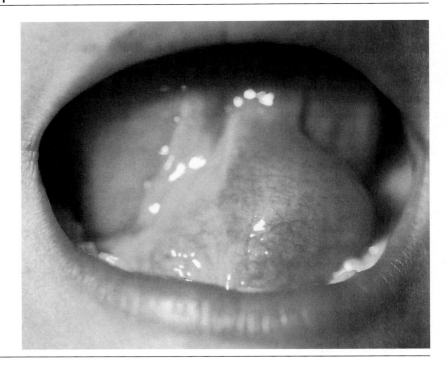

Figure 19–2. *Cyst beneath tongue. (See also color plate.)*

4. The optimal management is:
   A. Excision
   B. Marsupialization
   C. A CT scan, excision
   D. Magnetic resonance imaging (MRI) scan, marsupialization
   E. Needle aspiration; watchful waiting

5. A 3-week-old male infant comes to your office with a mass in the right side of his neck (Figure 19–3; see also color plate). There is no erythema. On palpation, it is firm, nontender, and seems to be located within the right sternocleidomastoid muscle. The diagnosis is:
   A. Branchial cleft cyst
   B. Thyroglossal duct cyst
   C. Cervical lymphadenitis
   D. Torticollis
   E. Cystic hygroma

6. Optimal management is:
   A. Biopsy, frozen section, excision
   B. Biopsy without frozen section
   C. Division of the sternocleidomastoid muscle
   D. Ultrasound, watchful waiting
   E. Stretching and range-of-motion exercises

ANSWERS AND DISCUSSION

1. **C** The diagnosis is dermoid cyst of the brow. The term "dermoid" is a kind of colloquial term for a choristomatous nodule of ectoderm, which is trapped during development along a suture line between cranial bones. The most common site is the lateral brow over the

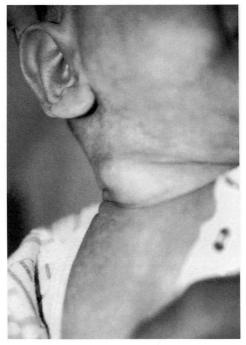

Figure 19–3. *Mass in lateral neck. (See also color plate.)*

frontal-zygomatic suture. Usually there is deep attachment to carti-lage. Dermoids are found less commonly along the occipital suture line or at the glabella. Lipoma (**A**), a fatty tumor, and osteoma (**B**), a bony tumor, rarely occur at this location. The calcifying epithelioma (**D**), a unique soft-tissue mass in children, originates from skin structures. Usually, there is an overlying dimple. On palpation, it feels like a disc-shaped fragment of eggshell under the skin. Nonaccidental trauma (**E**) (ie, child abuse) may present with bruises of various ages and lumps from healing fractures on ribs and other bones, but the lateral brow would be an unusual site.

2. **E** Excision is the treatment for a dermoid cyst of the lateral brow. The incision is made through the eyebrow, without shaving the eye-brow, for the best cosmetic result. The deep cartilaginous attach-ment should be removed completely. In a typical case, adjunctive measures are neither necessary nor cost effective. The probability that a dermoid of the lateral brow might extend through the skull into the epidural or subdural space approaches zero. Skull films (**A**) are unlikely to show a defect in the cranial bones. A CT scan (**B**) or neurosurgical consultation (**C**) might be reassuring for management of a glabellar dermoid, which has a small risk of "dumbbell" in-tracranial extension, but it is not needed for a dermoid of the lateral brow. Ophthalmologic consultation (**D**) is likewise not necessary.

3. **E** The diagnosis is ranula, a cystic enlargement of an accessory sali-vary gland in the floor of the mouth. Cystic hygroma (**A**) usually oc-curs in the neck or axilla. Rarely, it may occur in other locations (retroperitoneum, extremities), but it would not present as an iso-lated cyst beneath the tongue in a 4-year-old child. Cystic lymphan-gioma (**B**) is no different from cystic hygroma; the latter is a more colloquial term. A cystic teratoma (**C**) may occur at the base of the tongue in a neonate, but it would be most unlikely in a 4-year-old child. Thyroglossal duct cyst (**D**) typically presents as a midline neck mass. In its rare presentation as a midline cyst of the tongue, it would be located on the dorsum of the tongue (the site of the fora-men cecum), rather than beneath the tongue.

4. **B** Marsupialization is the optimal management of the ranula. Because the cyst is lined with normal mucosa, the deep portion can be left in situ without risk. Complete excision (**A**) is not necessary and might produce excessive blood loss. A CT scan (**C**) is not needed, as the ranula does not have deep extensions. An MRI scan is a very good study for mapping the extent of a large cystic hygroma but is not needed for management of a ranula. Needle aspiration (**E**) would empty the cyst temporarily, but, since the lining remains in-tact, the fluid would soon reaccumulate.

5. **D** The diagnosis is congenital torticollis. The mass is within the sternocleidomastoid muscle, whereas branchial cleft cyst (**A**) is typi-cally located anterior to the muscle, and cystic hygroma (**E**) is lo-cated posterior to the muscle. Thyroglossal duct cyst (**B**) is located anteriorly in the midline. Cervical lymphadenitis (**C**), an inflamma-tory lesion, usually occurs in the first 2 years of life, but it is rare in the first month. The diagnosis of torticollis may be confirmed on physical examination by rotating the infant's head in both direc-

tions. Normally, when the sternocleidomastoid muscle contracts, the face turns toward the opposite side. Torticollis represents an exaggeration of the normal, with spastic contraction of the muscle. In this case of right-sided torticollis, the head turns preferentially to the left but meets resistance when turned to the right.

6. **E** Torticollis is treated by stretching and range-of-motion exercises designed to relieve the spasm and to balance the muscle pull on the two sides of the neck. This approach is successful in approximately 95% of cases diagnosed in infancy. Skeptics have argued that the mass will resolve spontaneously with or without the exercises, but there are no randomized trials to support either approach. Biopsy (**A, B**) is clearly unnecessary. Excision or division of the sternocleidomastoid (**C**) is indicated only in rare instances in which a child 12 to 18 months or older develops a chronic tilt of the head with facial asymmetry. Pathologic section, in such cases, shows fibrosis of the sternocleidomastoid. Ultrasound (**D**) is a good confirmatory study for diagnosis but is rarely needed.

BIBLIOGRAPHY

Beasley SW. Torticollis. In: O'Neill JA Jr, Rowe MI, Grosfeld JL, et al., eds. *Pediatric Surgery.* 5th ed. St. Louis: Mosby-Year Book 1998:773–778.

Fallat ME. Neck. In: Oldham KT, Colombani PM, Foglia RP, eds. *Surgery of Infants and Children: Scientific Principles and Practice.* Philadelphia: Lippincott-Raven; 1997:836, 850.

Quinn GE, Jockin YM. Tumors of orbit and lid. In: O'Neill JA Jr, Rowe MI, Grosfeld JL, et al. eds. *Pediatric Surgery.* 5th ed. St. Louis: Mosby-Year book; 1998:667.

Repka MX. Orbital and eyelid dermoid. In: Oldham KT, Colombani PM, Foglia RP, eds. *Surgery of Infants and Children: Scientific Principles and Practice.* Philadelphia: Lippincott-Raven; 1997:789.

A 7-YEAR-OLD BOY WITH ACUTE ABDOMINAL PAIN

HISTORY A 7-year-old boy presents to the emergency room with a 24-hour history of abdominal pain. The pain, initially periumbilical and crampy, has become localized and constant in the right lower quadrant. He has vomited three times and remains anorexic. He has had one loose stool. A sibling is recovering from an acute febrile illness with diarrhea and vomiting.

EXAMINATION A healthy male child is lying comfortably. Temperature is 38°C axillary. Abdomen is scaphoid with localized tenderness and voluntary guarding in the right lower quadrant. Groins clear; testicles descended and nontender. Rectal examination is normal.

LABORATORY White blood cell count (WBC) 13,000; urinalysis 1 to 5 red blood cells (RBC), 1 to 5 white blood cells. An abdominal x-ray is shown in Figure 20–1.

Please answer all questions before proceeding to discussion section.

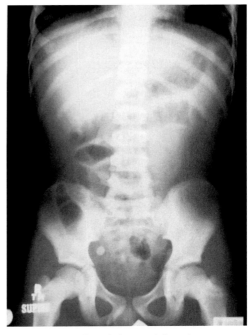

Figure 20–1. *This abdominal flat plate demonstrates a spheroid calcification in the right lower quadrant consistent with a fecalith of the appendix (appendicolith).*

✓ QUESTIONS

1. The most appropriate next "diagnostic" test would be:
   A. Ultrasound
   B. Computed tomography (CT) scan
   C. Urine culture
   D. Laparoscopic or open appendectomy

2. Fecaliths on abdominal x-ray are:
   A. Visible in 10% to 20% of all cases of appendicitis
   B. Visible in 50% of all cases of appendicitis
   C. Visible in 90% of all cases of appendicitis
   D. An absolute indication for appendectomy even in the absence of abdominal symptoms

3. Prior to operation, the boy should receive the following resuscitation:
   A. 20 mL/kg crystalloid (lactated Ringer's or normal saline)
   B. 20 mL/kg crystalloid plus intravenous second generation cephalosporin
   C. 20 mL/kg crystalloid, nasogastric tube, Foley catheter
   D. None (resuscitation to be done in operating room)

4. At operation, the appendix appears normal. You should:
   A. Remove the appendix and close
   B. Close the right lower quadrant incision, and explore the abdomen through a lower midline incision
   C. Extend the right lower quadrant incision, and explore as much of the abdomen and ileum as possible through that incision
   D. Perform laparoscopy

5. Inspection of the distal ileum demonstrates a segment of narrow, thickened, nonpliable intestine with mesenteric thickening and fibrosis and a "creeping fat" appearance. This process extends to the base of the cecum. You would:
   A. Biopsy the small intestine, remove the appendix, and close
   B. Resect the terminal ileum and cecum, and perform an ileo-ascending colon anastomosis
   C. Remove the appendix and close
   D. Close the abdomen

6. Treatment of perforated appendicitis consists of:
   A. Appendectomy, antibiotic wound irrigation with abdominal cavity drainage, skin incision left open, and 1 week of broad spectrum intravenous antibiotics
   B. Appendectomy, wound closure without irrigation or drainage, and 5 days of intravenous antibiotics
   C. Appendectomy, wound irrigation, delayed primary skin closure, and 48 hours of antibiotics
   D. All of the above

ANSWERS AND DISCUSSION

1. **D** This typical history with localized, right lower quadrant peritonitis on physical examination is sufficient for a clinical diagnosis of appendicitis. No other validating diagnostic tests are required.

   In cases where the diagnosis of appendicitis is not clear, then ultrasound and CT scan offer a high degree of diagnostic accuracy. The sonographic demonstration of an enlarged, noncompressible tubular structure that connects to the cecum, associated with some free fluid and "transducer" tenderness is virtually 100% sensitive and specific for appendicitis (Figure 20–2). Depending on availability and operator expertise, ultrasound is probably preferable to CT scan, in that it is less expensive and does not involve radiation. Compared to ultrasound, however, CT scanning offers a broader scope of diagnostic potential.

   The question of laparoscopic versus open appendectomy remains controversial. The clear benefit of a laparoscopic approach is the advantage conferred by complete peritoneal cavity examination, so it

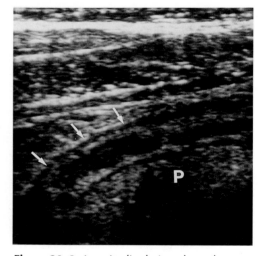

Figure 20–2. *Longitudinal view through a tender, noncompressible tubular structure (arrows), lying on top of the psoas muscle (P). The presence of this structure and demonstration of its connection to the cecum is virtually diagnostic of acute appendicitis.*

should be considered if the diagnosis is in doubt. Most studies show only marginal or no advantage of laparoscopic over open appendectomy with regard to length of hospitalization, postoperative analgesic use, length of time to full activity, and wound infection rate. Laparoscopic appendectomy is generally more expensive because of increase equipment costs not offset by earlier discharge.

2. **A** Fecaliths are visible on plain x-ray in 10% to 20% of all cases of appendicitis. Their radiographic existence in the presence of some abdominal symptoms, however mild, is considered an indication for appendectomy by most surgeons.

3. **B** All surgical patients must be appropriately resuscitated before surgery. A minimum of 20 mL/kg of crystalloid should be given to restore euvolemia and reasonable organ perfusion. Since most patients present with a short history of illness, their dehydration is usually easily reversed with one or two boluses of crystalloid given during the time it takes to get them into an operating room. In situations where a patient presents late, often with complicated appendicitis, it is far more important to restore intravascular volume adequately, correct electrolyte disturbances, and achieve adequate tissue and blood levels of broad spectrum antibiotics than it is to get their appendix out. In such instances, a patient may require admission for 6 to 8 hours of resuscitation, close monitoring of urine output, and correction of metabolic disturbances before surgery. Preoperative antibiotics are given to all patients with suspected appendicitis. Although the gold standard of antibiotic therapy for appendicitis, both for prophylaxis and treatment of complicated disease, is triple therapy (ampicillin, gentamicin, and either clinidamycin or metronidazole), most surgeons now use a single preoperative dose of a second or third generation cephalosporin (for example, cefotetan), for suspected, uncomplicated appendicitis.

4. **C** The answer to this question is somewhat controversial. The extent to which one tries to exclude other pathology if the appendix appears normal probably depends, in part, on how sick the child appears and how certain the surgeon is of the presence of peritonitis. In most instances, if the appendix appears completely normal, then a limited evaluation of the distal ileum through the same incision to exclude a Meckel's diverticulum or ileitis (viral, bacterial, or granulomatous) should be performed. If nothing is found, except perhaps some enlarged mesenteric lymph nodes in a relatively well child, then the likely diagnosis is mesenteric adenitis, and the normal appendix is removed. Most large series quote a negative laparotomy rate of 1% to 10% for presumed appendicitis. If, on the other hand, more convincing evidence of peritonitis exists (such as the presence of fibrin or pus) in a child who appears ill but has a normal appendix, then one should be more diligent in the search for explanatory pathology. If local exploration through the right lower quadrant incision is not revealing, then consideration should be given to a second incision or laparoscopy.

5. **D** This patient almost certainly has Crohn's disease. The appendix should not be removed if it or the cecum is involved in the disease process because removal is associated with a subsequent high inci-

dence of fistula formation. The involved small bowel should not be biopsied for the same reason.

6. **B** This is another controversial question that has no definite answer. Appendiceal perforation rates vary according to age and cultural and socioeconomic status of the patient population, and they are reported to range from 16% to 57%. When encountered in the operating room, the appendix should be removed, the pus drained, and the wound irrigated locally. The use of antibiotic irrigation solutions, peritoneal cavity versus local wound irrigation, drains, and the issue of primary or delayed skin closure are all options, none of which have any proven benefit over the other. The choice of antibiotics and duration of therapy after surgery is also controversial. Most centers would give 5 days of intravenous antibiotics, and then discharge if the patient has been afebrile for at least 24 hours, has a normal WBC, and a functioning gastrointestinal tract. Some would also give a course of oral antibiotics (Septra, Flagyl) postdischarge.

Complicated appendicitis presenting with an intra-abdominal abscess or as a palpable appendiceal phlegmon can also be managed by nonoperative means, provided the patient's condition is stable, and there are no signs of generalized peritonitis. If imaging studies (ultrasound, CT scan, or both) demonstrate a walled-off intra-abdominal or pelvic abscess, radiographically guided catheter drainage by either the percutaneous transabdominal or transrectal route may be performed. Patients with localized abscesses will often respond dramatically to catheter drainage and a course of intra-venous and oral antibiotics and may recover more quickly than if their initial therapy had consisted of appendectomy and abscess drainage. Similarly, patients with an appendiceal phlegmon, but no abscess, can be treated with intravenous fluids and antibiotics. In both patient groups, criteria for success or failure of nonoperative therapy must be clearly defined, and patients who do not respond promptly to nonoperative therapy should undergo appendectomy.

The need for routine, delayed, or "interval" appendectomy following successful nonoperative management of complicated appendicitis is unclear, since there are no large series of patients with long-term follow-up. The general recommendation at this time would be that children undergo routine elective appendectomy approximately 6 weeks after their initial nonoperative therapy.

BIBLIOGRAPHY

Anderson KD, Parry RL. Appendicitis. In: O'Neill JA, Rowe MI, Grosfeld JL, et al. eds. *Pediatric Surgery.* St Louis: Mosby-Year Book, 1998.

Blakely ML, Spurbeck W, Lakshman S, et al. Current status of laparoscopic appendectomy in children. *Curr Opin Pediatr.* 1998;10:315–317.

Blewett CL, Krummel TM. Perforated appendicitis: past and future controversies. *Semin Pediatar Surg.* 1995;4:234–238.

Gupta H, Dupuy DE. Advances in imaging of the acute abdomen. *Surg Clin North Am.* 1997;77:1245–1263.

ACUTE ABDOMEN IN A 5-DAY-OLD PREMATURE INFANT

HISTORY A 30-week, 1200 g premature male infant develops abdominal distention and blood-streaked stools on the fifth day of life. He has an episode of apnea and bradycardia, requiring mask ventilation, oxygen, and endotracheal intubation.

EXAMINATION He is a lethargic infant with mottled skin and circumoral cyanosis. Doppler blood pressure is 64/46; pulse is 178. Ventilator rate is 28 per minute. Breath sounds are present over the right side of the chest but markedly decreased on the left. The abdomen is moderately distended and tense without masses or cellulitis. Bowel sounds are absent. The testes are palpable in the inguinal canals bilaterally. Femoral pulses are full; posterior tibial and radial pulses are faint; dorsalis pedis pulses are absent. Urine output for the past 4 hours is 7 mL. An orogastric tube is placed and returns bilious fluid. X-rays are obtained (Figure 21–1).

Please answer all questions before proceeding to discussion section.

✓ QUESTIONS

1. The diagnosis of this infant is:
   A. Necrotizing enterocolitis (NEC) of the newborn
   B. Hirschsprung disease with enterocolitis
   C. Meconium ileus
   D. Meconium peritonitis
   E. Neonatal sepsis

2. Management of this infant should include all of the following *except:*
   A. An intravenous bolus of 30 mL/kg of normal saline or colloid solution
   B. Intravenous fluid rate at two to three times maintenance

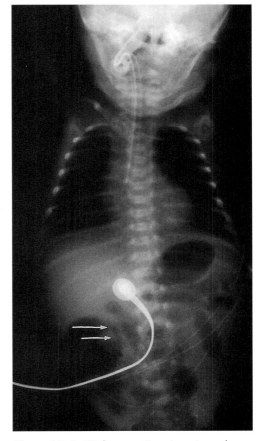

Figure 21–1. *"Babygram," supine view, showing dilated intestinal loops in the right side of the abdomen and pneumatosis intestinalis (arrows). The tip of the endotracheal tube is in the right mainstem bronchus.*

    C. Cultures of blood and cerebrospinal fluid (CSF)
    D. Intravenous antibiotics, including an aminoglycoside and a penicillin
    E. Abdominal x-rays every 6 to 8 hours for the next 24 hours

HOSPITAL COURSE The endotracheal tube is suctioned and pulled back 1 cm, after which the breath sounds are equal, and the circumoral cyanosis disappears. The infant stabilizes on medical supportive treatment and gradually improves. Feedings of an elemental formula are begun 10 days after the acute episode. He tolerates the feedings well but continues to pass stools that are intermittently positive for occult blood. Two and one-half weeks after the acute episode, he develops abdominal distention and vomiting, which resolves when feedings are stopped for 24 hours. A similar episode occurs 4 days later. He is afebrile, and his abdomen is soft. No abdominal mass is palpable. Abdominal films show a nonspecific gas pattern.

  3. Which *one* of the following studies is *most* likely to identify a potentially serious problem?
    A. Abdominal ultrasound
    B. Upper gastrointestinal (GI) series
    C. Barium enema
    D. Technitium scan for Meckel's diverticulum
    E. Cultures of blood and CSF

  4. Following a positive study (question 3), the optimal management of this infant is:
    A. Incision and drainage
    B. Ladd's procedure
    C. Resection and anastomosis
    D. Balloon dilation
    E. Temporary colostomy

  5. No single, specific cause has been discovered for NEC. All of the following factors nevertheless have been implicated in its pathogenesis *except:*
    A. Selective circulatory ischemia (the diving reflex)
    B. Immature barrier function of the neonatal gut
    C. Bacterial colonization of the GI tract
    D. Breaks in isolation technique by nursery personnel
    E. Intestinal ischemia in utero

  6. Which of the following perinatal conditions has a (statistically) *significant* association with NEC?
    A. Apneic spells
    B. Low Apgar scores
    C. Umbilical arterial catheterization
    D. Prematurity
    E. All of the above

  7. Which of the following radiographic findings is associated with the highest mortality?
    A. Severe pneumatosis intestinalis
    B. Pneumoperitoneum
    C. Portal venous gas

D. Both A and B

E. Both A and C

8. Prevention of NEC may be achieved by:
   A. Feeding of breast milk
   B. Oral administration of gentamicin and metronidazole
   C. Intravenous administration of triple antibiotics (ie, a penicillin, an aminoglycoside, and an antianaerobic agent, such as clindamycin)
   D. Intravenous administration of immunoglobulins A and G
   E. All of the above

ANSWERS AND DISCUSSION

1. **A** Necrotizing enterocolitis (NEC) of the newborn is the most likely diagnosis. The clinical signs of abdominal distention, ileus, and gastrointestinal bleeding in a sick premature infant are characteristic for NEC. The radiographic finding of pneumatosis intestinalis (air in the bowel wall) is pathognomonic. Infants with severe NEC may also develop pneumoperitoneum, portal venous gas, or both. Pneumatosis intestinalis is not found in the other conditions, all of which are included in the differential diagnosis of the acute abdomen in the neonate. The enterocolitis of Hirschsprung disease (**B**) is a life-threatening problem, which characteristically occurs in a term male infant who fails to pass meconium in the first 24 hours and becomes distended and toxic. Meconium ileus (**C**) is a mechanical bowel obstruction due to viscid meconium impacted in the baby's terminal ileum. It is associated with cystic fibrosis in virtually every case. Meconium peritonitis (**D**) is a chemical, sterile peritonitis resulting from prenatal intestinal perforation, in contrast to the peritonitis of NEC, which is a bacterial peritonitis from postnatal perforation. In meconium peritonitis, abdominal films classically show intraperitoneal calcifications. Most, but not all, of the infants prove to have cystic fibrosis. Neonatal sepsis (**E**) is incorrect because it is not the primary problem, although sepsis is associated with NEC in 30% to 35% of cases.

2. **B** Although the infant is hypovolemic, as manifested by tachycardia and mottling, his blood pressure and urine output have not yet decreased. He needs a bolus of fluid to restore perfusion; however, 30 mL/kg (total 36 mL) is too much for a 1.2 kg infant. A more appropriate initial bolus would be 10 to 20 mL/kg (12 to 24 mL), which should be repeated after a few minutes if perfusion does not improve. All of the other statements are true. Intravenous fluid requirements are two to three times maintenance (**A**) because of "third spacing" (ie, sequestration of fluid in the bowel lumen, bowel wall, and peritoneal cavity [ascites]). A septic work-up, including cultures of blood and CSF, is indicated at onset of NEC (**D**). The clinical presentation of NEC may be indistinguishable from that of neonatal sepsis (**E**). Further, blood cultures are positive in 30% to 35% of infants with severe NEC. The specific antibiotics vary in different nurseries, depending on the local pathogens of neonatal sepsis, but a penicillin and an aminoglycoside (**C**) are a standard combination. A third agent that is effective against anaerobic bacteria (eg, clin-

damycin) may be added. Abdominal x-rays should be obtained (usually supine and left lateral decubitus views) every 6 to 8 hours (**E**) for about 24 hours to identify changes that may signify improvement (eg, resolution of pneumatosis intestinalis) or deterioration (eg, pneumoperitoneum). The left lateral decubitus view is particularly helpful for identification of pneumoperitoneum. After the first 24 hours, abdominal films are less helpful because most of the intestinal air has been removed by gastric suction, and films should be ordered less frequently.

3. **C** This infant has early signs of intestinal stricture, a complication that occurs in 20% to 25% of infants who recover from acute NEC. The stricture occurs at a site of bowel injury, which retains some viable elements. Intermittent blood in the stool is a clue to diagnosis. The injured mucosa is ulcerated. Ultimately, the bowel may heal by formation of circumferential scar, producing intestinal obstruction. The colon is the most common location, hence the barium enema (Figure 21–2). Upper GI series (**B**) will occasionally identify a stricture of the small intestine. Abdominal ultrasound (**A**) is generally not helpful for diagnosis of intestinal obstruction, although it is the imaging study of choice for diagnosis of pyloric stenosis. Meckel's diverticulum with ectopic gastric mucosa (**D**) may cause GI hemorrhage in infants or children, but rarely presents in the neonatal period. The signs of neonatal sepsis (**E**) are nonspecific and include lethargy, poor feeding, vomiting, abdominal distention, cyanosis, and temperature instability. Fever is uncommon. The premature infant in this case should receive a work-up for sepsis, but intestinal stricture is still the more likely diagnosis.

4. **C** Resection and anastomosis is usually the treatment of choice for colonic stricture, unless the infant has acute intestinal obstruction, a

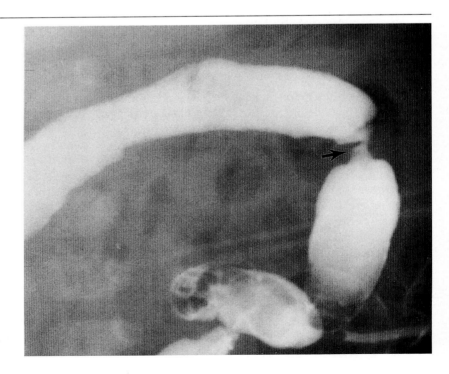

Figure 21–2. *Barium enema showing a stricture (arrow) at splenic flexure of colon following necrotizing enterocolitis (NEC).*

situation that might require a temporary colostomy (**E**). Incision and drainage (**A**) is the treatment for abscess, which this infant does not have. Ladd's procedure (detorsion of midgut volvulus, lysis of congenital duodenal and jejunal bands) is the treatment for midgut volvulus, a condition that is less likely than stricture in this infant. Balloon dilation (**D**) is a good option for treatment of focal colonic strictures distal to an enterostomy, but it would risk sepsis or perforation of colon, which is still in the fecal stream.

5. **E** Intestinal ischemia in utero results in sterile necrosis, which is manifested at birth as intestinal atresia not NEC. Selective circulatory ischemia (**A**) of the gastrointestinal tract, a normal physiologic reflex triggered by stress, may produce ischemic changes in the gut, leading to necrosis and perforation. Mucosal immunity is not well developed (**B**) in the neonatal gut, particularly if the infant has not received maternal colostrum or breast milk. The premature gut may be vulnerable to invasion from its own bacterial flora or to damage from antigenic substances in its lumen. Bacterial colonization of the gastrointestinal tract (**C**) is necessary for the development of NEC, which does not occur prenatally or in germ-free animals. An epidemiologic study by Book and colleagues documented clustering of cases of NEC during periods in which viral infections were increased in the nursery personnel. Breaks in isolation technique (**D**), especially handwashing, were implicated.

6. **D** Although stressful perinatal events, such as apneic spells (**A**), low Apgar scores (**B**), and umbilical arterial catheterization (**C**), are frequently documented in infants who develop NEC, case-control studies have failed to show statistical significance with any factor except (**D**) prematurity. Ninety percent of infants with NEC are premature.

7. **E** A study from New Mexico of 147 infants with NEC demonstrated that outcomes of NEC can be predicted by the initial radiographic findings. Pneumatosis intestinalis was graded as mild, moderate, or severe by a pediatric radiologist. The mortality rates associated with specific abnormalities were: mild or moderate pneumatosis intestinalis, 19%; severe pneumatosis intestinalis, 63%; pneumoperitoneum, 47%; and portal venous gas, 65%. The highest mortality rate (86%) was associated with the combination of severe pneumatosis and portal venous gas.

8. **A** Breast milk is protective against the development of NEC. The British multicenter study documented a low incidence of NEC among premature infants who received breast milk as their only feeding. Necrotizing enterocolitis was six to ten times more common among infants who were fed formula only, and three times more common among infants who received a combination of formula and breast milk. None of the other factors has proved to be protective against NEC. Prophylactic antibiotics, either oral (**B**) or parenteral (**C**), serve only to select out resistant strains of bacteria but do not prevent NEC. A study from Vienna showed a protective effect of oral (not parenteral) administration of a preparation of immunoglobulins A and G (**D**) to infants at risk for NEC, but other investigators have been unable to duplicate this result.

HOSPITAL COURSE The infant receives a barium enema (Figure 21–2). The stricture is resected, and primary anastomosis is done. He makes a good recovery and is discharged at 7 weeks of age.

BIBLIOGRAPHY

Ball WS Jr, Kosloske AM, Jewell PF, et al. Balloon catheter dilatation of focal intestinal strictures following necrotizing enterocolitis. *J Pediatr Surg.* 1985;20:637–639.

Book LS, Overall JC, Herbst JJ, et al. Interruption of necrotizing enterocolitis clustering by infection-control measures. *New Engl J Med.* 1977; 297:984–986.

Eibl MM, Wolf HM, Furnkranz H, et al. Prevention of necrotizing enterocolitis in low-birth weight infants by IgA-IgG feeding. *New Engl J Med.* 1988;319:1–7.

Israel EJ. Neonatal necrotizing enterocolitis: a disease of the immature intestinal mucosal barrier. *Acta Paediatr Suppl.* 1994;396:27–32.

Kliegman RM, Fanaroff AA. Necrotizing enterocolitis. *New Engl J Med.* 1984;310:1093–1103.

Kosloske AM. The epidemiology and pathogenesis of necrotizing enterocolitis. *Semin Neonatol.* 1997;2:231–238.

Kosloske AM. Necrotizing enterocolitis. In: Oldham KT, Colombani PM, Foglia RP, eds. *Surgery of Infants and Children: Scientific Principles and Practice.* Philadelphia: Lippincott Raven; 1997:1201–1214.

Kosloske AM, Musemeche CA, Ball WS Jr, et al. Necrotizing enterocolitis: value of radiographic findings to predict outcome. *AJR.* 1988;151: 371–392.

Lloyd JR. The etiology of gastrointestinal perforations in the newborn. *J Pediatr Surg.* 1969;4:77–84.

Lucas A, Cole TJ. Breast milk and neonatal necrotizing enterocolitis. *Lancet.* 1990;336:1519–1523.

Stoll BJ, Kanto WP, Glass RI, et al. Epidemiology of necrotizing enterocolitis: a case control study. *J Pediatr.* 1980;96:447–451.

A NEWBORN GIRL WITH IMPERFORATE ANUS

HISTORY You are called by the neonatologist about a newborn girl found to have imperforate anus (Figure 22–1; see also color plate) at a screening examination in the well baby nursery. The nurse reports that the baby's diaper is full of meconium. The infant is breast feeding well without abdominal distention or vomiting.

EXAMINATION The baby is 3850 g and appears healthy and vigorous. Vital signs are normal. Breath sounds are clear and equal. Heart tones are normal without a murmur. The abdomen is soft, nondistended, and nontender in all quadrants, with no masses or hepatosplenomegaly.

The perineal examination reveals an imperforate anus with meconium within the fourchette. The vagina and urethra appear normal. The back is normal.

LABORATORY Hemoglobin is 15.8; hematocrit is 51; white blood cell count is 7.8. A chest x-ray reveals normal heart and lung shadows. Abdominal film shows several hemivertebrae in the lumbar spine.

Please answer all questions before proceeding to discussion section.

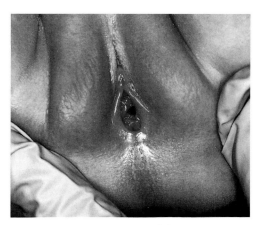

Figure 22–1. *Appearance of the perineum in a newborn girl with imperforate anus. (See also color plate.)*

✓ QUESTIONS

1. The most common anatomic abnormality accounting for these findings is:
   A. Persistent cloaca
   B. Imperforate anus with rectovestibular fistula
   C. Imperforate anus with low vaginal fistula
   D. Imperforate anus with high vaginal fistula
   E. C or D

2. On physical examination, you diagnose the most common type of anomaly. Management options at this point include:
   A. Immediate colostomy
   B. Calibration or dilation of the fistula, discharge home, and plan for repair in the future
   C. Repair at age 4 months without protective colostomy
   D. All of the above
   E. Retrograde contrast study through the fistula

3. You decide to admit the baby to the hospital at 3 weeks of age to do a colostomy. You examine the baby prior to induction and hear a systolic heart murmur. The baby's mother tells you she has fed poorly over the past week. Which of the following is true?
   A. Serious structural heart disease has been ruled out based on the absence of a murmur at birth and a normal chest x-ray
   B. A new murmur is highly suspicious for the development of endocarditis secondary to bacteremia from the anorectal malformation
   C. As long as the lungs are clear and the capillary refill is normal, you should proceed with colostomy
   D. All babies with anorectal malformations should have an echocardiogram in the newborn period to look for associated cardiac abnormalities
   E. The baby probably has a ventricular septal defect

4. At 4 months of age, you repair the imperforate anus by means of posterior sagittal anorectoplasty. The baby makes an uneventful recovery. Success of your repair is most dependent on:
   A. Delay of at least 12 weeks prior to colostomy closure
   B. Reliable performance of postoperative rectal dilation
   C. Avoidance of urinary sepsis
   D. Daily use of laxatives beginning as soon as the colostomy is closed

5. You see the child again at 9 months of age. She is eating a variety of table foods. Her mother tells you she appears to be doing well. She passes stool every 3 days or so, and her stool is formed and hard. On examination, the neoanus appears to be perfectly placed in the muscle complex. The opening is nicely puckered by the muscle complex. The opening easily accepts your little finger with no evidence of stricture. There is some stool in a slightly dilated rectal vault. Which of the following is true?
   A. The child is at risk for progressive bowel dilation and fecal retention; treatment with dietary changes or laxatives should begin immediately
   B. The child is doing very well and should be seen again in 1 year
   C. Prognosis is primarily related to the anatomic accuracy of the anoplasty
   D. You should explain to the mother that vaginoplasty will probably be required around the time of puberty
   E. All of the above

6. The child is lost to follow-up for several years. She returns at age 8 years complaining of fecal incontinence. She has never had a voluntary bowel movement. She soils frequently while at school. On phys-

ical examination she has a distended abdomen. There is a doughy mass filling the pelvis. Perineal examination reveals dried stool on the buttocks. The anus is widely patent without stricture. The rectal vault is full of stool. You order a contrast enema (Figure 22–2). Which of the following is true?

A. This patient appears to be one of the few unfortunate patients born with rectovestibular fistula who are physiologically incontinent

B. This patient can almost certainly be treated successfully with a constipating diet

C. This patient can almost certainly be treated successfully with a program of laxatives and enemas

D. The most common etiology of this problem is a missed spinal dysraphism

E. Treatment will likely involve resection of the sigmoid colon

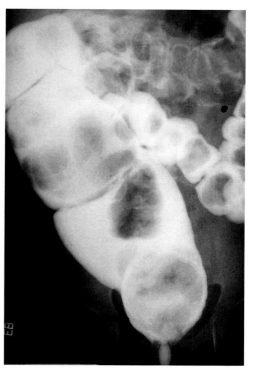

Figure 22–2. *Contrast enema in an 8-year-old girl who underwent repair of imperforate anus with rectovestibular fistula in infancy.*

ANSWERS AND DISCUSSION

1. **B** An imperforate anus in a female infant almost always results in a fistula to the perineum or the vagina. A fistula to the posterior fourchette (immediately posterior to vagina) occurs in 70% to 80% of girls with imperforate anus. Physical examination can be confusing for the inexperienced observer. Since the fistula is inside the labia minora, this abnormality is frequently misdiagnosed as a vaginal fistula. To visualize this lesion accurately, the examiner should spread the labia widely and gently retract the protruding vaginal mucosa anteriorly. The fistula is then readily identified. If no opening is seen here, then the diagnosis of vaginal fistula should be considered. Vaginal fistulae are quite uncommon. Examination under anesthesia may be required to confirm the diagnosis. A persistent cloaca presents with a single perineal opening. Hypoplastic appearing labia commonly accompany this abnormality.

2. **D** In the male infant, imperforate anus usually presents as a complete bowel obstruction requiring prompt surgical attention. In contrast, female infants with imperforate anus almost always have an external fistula. Unless this fistula is uncommonly narrow, these babies usually pass stool normally during the first few months of life. If the opening is narrow, it will usually enlarge readily with gentle passage of dilators. Therefore, operative repair of this defect is not urgent. Most surgeons do a colostomy sometime in the first 2 months of life followed by a repair at 3 to 6 months of age. Some surgeons recommend repair of this defect without a colostomy. While this has been done successfully, infection at the repair site and pelvic sepsis have been reported. If infection occurs, the delicate anal sphincter mechanism can be irreparably damaged. Contrast studies of the bowel are not necessary when the fistula is external.

3. **E** Structural heart disease is a part of the VATER (vertebral, anorectal, tracheoesophageal, renal, limb, and cardiac) association of anomalies that occurs with imperforate anus. The most common defects are ventricular and atrial septal defects. These defects are often silent at birth because systemic and pulmonary arterial pressure is about equal. The normal physiologic drop in pulmonary

pressure during the first few weeks of life can allow these shunts to become clinically apparent. This baby's poor feeding may be a manifestation of early congestive heart failure. Physical examination for hepatomegaly and a chest x-ray would provide useful information. The elective operation should be delayed until the child's cardiac status is fully evaluated. Endocarditis is exceedingly rare in this setting. Babies with external fistulae are not at risk for episodes of bacteremia. Echocardiographic examination of all children with anorectal malformations is not necessarily indicated. As long as the child receives close medical follow-up, those with heart disease will develop clinical evidence of disease. If experienced medical follow-up may not be available or compliance with care may be poor, then an echocardiogram in the nursery can effectively rule out structural heart disease.

4. **B** A regimen of postoperative rectal dilations is absolutely essential to the success of anoplasty. As the circumferential anoplasty heals by the normal process of wound contraction, stricture is the inevitable consequence. Gentle twice daily dilation prevents stricture formation and allows the neoanus to heal to appropriate caliber. Stricture is far easier to prevent than to treat. Once a stricture forms, it usually consists of dense scar tissue. Dilation at this point tends to induce tearing and formation of denser scar tissue. Colostomy closure is generally recommended at about 6 weeks following anoplasty. Urinary sepsis is generally not a problem in patients without associated urinary tract abnormalities. Laxatives should be used only when indicated and are rarely necessary in infancy.

5. **A** All patients born with imperforate anus will have a tendency to constipation, regardless of the anatomic correctness of the repair. Understanding this concept is essential for successful management of these children. Parents of these children should be taught to avoid constipation aggressively. In children without anorectal malformations, constipation is usually benign and self-limited. In children with corrected imperforate anus, constipation leads to a vicious cycle of stool retention, fecal impaction, and bowel dilation. This process generally begins around 9 to 12 months of age when the child begins table food. This child's stool habits are abnormal. Her stools are infrequent and hard. This is the ideal time to begin a bowel regimen that ensures that the child has a stool every day. This can often be done with dietary modification alone. Sometimes laxatives are required. The child should be seen frequently during this period to ensure that the bowel program is working effectively. Vaginoplasty is rarely required for this defect.

6. **E** The barium enema shows massive dilation of a stool-filled rectosigmoid. This is the consequence of inattention to the issues discussed in the preceding question. This patient has had years of fecal retention and bowel dilation that could have been prevented but now is very difficult to treat. She does not have true incontinence but rather pseudoincontinence secondary to severe constipation. Her massively dilated sigmoid and rectum "overflows" periodically, resulting in soiling. Pena has reported that once the sigmoid becomes massively dilated, it loses function and will not return to normal. It should be resected. This problem may be partially due to an

anatomically incorrect anoplasty. Evaluation should include examination in the operating room with a nerve stimulator to confirm that there is reasonable bilateral muscle contraction and that the anus is properly located. Occult spinal dysraphism can present in this manner and must be ruled out. It is, however, found in a minority of cases. A detailed approach to this problem can be found in the references.

BIBLIOGRAPHY

Husberg B, Lindahl H, Rintala R, et al. High and intermediate imperforate anus: results after surgical correction with special respect to internal sphincter function. *J Pediatr Surg.* 1992;27:185–189.

Javid PJ, Barnhart DC, Hirschl RB, et al. Immediate and long-term results of surgical management of low imperforate anus in girls. *J Pediatr Surg.* 1998;33:198–203.

Moss RL. The failed anoplasty: successful outcome after reoperative anoplasty and sigmoid resection. *J Pediatr Surg.* 1998;33:1145–1147.

Pena A. Atlas of surgical management of anorectal malformations. New York: Springer-Verlag; 1990.

Pena A, El Behary M. Megasigmoid: a source of pseudoincontinence in children with repaired anorectal malformations. *J Pediatr Surg.* 1993;28: 199–203.

Pena A, Guardino K, Tovilla JM, et al. Bowel management for fecal incontinence in patients with anorectal malformations. *J Pediatr Surg.* 1998; 33:133–137.

PNEUMOPERITONEUM IN A 650-GRAM PREMATURE INFANT

HISTORY This 25-week-old, 650-g male infant is born to a 16-year-old woman who had no prenatal care. One minute Apgar score is 4. He in intubated in the delivery room and transported to the neonatal intensive care unit.

EXAMINATION He is a very immature infant who moves all four extremities. Temperature is 97.2°F, Doppler blood pressure is 60/42, pulse is 170. Ventilator settings are rate 22/min; pressures 18/4; Fio_2 50%. His skin is shiny and transparent. No anomalies of head, eyes, ears, or palate are apparent. The chest moves symmetrically; breath sounds are good bilaterally. Heart rate is rapid and regular; no murmur is audible. The abdomen is soft, with the liver edge just below the right costal margin. The testes are palpable in the inguinal canals bilaterally. The extremities are slightly mottled, but peripheral pulses are palpable, and capillary refill is normal.

LABORATORY Hemoglobin 16 gm; hematocrit 63%; white blood cell count 18,000, with segmented neutrophils 59, bands 4, lymphocytes 30, monocytes 6, eosinophils 1. Urinalysis is normal. Arterial blood gas: pH 7.28, Pco_2 50, Po_2 135. Serum electrolytes; blood, urea, and nitrogen; and creatinine are normal.

HOSPITAL COURSE Umbilical arterial and venous lines are placed, and he receives an intravenous bolus of 6.5 mL of normal saline. Ventilator adjustments are made. His vital signs and respiratory status stabilize. He receives nutrition by peripheral IV, starting with a solution of 2.5% dextrose, amino acids, and electrolytes. The dextrose is gradually increased to 5%, and a lipid solution is added. Drip feedings by orogastric tube are begun on the tenth day of life, using a special formula for premature infants, starting at 1 mL/h. These are gradually increased to 2.5 mL/h by the 20th day. He regains his birth weight on the 21st day.

On the 22nd day, however, he becomes lethargic and develops abdominal distention. Feedings are stopped; a gastric aspirate of 9 mL of thick, bile-stained liquid is obtained. The extremities are mottled and flaccid. He receives a work-up for sepsis and is begun on intravenous antibiotics. The "babygram" is shown in Figure 23–1. A gastric tube is placed to suction intermittently. He improves on this medical supportive treatment. The following morning, a generalized, erythematous rash appears, with peeling of the skin of the hands and feet (Figure 23–2A and B; see also color plates). The laboratory calls in the afternoon with the report of a positive blood culture.

Please answer all questions before proceeding to discussion section.

✓ QUESTIONS

1. Which of the following is the most likely pathogen in this infant?
   A. *Escherichia coli*
   B. *Klebsiella pneumoniae*
   C. *Staphylococcus epidermidis*
   D. *Streptococcus fecalis* (enterococcus)
   E. *Candida albicans*

2. Which of the following is a portal of entry for infection in the very low birth weight (VLBW) infant?
   A. Skin
   B. Vascular catheters
   C. Urinary catheter
   D. Endotracheal tube
   E. All of the above

HOSPITAL COURSE (CONT.) That evening, the abdominal distention suddenly increases. A left lateral decubitus film (Figure 23–3) is taken. Aterial blood gases now are pH 7.12, P_{CO_2} 71, P_{O_2} 38, F_{IO_2} 60%.

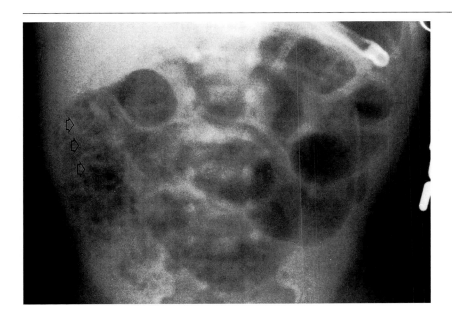

Figure 23–1. *Abdominal x-ray, supine view, showing moderate pneumatosis intestinalis (arrows) and diffuse bowel dilation.*

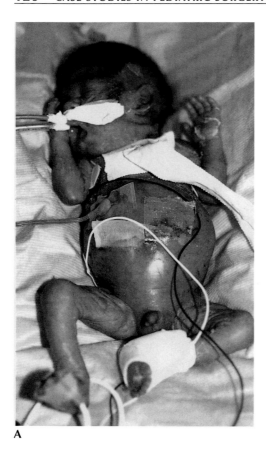

A

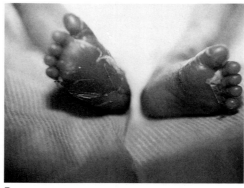

B

Figure 23–2. A. *Premature infant (650 g) with*
Staphylococcus epidermidis *sepsis and necrotizing enterocolitis (NEC). Portals of entry for
infection are thin, cracked skin and catheters
in vascular, urinary, gastrointestinal (GI), and
respiratory systems.* **B.** *The rash, with peeling
of the skin of the hands and feet, is a manifestation of a staphylocccal toxin. (See also color
plates.)*

3. Which of the following is the emergency treatment of choice for this infant?
   A. Immediate laparotomy
   B. Dopamine at 10 µg/kg/min, administered directly into the umbilical arterial catheter
   C. Peritoneal drainage
   D. An intravenous bolus of 10% dextrose in Ringer's lactate
   E. All of the above

4. Which of the following statements is true regarding "spontaneous" intestinal perforation in the VLBW infant?
   A. The infant has a better survival rate than the VLBW infant with perforated necrotizing enterocolitis (NEC)
   B. Bluish discoloration of the abdomen is characteristic
   C. Optimal surgical management is closure of the perforation in two layers
   D. A and B
   E. A, B, and C

5. Which of the following statements is true regarding peritoneal drainage for perforated NEC in the VLBW infant?
   A. The infant's respiratory status often improves after this procedure
   B. *Candida albicans* is often cultured from the peritoneal fluid
   C. This procedure is widely considered definitive surgical management of NEC in the VLBW infant
   D. A and B
   E. A, B, and C

6. During laparotomy for NEC, a 28-week, 900 g premature infant develops an expanding hematoma beneath the capsule of the right lobe of the liver. Gentle pressure is applied, whereupon the hematoma ruptures. The optimal management now is:
   A. Intravenous fresh frozen plasma (FFP) and factor 8; direct cautery and compression until bleeding stops
   B. Intravenous FFP and factor 8; liberal application of fibrin glue to the liver; continue operation *only* after bleeding stops
   C. Rapid administration of inotropes
   D. Pack the liver and "run"
   E. Right hepatic lobectomy

7. Which of the following statements regarding the outcome of NEC is true?
   A. The survival rate of NEC has improved in the last decade
   B. The proportion of VLBW infants with NEC has increased in the past decade
   C. The long-term outcome of premature infants suriving NEC is similar to that of premature infants without NEC, when matched for birth weight and gestational age
   D. Following resection for NEC, long-term growth and survival of infants who lose the ileocecal valve is similar to that of infants who retain the ileocecal valve
   E. All of the above

ANSWERS AND DISCUSSION

1. **C** *Staphylococcus epidermidis* is the most common pathogen of neonatal sepsis in the newborn infant and may be associated with NEC. This organism of normal skin, once considered a contaminant of blood cultures, may invade through breaks in the thin, fragile skin of premature infants or along the path of indwelling devices (eg, umbilical catheters, central venous lines). Vancomycin is the antibiotic treatment of choice. The enteric bacteria (eg, *E. coli* [**A**], *Klebsiella* [**B**], enterococcus [**D**]), are also good choices, as they are often cultured from the peritoneal fluid or blood of infants with NEC. A clue to the organism in this infant, however, is the generalized rash, with peeling of the skin of the hands and feet (Figure 23–2B), which is due to a staphylococcal toxin similar to that found in toxic shock syndrome. Since about 20% of infants with severe NEC have a positive blood culture, it is sometimes difficult to decide which came first, the sepsis or the NEC. *Candida* (**E**) or other fungi are pathogens of neonatal sepsis, especially in infants who receive prolonged courses of antibiotics.

2. **E** All of the portals—skin, mucosa, vascular catheters, urinary catheters, and endotracheal tubes—provide pathways for infection by bacteria or fungi (Figure 23–2A and B; see also color plates). Very low birth weight (VLBW) infants, also known as "micropremies," are defined by a birth weight of less than 1000 g, gestational age of 28 weeks or less, or both. Barrier function of both skin and mucosa is immature in such infants. Lack of secretory immunoglobulins in the first 2 to 3 weeks of life may allow translocation of bacteria and antigens across the premature gut.

3. **C** Peritoneal drainage is a good choice for initial management of this critically ill, 650 g infant. He is unstable, and immediate laparo-

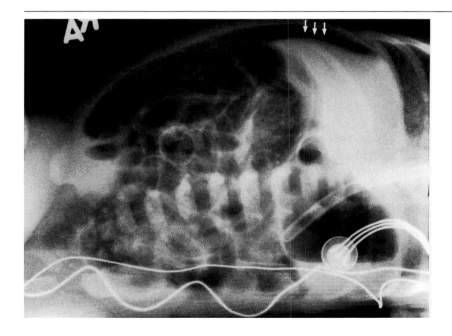

Figure 23–3. *Abdominal x-ray, left lateral decubitus view (taken several hours after Figure 23–1). Pneumatosis intestinalis is again seen in right side of abdomen, and pneumoperitoneum (arrows) is now present.*

tomy (**A**) might be the final event of a short life. Peritoneal drainage will deflate his distended abdomen, allowing better movement of the diaphragm and improved respiration. Removal of feculent fluid may also diminish the systemic effects of sepsis syndrome. The infant should be prepared for laparotomy within 24 to 48 hours. (More about peritoneal drainage is in answer 5.) An infusion of dopamine (**B**) may enhance renal perfusion, but it should be started at low dose (5 μg/kg/min), not at 10 μg. Vasoactive drugs are preferably given via a central venous catheter, not the umbilical arterial catheter. A bolus of 10% dextrose (**D**) will likely produce hyperglycemia and hyperosmolality in this infant. Hyperosmolar solutions should not be given to VLBW infants because of the risk of intraventricular hemorrhage from the fragile vessels of the choroid plexus. A better choice for a bolus would be 10 to 13 mL of Ringer's lactate, normal saline, or 5% albumin.

4. **D** Does "spontaneous" intestinal perforation exist as a separate disease? Or is it just a focal form of NEC with a better survival rate? There are lumpers and splitters on this issue. One splitter study (**A**) reported a better survival (88%) for spontaneous perforation compared with 56% for NEC. Bluish discoloration of the abdomen is characteristic of spontaneous perforation (**B**). The optimal surgical management, however, is exteriorization, not closure of the perforation (**C**). These infants have a way of developing second perforations about 2 to 3 days after the first. Exteriorization is the most conservative operation, as there is no risk of sepsis and death from a leaking suture line.

5. **D** Most pediatric surgeons do not consider peritoneal drainage as definitive therapy for perforated NEC (**C**), but rather as an useful adjunct to resuscitation of the VLBW infant prior to laparotomy. Several recent reports, however, suggest that peritoneal drainage may serve as definitive therapy. Insertion of a drain may improve ventilation (**A**) by relieving the pressure effects of pneumoperitoneum and removes infected fluid from the peritoneal cavity. The procedure, which originated in Toronto, was intended to help stabilize critically ill infants under 1000 g prior to laparotomy. As a bonus, 31% to 33% of infants improved so much that they never required laparotomy. A group from Stanford reported a remarkable 74% of survivors required no further operative procedure and recommended peritoneal drainage as the primary procedure for perforated NEC in the VLBW infant population. *Candida albicans* (**B**) is commonly found in culture material from VLBW infants, virtually all of whom have received courses of antibiotic therapy since birth.

6. **D** Major hemorrhage from the liver during laparotomy for NEC, a life-threatening emergency, is a manifestation of coagulopathy in the septic, VLBW infant. The typical scenario is that after minimal (or no) retraction of the liver, a subcapsular "blood-blister" develops, which swells and ruptures spontaneously. Within minutes, the infant dies of uncontrollable hemorrhage. In this situation, the usual techniques for surgical hemostasis (**A** or **B**) are futile; the bleeding will *never* stop until the coagulopathy is controlled, which may take hours. (In the meantime, the patient dies.) Stone outlined the management of this emergency (in adults) more than a decade ago.

Stone recommended packing the liver, clipping out any obviously dead bowel (with ligatures above and below), dropping the ligated bowel ends back into the abdomen, closing rapidly in one layer, and coming back another day to finish the operation, after the coagulopathy is corrected. This approach works in neonates. Although additional measures (eg, administration of inotropes [C], avoiding fluid overload) are recommended, the few survivors of this catastrophe have occurred after packing (and running). Hepatic lobectomy (E), a terrible choice, would only worsen the hemorrhage.

7. **E** All of the statements are true. Although the proportion of VLBW infants who survive (and develop NEC) has increased in the past decade (B), the overall survival of NEC has nevertheless improved (A). The surgical mortality is 23% to 50%. Virtually all of medically treated infants survive NEC, although they may die later from other problems of prematurity. Long-term outcome of NEC is surprisingly good. Studies comparing growth and neurodevelopmental outcome (D) of premature infants who survive NEC to premature infants who never had NEC showed that morbidity was no higher among NEC survivors. Loss of the ileocecal valve in the neonatal period (E) has little long-term effect on growth and survival. In a large series from Grosfeld and colleagues, there was no difference in growth and survival between infants who lost the valve and those who retained it after resection for NEC. Loss of the ileocecal valve may have an effect only following massive resection, when residual length of small bowel is 20 cm or less, which, fortunately, is a rare situation.

HOSPITAL COURSE (*CONT.*) Peritoneal drainage is carried out with evacuation of a puff of air and a small amount of feculent fluid. The respiratory status improves, and with continued medical support, the vital signs stabilize. Laparotomy is performed 24 hours later. A perforated, necrotic segment of ileum is resected, and double enterostomy performed. The infant makes a gradual recovery, and 2.5 months later, after closure of the ileostomy, he is discharged from the hospital.

BIBLIOGRAPHY

Abbasi S, Pereira GR, Johnson L, et al. Long-term assessment of growth, nutritional status, and gastrointestinal function in survivors of necrotizing enterocolitis. *J Pediatr.* 1984;104:550–554.

Bhattacharyya N, Kosloske AM, Macarthur C. Nosocomial infection in pediatric surgical patients: a study of 608 infants and children. *J Pediatr Surg.* 1993;28:338–344.

Ein SH, Shandling B, Wesson D, et al. A 13-year experience with peritoneal drainage under local anesthesia for necrotizing enterocolitis perforation. *J Pediatr Surg.* 1990;25:1034–1037.

Grosfeld JL, Cheu H, Schlatter M, et al. Changing trends in necrotizing enterocolitis: Experience with 302 cases in 2 decades. *Ann Surg.* 1991;214: 300–306.

Kosloske AM. Sepsis and infection in the neonate. In: Fonkalsrud EW, Krummel TM, eds. *Infection and Immunologic Disorders in Pediatric Surgery.* Philadelphia: Saunders; 1993.

Kosloske AM. Management of subcapsular hematoma of the liver during neonatal laparotomy. Presented at the Meeting of the Pacific Association of Pediatric Surgeons; May 1995; Oaxaca, Mexico.

Mintz AC, Applebaum H. Focal gastrointestinal perforations not associated with necrotizing enterocolitis in very low birth weight neonates. *J Pediatr Surg.* 1993;28:857–860.

Mollitt DL, Tepas JJ, Talber JL. The role of coagulase-negative *Staphylococcus* in neonatal necrotizing enterocolitis. *J Pediatr Surg.* 1988;23:60–63.

Morgan LJ, Shochat SJ, Hartman GE. Peritoneal drainage as primary management of perforated NEC in the very low birth weight infant. *J Pediatr Surg.* 1994;29:30–34.

Rescorla FJ, Ladd AP. Necrotizing enterocolitis. In: Stringer MD, Oldham KT, Mouriquand PDE, et al. eds. *Pediatric Surgery and Urology: Long Term Outcomes.* London: Saunders; 1998.

Rowe MI, Reblock KK, Kurkchubasche AG, et al. Necrotizing enterocolitis in the extremely low birth weight infant. *J Pediatr Surg.* 1994;29:987–991.

Snyder CL, Gittes GK, Murphy JP, et al. Survival after necrotizing enterocolitis in infants weighing less than 1,000 grams: 25 years' experience at a single institution. *J Pediatr Surg.* 1997;32:434–437.

Stone HH, Strom PR, Mullins RJ. Management of the major coagulopathy with onset during laparotomy. *Ann Surg.* 1983;197:532.

Uceda JE, Laos CA, Kolni HW, et al. Intestinal perforations in infants with a very low birth weight: a disease of increasing survival? *J Pediatr Surg.* 1995;30:1314–1316.

VanderKolk WE, Kurz P, Daniels J, et al. Liver hemorrhage during laparotomy in patients with necrotizing enterocolitis. *J Pediatr Surg.* 1996;31:1063–1067.

A 9-MONTH-OLD BOY WITH AN ABDOMINAL MASS AND CONSTIPATION

HISTORY   A 9-month-old boy is brought to your office by a worried mother because a right lower quadrant abdominal mass was noted when his pediatrician was evaluating the child for progressive constipation of 3 months' duration. He has not been gaining weight and has become a fussy eater. From behind your desk you can see the mass when the mother lifts up his shirt.

EXAMINATION   His vital signs are normal, he seems indifferent to examination, which discloses a paucity of subcutaneous fat. A firm right lower quadrant mass arises to the level of the umbilicus. Examination of the perineum shows an obvious asymmetric bulge where the mass appears to be pushing the skin inferiorly. Rectal examination is tight because of compression by a mass in the posterior midline. A small Hegar dilator can be passed and elicits evacuation of liquid stool.

LABORATORY   An abdominal computed tomography (CT) scan is seen in Figure 24–1. Routine blood work is normal, including his creatinine. Abdominal ultrasound demonstrates mild bilateral hydronephrosis and an elongated but normal-appearing bladder that has been pushed up out of the pelvis into the abdomen.
   Please answer all questions before proceeding to discussion section.

✓ QUESTIONS

   1. Of the further investigations listed, which would be *least* useful?
      A. Bone marrow biopsy
      B. Serum catecholamines, vanillylmandelic acid (VMA), and homovanillic acid (HVA)

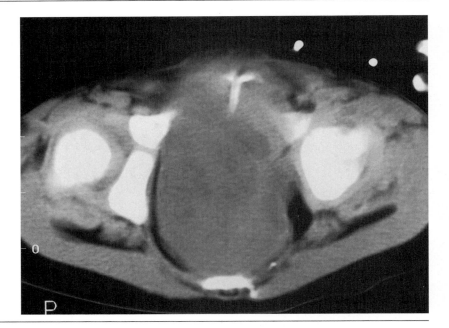

Figure 24–1. *Computed tomography (CT) scan of upper pelvis showing contrast in a bladder catheter. The bladder is pushed up and out of the field by a large heterogeneous mass. On this cut, no calcifications can be seen. Although contrast was present in the rectum, it is so compressed by the tumor that it is not visible on this cut.*

C. Alpha-fetoprotein (AFP) and beta-human chorionic gonadotropin (beta-hCG) levels
D. Metastatic work-up of the chest
E. Metastatic work-up of the brain

2. His chest x-ray is normal, the bone marrow biopsy is normal, his beta-hCG is mildy elevated, his AFP is 54,000, and the serum catecholamine levels go off to Tennessee and won't be back for a week. Reviewing the AFP, imaging, and physical exam, you suspect a:
A. Lymphoma
B. Sacrococcygeal teratoma
C. Rhabdomyosarcoma
D. Primitive neuroectodermal tumor
E. Ewing's sarcoma

3. Concerning AFP and beta-hCG:
A. Alpha-fetoprotein (AFP) is produced early in gestation and falls to its normal level by about 4 months of life
B. Alpha-fetoprotein (AFP) is the fetal equivalent of albumin—it serves as the principal serum binding protein
C. Alpha-fetoprotein (AFP) is elevated in the presence of hepatoblastoma, yolk sac tumors, endodermal sinus tumors, and sacrococcygeal teratomas with or without malignant components
D. The half lives are, respectively: AFP—1 week; beta-hCG—1 day
E. Markedly elevated beta-hCG indicates the presence of syncytiotrophoblasts associated with choriocarcinoma, seminomas, dysgerminomas, and sacrococcygeal teratomas

4. If this is a teratoma, it would be Altman stage:
A. I
B. II
C. III
D. IV
E. V

5. Which of the following is *false?*
   A. Teratomas are the most common type of childhood germ cell tumor
   B. They may be classified as mature, immature without malignancy, and malignant
   C. By definition they contain at least two of three embryonic germ layers
   D. "Teratoma" derives from Greek words meaning "monster" and "tumor"
   E. Teratomas may originate from totipotent cells of the primitive streak, primitive germ cells arising after the first meiotic division, or failed twinning

6. Were the tumor large and detected on antenatal ultrasound, which is *false?*
   A. Solid lesions are more dangerous than the cystic ones
   B. If the tumor's dimensions approach those of the baby's head, cesarean delivery should be considered
   C. Indications for fetal surgery include a large, solid tumor with evidence of polyhydramnios or critical vascular shunting
   D. Fetal surgery consists of resection or radiofrequency ablation of the bulk of the tumor with completion of resection after birth
   E. The blood supply to a large tumor may be as much as a quarter of cardiac output

7. Which is *false,* concerning sacrococcygeal teratomas (SCTs) and the risk of malignancy?
   A. It correlates with the size of tumor
   B. Seventeen percent exhibit malignant features
   C. It correlates with the age of the child
   D. It correlates with the stage
   E. It correlates with the elevation of AFP above expected levels

8. Principles of surgery do not include:
   A. Control the median sacral artery early—it or internal iliac branches feed the tumor, and it may even be worth laparotomy (prior to perineal resection) to obtain control
   B. Prepare the entire lower torso and use an inverted chevron-shaped excision on the perineum
   C. Remove the coccyx
   D. Reattach the levators at the end of the procedure
   E. Early, complete excision is the mainstay of therapy, unless there are malignant elements—in which case the tumor is very dangerous and excision may include exenteration

9. In this patient you perform cystoscopy (no evidence of tumor), central line insertion, and laparotomy that, combined with a perineal incision, enable you to remove grossly the entire tumor, coccyx, and lymph nodes. The pathology shows malignant degeneration with yolk sac and endodermal sinus elements. Concerning the future, you would *not* recommend:
   A. Close follow-up for many years will be necessary
   B. Optimal follow-up involves the use of rectal examination, magnetic resonance imaging (MRI) scanning, and AFP levels

C. Formerly, 10% of children with malignancy survived; now, using high-dose platinum added to bleomycin and etoposide the cure rate may exceed 90%

D. Low-dose pelvic radiation is used for local control

E. The AFP levels that rise after a dose of chemotherapy are not alarming

ANSWERS AND DISCUSSION

1. **E** The differential diagnosis of this large pelvic and abdominal mass includes rhabdomyosarcoma, sacrococcygeal teratoma (SCT), neuroblastoma, and primitive neurectodermal tumor, among other less common lesions. All of the investigations listed are appropriate. Bone marrow examination is essential in rhabdomyosarcoma, which often spreads to the marrow. Serum catecholamines and their urinary by-products may be abnormal in neuroblastoma. The AFP level is commonly elevated in SCT. Lung metastases are seen in all of these lesions. Head scanning would (initially) be the least helpful, although rare brain metastases are reported.

2. **B** The marked elevation in AFP strongly suggests the diagnosis of sacrococcygeal tumors. This is even more likely given radiographic evidence of coccygeal involvement by tumor and the absence of involvement of the bladder and bowel. Macrocalcifications, not present in this case, result from teeth and pieces of bone, which often help in the diagnosis of SCT. The remainder of the choices form a group of pediatric tumors known as "round blue cell tumors." This name derives from their similar histologic appearance. With the exception of SCT, where the elevated serum AFP is typically diagnostic, biopsy with immunohistochemistry is often necessary to differentiate between these tumors.

3. **B** The half-life (T1/2) of AFP is actually quite a complicated affair. As shown in Table 24–1, the levels are very high at birth and decay to normal by 8 months of age. The decay is not linear because the T1/2 is variable during the first year of life, settling ultimately at about 1 week. The T1/2 of beta-hCG is correct as given. The AFP is elevated in all the conditions of (**C**) except a mature SCT—the hormone is only produced by malignant tumor cells. **E** is true for all but SCT—in this disease AFP is a much better marker.

4. **C** See Figure 24–2. There is no such thing as stage V.

5. **C** By definition teratomas must contain all three germ cell layers: endoderm, mesoderm, and ectoderm. Heterogeneous postulates about SCT etiology are used to explain partial twinning, *fetu-in-fetu*, and Siamese twins—all poorly understood anomalies.

6. **E** Lesions may be solid or cystic; the former is associated with a 67% incidence of death in utero (if nothing is done) and the overall mortality approaches 100%. **B** is intuitive—provoking bleeding in a large lesion may easily be a terminal event. **E** is false since these tumors may be larger than the child and have blood flow that is greater than systemic requirements. Hydrops fetalis due to high output fetal

Type I Type II
Type III Type IV

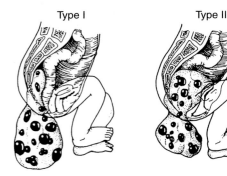
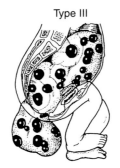
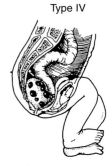

Figure 24–2. *Altman staging of sacrococcygeal teratoma. Reprinted with permission from Pizzo P, Poplack DG.* Principles and Practice of Pediatric Oncology, *3rd ed. Lippincott-Raven; 1997:938.*

Table 24–1 ALPHA-FETOPROTEIN LEVELS FROM BIRTH TO 8 MONTHS OLD

Age	No. pts.	Mean ± SD (ng/mL)
Premature	11	134,734 ± 41,444
Newborn	55	48,406 ± 34,718
Newborn–2 wk	16	33,113 ± 32,503
2 wk–1 mo	12	9452 ± 12,610
2 mo	40	323 ± 278
3 mo	5	88 ± 87
4 mo	31	74 ± 56
5 mo	6	46.5 ± 19
6 mo	9	12.5 ± 9.8
7 mo	5	9.7 ± 7.1
8 mo	3	8.5 ± 5.5

SD, standard deviation.
Reprinted with permission from Pizzo P, Poplack DG. *Principles and Practice of Pediatric Oncology,* 3rd ed. Lippincott-Raven; 1997:929.

congestive heart failure is an extremely poor prognostic sign and mandates consideration of fetal intervention.

7. **A** Tumor size does not relate to the risk of malignancy. Age does, and this is very significant. In children less than 2 months of age, the risk of malignancy is 10% to 20%. After 2 months, it is 67%. Fortunately, almost 80% of these tumors are diagnosed within the first 2 months of life. The greater the stage, the higher the risk of malignancy. Elevations of AFP in the neonatal period are difficult to interpret because of the high levels at birth. It becomes a very useful marker after tumor excision (or at an older age) where an upward trend is an ominous sign of recurrence.

8. **E** Intraoperative death (5%) is almost always because of uncontrolled bleeding. If rapid vascular control is required or a low tumor seems stuck to upper pelvic structures, prepping the entire torso permits timely laparotomy. Recurrence rates are unacceptably high (~30%) when the coccyx is not removed. If one fails to reattach the levators, the natal cleft will be lost. The sacrifice of vital organs in malignant, untreated SCTs has not proven beneficial.

   Figure 24–3 (see also color plate) shows the typical appearance of a large sacrococcygeal teratoma in a newborn. The tumor may weigh as much or even more than the baby.

9. **D** Benign SCTs have a significant recurrence rate mandating close follow-up for more than 3 years. Magnetic resonance imaging (MRI) scanning is superior to CT and ultrasound, initially because it detects intraspinal invasion and soft-tissue infiltration. On newer regimens, survival is much improved. Radiation is rarely used in this disease. Local control with surgery and chemotherapy is usually sufficient. Because AFP is produced by tumor cells and because chemotherapy causes tumor cell lysis, it is common to have a transient rise in AFP following chemotherapy, which should continue to decline before the next cycle. A significant proportion of children will have long-term difficulty with bladder and bowel control related to the pelvic dissection.

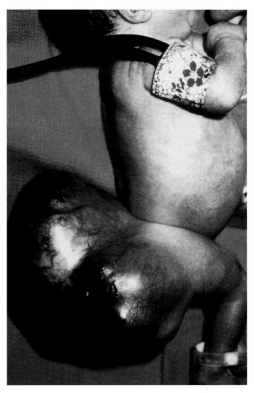

Figure 24–3. *Newborn with a large sacrococcygeal teratoma. (See also color plate.)*

BIBLIOGRAPHY

Chisholm CA, Heider AL, Kuller JA, et al. Prenatal diagnosis and perinatal management of fetal sacrococcygeal teratoma. *Am J Perinatol.* 1999; 16:89–92.

Ein SH, Mancer K, Adeyemi SD. Malignant sacrococcygeal teratoma—endodermal sinus, yolk sac tumor in infants and children: a 32-year review. *J Pediatr Surg.* 1985;20:473–477.

Holterman AX, Filiatrault D, Lallier M, Youssef S. The natural history of sacrococcygeal teratomas diagnosed through routine obstetric sonogram: a single institution experience. *J Pediatr Surg.* 1998;33:899–903.

Pizzo P, Poplack DG. *Principles and Practice of Pediatric Oncology.* 3rd ed. Lippincott-Raven; 1997:928–939.

A 2-WEEK-OLD BOY WITH A MIDLINE ABDOMINAL MASS

HISTORY A 2-week-old term male infant is sent to you because of a midline abdominal mass noted on routine examination. The baby required oxygen for 1 week after birth for unknown reasons but otherwise has been doing well. The mother relates a history of oligohydramnios during pregnancy.

EXAMINATION The baby appears healthy. Heart and lung examination is normal. There is a firm mass in the midline arising out of the pelvis that seems to be a bit tender.

LABORATORY None available.
Please answer all questions before proceeding to discussion section.

✔ QUESTIONS

1. The differential diagnosis includes:
   A. Mesenteric cyst
   B. Neuroblastoma
   C. Urinary retention
   D. All of the above
   E. None of the above

2. You order an abdominal ultrasound, which is shown in Figure 25–1. The cause of this abnormality is most likely:
   A. Occult spinal cord lesion with neurogenic bladder
   B. Pelvic rhabdomyosarcoma causing bladder outlet obstruction
   C. Pelvic neuroblastoma causing bladder outlet obstruction
   D. Posterior uretheral valves
   E. Prune belly syndrome

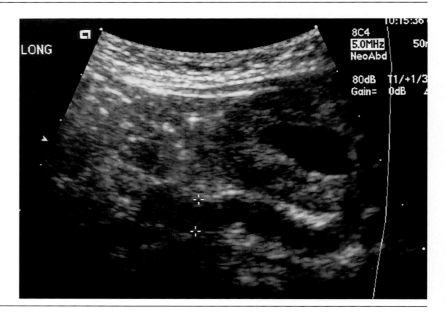

Figure 25–1. *Ultrasound image of the pelvis oriented in a transverse direction. The patient's head is to the left and feet to the right.*

3. Appropriate management options at this time include:
   A. Foley catheter decompression of the urinary tract
   B. Abdominal computed tomography (CT) scan with oral and intravenous contrast
   C. Magnetic resonance imaging (MRI) of the spinal cord
   D. Antibiotic prophylaxis for vesicoureteral reflux
   E. A and B

4. Definitive diagnosis of this condition may be made by:
   A. Voiding cystourethrography
   B. Cystoscopy
   C. Nuclear medicine renal scan
   D. Abdominal ultrasound
   E. A and B

5. Antenatal urinary obstruction may prove fatal in the first few days after birth because of
   A. Intractable renal failure
   B. Progressive acidosis
   C. Pulmonary hypoplasia
   D. Sepsis

6. Prenatal intervention for urinary obstruction is considered in which of the following situations:
   A. When there is severe bilateral hydronephrosis
   B. When other anomalies are present
   C. When the bladder size is greater than 4 cm in its longest dimension
   D. When a fetus has bilateral hydronephrosis and develops progressive oligohydramnios
   E. All of the above

ANSWERS AND DISCUSSION

1. **D** All of the listed lesions may cause an abdominal mass in the newborn. A mesenteric cyst is a congenital collection of lymphatic fluid within the mesentary of the bowel. Usually these are quite mobile. A neuroblastoma is the most common abdominal tumor of the newborn. It most often occurs in the adrenal. Neuroblastoma may be widely metastatic in the newborn and may be most palpable in the liver. The most common midline abdominal mass is an enlarged bladder. Abdominal ultrasound is an excellent initial test. It will reveal whether the lesion is solid or cystic and whether or not it is separate from the urinary tract.

2. **D** The ultrasound shows marked thickening of the bladder wall (right side of the image) with hydroureteronephrosis (cursors are measuring the dilated ureter). This is virtually diagnostic of bladder outlet obstructions secondary to posterior urethral valves. These valves are caused by an extension of tissue at the level of the prostatic verumontanum. They cause bladder outlet obstruction with a wide spectrum of clinical presentations. In some cases, the lesion causes destruction of the kidneys in utero, while in others the child presents at school age with voiding difficulties or enuresis.

   Occult spinal cord lesions may present with urinary retention, but this is uncommon in the newborn period. In addition, bilateral hydronephrosis would not typically be present. Pelvic tumors can cause bladder outlet obstruction. Rhabdomyoscarcoma of the prostate often presents in this fashion, but it is not a tumor seen in newborns. Neuroblastoma would be extremely unlikely to obstruct the bladder. Prune belly syndrome is associated with a vesicoureteromegaly and hydronephrosis. An ultrasound may appear very similar to this patient's. These children, however, lack abdominal wall musculature, and the diagnosis is clinically apparent.

3. **A** Immediate decompression of the urinary tract is crucial to avoid further renal damage and prevent urosepsis. Simple placement of a Foley catheter is adequate initial treatment. Abdominal CT scan is not necessary. Posterior urethral valves may be diagnosed in other ways. Furthermore, intravenous contrast is contraindicated in a baby who is likely to have compromised renal function. An MRI of the spinal cord has no role. Antibiotic prophylaxis for vesicoureteral reflux is only indicated if reflux is present after diagnosis and treatment of the primary problem.

4. **E** Posterior urethral valves are best diagnosed by voiding cystourethrography (Figure 25–2). Some authors have reported the use of cystoscopy followed by treatment under the same anesthetic. This is appropriate in experienced hands. A nuclear medicine renal scan may be appropriate to assess renal function in these patients but will not help diagnose the valves.

5. **C** Renal insufficiency in the fetus manifests as oligohydramnios (decreased amniotic fluid volume) and pulmonary hypoplasia. The etiology of the pulmonary hypoplasia is not entirely clear. Some experts believe it is simply due to mechanical compression on the

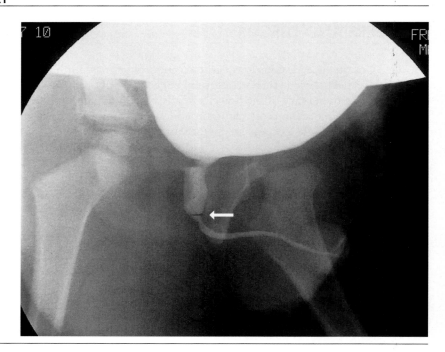

Figure 25–2. *This voiding cystourethrogram shows a dilated proximal urethra. The filling defect (arrow) caused by the valve is seen as the urethra changes to normal caliber below the obstruction.*

developing chest by the uterus in the absence of adequate amniotic fluid. In any event, affected infants may require aggressive ventilatory support or extracorporeal membrane oxygenation (ECMO), and many do not survive.

6. **D** Over 90% of fetuses diagnosed prenatally with urinary obstruction do not require treatment until after birth. The most established indication of fetal intervention is in the patient with bilateral hydronephrosis who develops oligohydramnios, and lung maturity will not allow early delivery. The role of fetal intervention for obstruction uropathy is not yet clear. This is due in part to the limited accuracy of prenatal diagnostic tests.

BIBLIOGRAPHY

Abbott JF, Levine D, Wapner R. Posterior urethral valves: inaccuracy of prenatal diagnosis. *Fetal Diagn Ther.* 1998;13:179–183.

Chevalier RL, Klahr S. Therapeutic approaches in obstructive uropathy. *Semin Nephrol.* 1998;18:652–658.

Dejter S, Gibbons MD. The newborn valve. In: Gonzales ET, Roth D, eds. *Common Problems in Pediatric Urology.* St. Louis: Mosby; 1991:76–84.

Drozdz D, Drozdz M, Gretz N, et al. Progression to end-stage renal disease in children with posterior urethral valves. *Pediatr Nephrol.* 1998;12:630–636.

A NEWBORN WITH FETAL POLYHYDRAMNIOS AND BILIOUS VOMITING

HISTORY   A 3.2 kg, 37-week male infant was born following premature rupture of membranes. The prenatal history was remarkable for polyhydramnios beginning at 28 weeks, and a sonogram demonstrated, in addition, a dilated fluid-filled stomach and duodenum. Amniocentesis and fetal echocardiogram were normal. Shortly after birth, a nasogastric tube was placed, which drained 35 mL of bile-stained fluid. The infant passed mucous plugs per rectum but no meconium.

EXAMINATION   Healthy male infant with no dysmorphic features. Cardiac examination normal. Nasogastric tube draining bile-stained mucus. Abdomen soft and scaphoid with no masses palpable. Anus patent.

LABORATORY   Supine and decubitus abdominal radiographs are shown in Figure 26–1.
   Please answer all questions before proceeding to discussion section.

✓ QUESTIONS

1. Congenital duodenal obstruction results from:
   A. An in utero vascular accident
   B. A failure of foregut vacuolization
   C. An associated foregut malformation (eg, annular pancreas)
   D. None of the above

2. Prenatal diagnosis reduces postoperative morbidity associated with duodenal atresia:
   A. True
   B. False

3. The level of obstruction is postampullary in what percentage of cases?

135

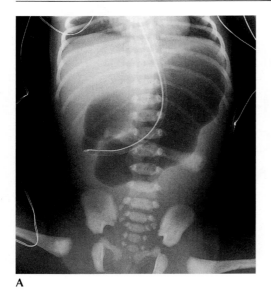

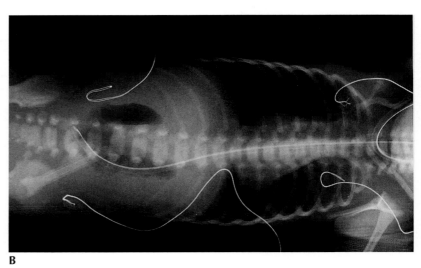

A   B

Figure 26–1. A. *Supine and* **B.** *left lateral decubitus x-rays of a newborn with bilious nasogastric tube output. The stomach and duodenum are markedly dilated and air filled. There is no distal gas. This is an example of a "double buble sign" that occurs when there is complete duodenal obstruction from duodenal atresia. If any gas is identified distal to the double bubble then the diagnosis is either duuodenal stenosis or malrotation with midgut volvulus.*

    A. Ten percent
    B. Thirty percent
    C. Fifty percent
    D. Eighty-five percent

4. The most frequently associated malformations are:
    A. Down syndrome (30%), congenital heart disease (30%), malrotation (30%), and annular pancreas (30%)
    B. Down syndrome (70%), congenital heart disease (10%), malrotation (30%), and annular pancreas (70%)
    C. Down syndrome (30%), congenital heart disease (10%), malrotation (10%), and annular pancreas (70%)
    D. Down syndrome (10%), congenital heart disease (30%), malrotation (30%), and annular pancreas (50%)

5. The most common variant of congenital duodenal obstruction is:
    A. Duodenal stenosis
    B. Type I atresia
    C. Type II atresia
    D. Type III atresia

6. Surgical treatment of congenital duodenal obstruction may involve:
    A. Duodenoduodenostomy
    B. Duodenojejunostomy
    C. Duodenotomy and web excision
    D. All of the above

7. Mortality associated with duodenal atresia is rare but usually results from:
    A. An associated cardiac malformation
    B. Anastomotic leak
    C. Fulminant pancreatitis
    D. None of the above

ANSWERS AND DISCUSSION

1. **B** Intrinsic congenital duodenal obstruction is thought to result from a failure of coalescent vacuolization of the solid cord stage (and hence recanalization of the lumen) of the distal foregut between the eighth and tenth week of gestation. Simultaneously, the extrahepatic biliary tree and pancreas develop from primordial foregut buds as intestinal rotation occurs. This concurrent organogenesis explains in part the association of other foregut malformations that may contribute to extrinsic duodenal obstruction. These include annular pancreas (30%), malrotation (30%), and preduodenal portal vein (5%).

2. **B** The diagnosis of duodenal atresia is suspected antenatally when polyhydramnios is present (approximately one third of cases) and can be confirmed by fetal sonography, which demonstrates a dilated, fluid-filled stomach and proximal duodenum (sonographic "double bubble"). Although prenatal diagnosis of duodenal atresia may lead to the fortuitous diagnosis of an associated malformation, such as Down syndrome or a life-threatening cardiac malformation, it probably does not alter outcome. There is evidence to suggest that delayed postnatal diagnosis is associated with poorer preoperative condition and hence greater nenonatal morbidity than when the diagnosis is made prenatally.

3. **D** In 85% of cases, the obstruction is below the ampulla of Vater, meaning that the nasogastric aspirate is typically bile stained.

4. **A** Approximately one third of babies with congenital duodenal obstruction have Down syndrome. Of these, *approximately 70%* have a cardiac malformation, most commonly an endocardial cushion defect. The association of other gastrointestinal anomalies (annular pancreas, malrotation) probably relates to concurrent disorders of foregut embryogenesis.

5. **B** The most common form of congenital duodenal obstruction is a type I or intraluminal membranous atresia. With windsock variants, the membrane takes its origin proximal to the point of apparent obstruction as judged by the external caliber of the duodenum. At operation, the origin of the web can usually be identified by passing a gastric tube down to the level of the obstruction and watching for proximal indentation of the duodenal wall. Duodenal stenosis is often diagnosed late, but it should be suspected in any infant or child with symptoms of partial obstruction.

6. **D** Choice of surgical procedure is determined by the nature and location of the obstruction and the surgeon's preference. After exposure and mobilization of the duodenum above and below the point of obstruction, most surgeons employ a duodenoduodenostomy in a side-to-side or proximal transverse to distal longitudinal (diamond-shaped) fashion. Others prefer a loop duodenojejunostomy, particularly if the obstruction is more distal in the duodenum. Windsock variants can be treated by a carefully placed duodenotomy and partial web excision. It is important to preserve the medial portion of

the web since, in most cases, it contains the papilla of Vater. In all cases, prior to duodenal anastomosis or closure, it is important to pass a small catheter into the distal duodenum to exclude the presence of a second atresia, which is present in 1% to 3% of cases. In instances where the proximal duodenum is significantly dilated, some authors recommend a tapering, antimesenteric duodenoplasty or plication to reduce the subsequent development of megaduodenum and duodenal hypomotility.

7. **A** Most large series report a survival rate of 90% to 95% for all infants with congenital duodenal obstruction, with almost all deaths resulting from complex cardiac defects. Late complications are reported to occur in approximately 15% of cases and include blind loop syndrome with bacterial overgrowth (particularly in those treated with duodenojejunostomy), megaduodenum with hypomotility, duodenogastric reflux, gastritis, peptic ulcer disease, and biliary-pancreatic conditions.

BIBLIOGRAPHY

Grosfeld JL, Rescorla FJ. Duodenal atresia and stenosis: reassessment of treatment and outcome based on antenatal diagnosis, pathologic variance and long-term follow-up. *World J Surg.* 1993;17:301–309.

Kimura K, Mukohara N, Nishijima E, et al. Diamond-shapted anastomosis for duodenal atresia: an experience with 44 patients in 15 years. *J Pediatr Surg.* 1990;25:977–979.

Romero R, Ghidini A, Costigan K, et al. Prenatal diagnosis of duodenal atresia: does it make a difference? *Obstet Gynecol.* 1988;71:739–741.

Spigland N, Yazbeck S. Complications associated with surgical treatment of congenital intrinsic duodenal obstruction. *J Pediatr Surg.* 1990;25:1127–1130.

A NEWBORN BOY WITH AN ABDOMINAL WALL DEFECT

HISTORY   A 2800 g boy is born via vaginal delivery at 36 weeks' gestation with an abdominal wall defect shown in Figure 27–1 (see also color plate). The baby is healthy and vigorous at birth. He is born at a small community hospital without experience in caring for such problems.

EXAMINATION   Vital signs are temperature 37.0°C, heart rate 158, blood pressure 80/50, respiratory rate 40. Breath sounds are clear and equal on both sides. The heart tones are normal without a murmur. The bowel is thickened, edematous, and friable. The left testis is nonpalpable.

Please answer all questions before proceeding to discussion section.

✓ QUESTIONS

1. What kind of defect is this?
   A. Gastroschisis
   B. Omphalocele
   C. Could be either gastroschisis or a ruptured omphalocele
   D. Pentalogy of Cantrell

2. The community hospital wishes to arrange transport to your institution for further care. Which of the following interventions should be made prior to transfer?
   A. Placement of a nasogastric tube
   B. Administration of an intravenous fluid bolus
   C. Coverage of the intestine with a plastic wrap
   D. All of the above
   E. A and C

3. When this lesion is diagnosed by means of prenatal ultrasound:
   A. The prognosis is much worse when diagnosed prior to 20 weeks' gestation

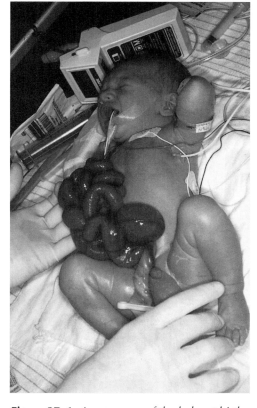

Figure 27–1. *Appearance of the baby at birth. (See also color plate.)*

    B. Labor should be induced at 36 weeks' gestation

    C. The baby should be delivered by cesarean section to prevent damage to the intestine

    D. Fetal echocardiogram must be done to look for structural heart disease

    E. None of the above

4. All of the following are true regarding early management *except:*
   - **A.** The baby is at considerable risk of heat loss through the exposed bowel
   - **B.** The patient must undergo endotracheal intubation because of associated respiratory problems
   - **C.** Failure to place a nasogastric tube immediately may lead to gaseous distention of the bowel, which can compromise the chance of primary reduction
   - **D.** Delivery by cesarean section is of no proven benefit

5. The baby arrives at your institution in good condition. During evaluation, you find that the bowel is somewhat thickened and matted. Which of the following is true of your management options?
   - **A.** Primary reduction may be attempted in the operating room
   - **B.** A silastic silo may be placed in the operating room
   - **C.** A silastic silo may be placed under local anesthesia in the neonatal intensive care unit
   - **D.** You may elect to observe the bowel "as is" and plan an attempt at reduction in 24 to 48 hours
   - **E.** A, B, and C

6. Gastroschisis is most strongly associated with which of the following anomalies?
   - **A.** Congenital heart disease
   - **B.** Chromosomal abnormalities
   - **C.** Cleft lip and palate
   - **D.** Intestinal atresia
   - **E.** Renal malformations

7. You have been able to repair the defect primarily, and the baby was started on parenteral nutrition. Three weeks later, the nasogastric output is still bilious and draining at the rate of about 60 mL per day. The baby has not yet passed meconium. Appropriate management includes:
   - **A.** Observation without intervention
   - **B.** Upper gastrointestinal series with barium
   - **C.** Upper gastrointestinal series with water soluble contrast
   - **D.** Contrast enema
   - **E.** Radionucleotide gastric emptying study

8. The most likely long-term complication after recovery from this condition is:
   - **A.** Midgut volvulus
   - **B.** Necrotizing enterocolitis
   - **C.** Small bowel obstruction
   - **D.** Parenteral nutrition associated cholestasis
   - **E.** Central venous catheter sepsis

ANSWERS AND DISCUSSION

1. **A** The defect pictured is gastroschisis. In gastroschisis, the defect occurs adjacent to a normal umbilical cord. This opening is almost always on the right, but left-sided gastroschisis has been reported. The stomach and intestine are frequently outside the abdominal cavity, but the liver is rarely involved. The appearance of the intestine varies markedly between cases. Typically, the bowel is somewhat thickened and matted. In some cases, it may appear nearly normal, while in others it appears intensely inflamed and presents as a single congealed mass of bowel where individual loops are indistinguishable.

2. **D** Proper immediate management of the infant with gastroschisis has an important impact on long-term outcome. After the ABCs of resuscitation have been addressed, the first intervention should be to place an orogastric tube. This will prevent vomiting and aspiration of gastric contents. In addition, it will prevent gaseous distention of the bowel due to air swallowing. If bowel distention occurs, the opportunity for primary reduction of the intestine may be lost.

   The exposed intestine in gastroschisis can cause large and rapid loss of heat and fluid. Hypothermia and hypovolemia may occur rapidly and cause severe circulatory compromise. Placement of the intestine in a plastic enclosure will markedly diminish these losses. A simple solution is to place the infant's entire lower body, including the exposed intestine, in a "bowel bag." If this is not available, the intestine may be wrapped in gauze soaked with warm saline and then plastic wrap. Initial fluid requirements in infants with gastroschisis may be considerable. An intravenous line should be started, and a moderate fluid bolus given. Further fluid resuscitation may be based on clinical grounds. With proper protection of the intestine, fluid requirements may be minimized. Overhydration can result in bowel edema that can compromise closure.

3. **E** Prenatal ultrasound is very useful in the diagnosis of abdominal wall defects. It allows for the baby to be delivered in a center that is prepared for the postnatal care. Ultrasound is highly accurate at identifying gastroschisis and differentiating it from omphalocele. Beyond this, the ultrasound has little prognostic value. There is no evidence to suggest that the gestational age at diagnosis or the appearance or size of the bowel predicts outcome. Recommendations are for vaginal delivery. This does not result in damage to the intestine. Some surgeons speculate that early delivery via cesarean section may reduce the inflammatory peal on the bowel and lead to earlier bowel function. This question has not yet been studied. Omphalocele, not gastroschisis, is associated with congenital heart disease.

4. **B** This patient, as well as most babies with gastroschisis, is quite stable. Endotracheal intubation is not necessary in the absence of respiratory compromise.

5. **E** Any of the first three options are acceptable. Primary reduction of the bowel into the abdomen is preferred if it is technically possible

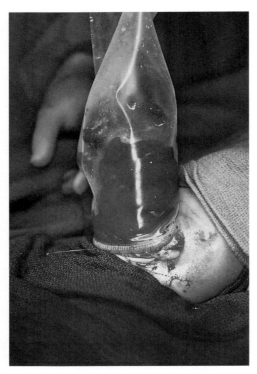

Figure 27–2. *Baby with gastroschisis in an abdominal silo. The top of the silo will be serially compressed in order to reduce the bowel into the abdominal cavity gradually. At a second operation, the silo will be removed, and the abdomen closed. (See also color plate.)*

and can be done safely. Reduction of bowel to create too high an intra-abdominal pressure can result in bowel injury or respiratory compromise. How much pressure is too high is debatable. Some surgeons use clinical judgment, while others recommend monitoring bladder pressure as an objective gauge of intra-abdominal pressure. Alternatively, the bowel may be suspended and protected in a silastic silo. Figure 27–2 (see also color plate) shows a silo in place. The bowel is protected from heat and water loss and resides in a sterile environment. The silo is gradually tightened over several days allowing reduction of the bowel.

6. **D** Gastroschisis is not associated with other congenital anomalies. Most babies with gastroschisis are otherwise entirely healthy. In 10% of cases, bowel abnormalities, such as atresias or stenoses, are seen. These abnormalities are thought to be related to bowel trauma or position in utero.

7. **A** The mean time from operation to initiation of oral feedings in gastroschisis is 3 to 6 weeks. This period of ileus is expected and does not justify investigation.

8. **C** Patients with repaired gastroschisis typically have considerable intraperitoneal adhesions. The most common late complication is adhesive small bowel obstruction. This is treated in the same manner as adhesive obstruction from other causes. Gastroschisis is associated with nonrotation of the intestine, but the adhesions make volvulus a very rare event. The small subset of patients with gastroschisis who have short gut syndrome are at risk for parenteral nutrition cholestasis and central venous catheter related sepsis.

BIBLIOGRAPHY

Bianch A, Dickson AP. Elective delayed reduction and no anesthesia: minimal intervention management for gastrochisis. *J Pediatr Surg.* 1998; 33(9):1338–1340.

Langer JC. Gastroschisis and omphalocele. *Semin Pediatr Surg.* 1996; 5:124–128.

Molenaar JC, Tibboel D. Gastroschisis and omphalocele. *World J Surg.* 1993;17:337–341.

Philippart AI, Canty TG, Filler RM. Acute fluid volume requirements in infants with anterior abdominal wall defects. *J Pediatr Surg.* 1972;7:553.

Torfs CP, Lam PK, Schaffer DM, et al. Association between mothers' nutrient intake and their offsprings' risk of gastroschisis. *Teratology.* 1998; 58:241–250.

LEG SWELLING IN A 5-YEAR-OLD BOY

HISTORY   A 5-year-old boy is brought to the emergency room by his mother. His left leg has become swollen and tender over the last day and a half. He has had a fever up to 101.5°F. He is an otherwise healthy boy with no significant medical history. The boy's mother does not recall any history of trauma. The boy was on a long bicycle ride 2 days ago. The boy is crying and says that his leg hurts terribly.

EXAMINATION   The child appears toxic. He is somewhat agitated and confused and frequently wrestles free from his mother's arms and then returns to her. Temperature 38.2°C, heart rate 160, blood pressure 110/70, respiratory rate 38. His respirations are deep with clear breath sounds. Heart tones are normal. His abdomen is mildly distended, soft, and nontender.

His left leg is markedly swollen from midthigh down to and including the foot. There is no blanching erythema. The entire leg is "woody" with dense edema that is difficult to pit. The dorsalis pedis pulse is present and normal. The posterior tibial pulse is difficult to palpate. Neurovascular function in the foot is normal. There is a healing puncture wound on the plantar surface of the foot. There is no skin ulceration anywhere on the extremity. The leg is diffusely tender to direct pressure.

LABORATORY   Hemoglobin 9.8, hematocrit 29, white blood cell count (WBC) 18.2 with 76% neutrophils and 6% bands. Electrolytes are normal. X-ray of the pelvis is shown in Figure 28–1.

Please answer all questions before proceeeding to discussion section.

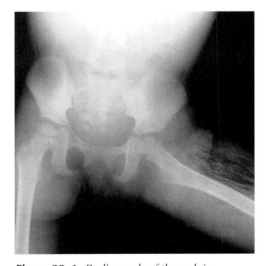

Figure 28–1. *Radiograph of the pelvis.*

✓ QUESTIONS

1. The next diagnostic maneuver should be:
   A. A radiolabeled white blood cell scan to localize the infection

B. An ultrasound of the leg to look for an abscess
C. A magnetic resonance image (MRI) of the leg to look for evidence of deep tissue infection or vascular thrombosis
D. A venous Doppler study of the leg to look for deep venous thrombosis
E. None of the above

2. Initial therapy should include:
A. Elevation of the leg
B. Placement of intermittent compression stockings
C. Administration of heparin
D. Immediate operation
E. None of the above

3. With respect to antimicrobial coverage:
A. It must include penicillin G
B. Cefazolin, gentamicin, and metronidazole is adequate
C. Subcutaneous injection of antibiotics will supplement the effectiveness of intravenous therapy
D. Antifungal coverage is indicated until wound cultures confirm the absence of fungal infection
E. Antibiotics should be withheld until culture results confirm infection

4. The most important prognostic factor determining outcome in this disease is:
A. Selection of antibiotics
B. Whether or not hyperbaric oxygen treatment is used
C. Rapidity of surgical therapy
D. Age of the patient
E. Presence or absence of positive blood cultures

5. Proper surgical therapy must include:
A. Radical excision of all nonviable tissue without regard for difficulty of wound closure
B. Regional anesthesia to avoid the systemic effects of anesthetic drugs
C. Strict avoidance of depolarizing neuromuscular blocking agents
D. Limited excision with frequent reoperation to evaluate tissue viability
E. Amputation

6. In the pediatric population, this disease is usually seen in:
A. Children with hematologic malignancies
B. Children with chronic granulomatous disease
C. Children receiving steroids
D. Children on antibiotics for an unrelated condition
E. None of the above

7. This disorder is most commonly caused by:
A. Clostridial species
B. Antibiotic resistant bacteria
C. Mixed aerobic and anaerobic flora
D. Beta lactamase producing streptococcus
E. *Escherichia coli* 0157

8. This disorder may be seen in which of the following locations?
   A. Around the umbilicus in a newborn
   B. In the perineum
   C. Around a chicken pox lesion
   D. Around the penis after circumcision
   E. All of the above

ANSWERS AND DISCUSSION

1. **E** This patient has clear clinical evidence of a necrotizing soft-tissue infection. This is the presumptive diagnosis until proven otherwise. Severe pain in the area is virtually always present in these infections and is the first clue to the diagnosis. Virtually all of these patients appear toxic and have an altered sensorium. The edema seen in these infections is very "woody" and has been described as *peau d' orange* (like an orange peel). This occurs due to obstruction of dermal lymphatics. Fever (40%) and tachycardia (70%) are not always present on presentation but are useful when seen.

   Laboratory evaluation is less useful. In one series, only 50% of patients had an elevated WBC, and 40% had an abnormal differential. Radiographs may reveal gas in the soft tissue as in Figure 28–1. This is present only 30% of the time but is absolutely diagnostic when seen. Radiographs are also important in the differential diangosis since a fracture in a young child can produce severe pain and marked swelling of the soft tissues.

   A radiolabeled WBC (**A**) scan is used to look for occult infection and takes 2 days to complete. An ultrasound (**B**) is a good study to look for an abscess, but an abscess is not the concern here. An MRI (**C**) has been occasionally used in necrotizing soft-tissue infections. It has not been found to yield any additional information to that found at operation and results in considerable delay in debridement, which is detrimental to outcome. Deep venous thrombosis is exceedingly rare in children and does not cause severe pain, fever, and gas in the soft tissue. Venous Doppler (**E**) is not indicated.

2. **D** Appropriate therapy for necrotizing fasciitis includes immediate administration of antibiotics, fluid resuscitation, and immediate operative exploration and debridement. Prompt debridement is absolutely essential. Any delay will adversely affect the outcome. Necrotic tissue is the "fuel feeding the fire" and must be removed. Elevation of the leg or placement of compression stockings will achieve nothing, and heparin will cause bleeding.

   The diagnosis of necrotizing soft-tissue infection is predominantly based on clinical grounds. At times, operative exploration is necessary to "rule out" the process. If clinical suspicion is strong, the patient should be taken to the operating room where an incision can be made and the site explored. In necrotizing fasciitis, the wound immediately oozes a large amount of watery brown fluid. The fat is pale and can be stripped off of the fascia easily by simply sweeping one's finger along this layer. Once an incision is made the findings are unmistakable. The skin over this extensive necrotic process is often viable, however, thereby obscuring the underlying process.

3. **B** The bacteriology of necrotizing fasciitis is highly variable. It is usually caused by mixed aerobic and anaerobic flora. It can be caused by group A beta-hemolytic streptococcus, clostridial species, or a variety of other organisms. Due to the common occurrence of gram-negative bacteria, anaerobes, and other organisms, antibiotic coverage should include a penicillin or cephalosporin, an aminoglycoside, and an agent active against anaerobes.

    Penicillin G (**A**) is the historically recommended therapy. It is still an effective drug when combined with the others listed. Other forms of penicillin and cephalosporins provide similar but broader coverage. Subcutaneous or topical antibiotics (**C**) are of no proven value. Invasive soft-tissue fungal infection is exceedingly rare in immunocompetent hosts. Fungi have not been implicated in necrotizing fasciitis in normal hosts. Broad-spectrum antibiotics are vital to therapy. They should not be withheld pending culture data. When cultures become available, coverage may be appropriately narrowed.

4. **C** Rapid surgical debridement is the key to patient survival. One series reported on 20 children with necrotizing fasciitis. A delay in surgical therapy was linked to all of the deaths. While antibiotic choice is important (**A**), it is secondary to the importance of prompt debridement of nonviable tissue. Hyberbaric oxygen (**B**) has been used in the treatment of these infections. There is no reliable data supporting its efficacy. Age (**D**) is an important factor. Even in the newborn population with necrotizing fasciitis due to omphalitis, however, prompt debridement is the most important factor determining survival. The presence (**E**) of positive blood cultures has not proven to be predictive of outcome.

5. **A** Complete and aggressive surgical debridement of all nonviable tissue is absolutely essential. All involved tissue should be resected back to healthy bleeding margins. This debridement must be done without concern for wound closure. Survival of the patient depends on adequate debridement and closure is a secondary issue. The patient should be returned to the operating room on a daily basis for examinations of the wound and further debridement where necessary. Figure 28–2 (see also color plate) shows a patient after five operative debridements and amputation of the foot in order to control the infection. Tissue has been excised down to muscle in over 35% of the body surface area. This area is now ready for skin grafting.

    There is no reason to prefer regional anesthesia (**B**) over general anesthesia. The use of neuromuscular blocking agents (**C**) has been questioned following burn injury but does not appear to be a problem here. Amputation (**E**) may be necessary if the deep tissues are involved.

6. **E** In the pediatric population, necrotizing faciitis is usually seen in normal healthy children without immune deficiencies. This is in contrast to adults, where necrotizing fasciitis tends to occur in diabetic, elderly, and debilitated people.

7. **C** Necrotizing fasciitis is usually caused by mixed flora. The bacteria involved do not appear to be unique strains or particularly virulent, but this is an area under research. Clostridia is certainly a cause of necrotizing soft-tissue infections but is found in a minority of cases. Most bacteria found on culture are sensitive to the usual antibiotics.

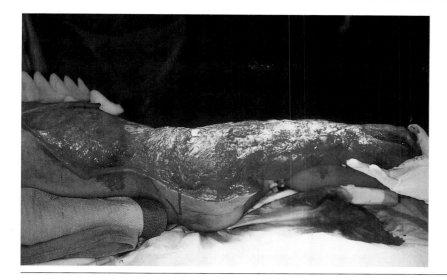

Figure 28–2. *This patient required five operative debridements and amputation of his right foot in order to control the infection. He required excision of all skin and subcutaneous tissue over 35% of his body surface area. He is shown here prior to skin grafting. This patient survived and is doing well. (See also color plate.)*

Streptococcus is frequently seen but less commonly as a single organism than as one of multiple. *Escherichia coli* 0157 causes gastroenteritis and is linked to hemolytic uremic syndrome, but it is not known to be associated with soft-tissue infections.

8. **E** Necrotizing fasciitis may be found in any of the mentioned locations. It can occur in any area of soft tissue. Frequently, it follows minor trauma or a surgical procedure, but often an inciting event is not known.

BIBLIOGRAPHY

Farrell LD, Karl SR, Davis PK, et al. Postoperative necrotizing fasciitis in children. *Pediatrics.* 1988;82:874–879.

Kosloske AM, Bartow SA. Debridement of periumbilical necrotizing fasciitis: importance of excision of the umbilical vessels and urachal remnant. *J Pediatr Surg.* 1991;26:808–810.

Kosloske AM, Cushing AH, Borden TA, et al. Cellulitis and necrotizing fasciitis of the abdominal wall in pediatric patients. *J Pediatr Surg.* 1981; 16:246–251.

Moss RL, Musemeche CA, Kosloske AM. Necrotizing fasciitis in children: prompt recognition and aggressive therapy improves survival. *J Pediatr Surg.* 1996;31:1142–1146.

Murphy JJ, Granger R, Blair GK, et al. Necrotizing fasciitis in childhood. *J Pediatr Surg.* 1995;30:1131–1134.

Sawin RS, Schaller RT, Tapper D, et al. Early recognition of neonatal abdominal wall necrotizing fasciitis. *Am J Surg.* 1994;167:481–484.

A 3-YEAR-OLD BOY WHO SWALLOWED A KEY

HISTORY This 3-year-old boy swallowed a key. He gulped once or twice but had no choking, vomiting, or respiratory distress. His mother gave him a sip of water, which went down, and brought him to the emergency room.

EXAMINATION He is a tanned, well-developed 3-year-old boy in no respiratory distress, who weighs 32 pounds. Pulse is 98/min; blood pressure is 92/68; tympanic membrane temperature is 37.8°C; respirations are 28/min. He is not drooling. Eyes and ears are unremarkable. The pharynx is normal, except for mild hypertrophy of the tonsils. The trachea is midline. No neck mass is palpable. The lungs are clear to auscultation. No cardiac murmur is audible. The remainder of his exam is normal.

LABORATORY Blood count and urinalysis were not done. The abdominal x-ray is shown in Figure 29–1.
Please answer all questions before proceeding to discussion section.

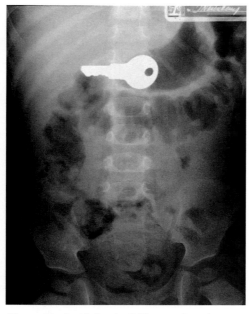

Figure 29–1. *Abdominal film, supine view, showing key in pylorus.*

✓ QUESTIONS

1. The optimal management of this child now is:
   A. Immediate gastroscopy
   B. Removal of the key under fluoroscopy, using a snare or a magnetic device
   C. A dose of intravenous metaclopramide
   D. Immediate ingestion of white bread and milk
   E. Watchful waiting

2. A 2-year-old boy swallows a foreign body, which reaches his stomach. Which of the following objects is *most* likely to cause complications?

A. A penny
B. A peso
C. An open safety pin 0.5 inch long
D. A 1.5-inch piece of lead from a mechanical pencil
E. A 3-inch broom bristle

3. A 2-year-old girl swallows a button battery from her grandfather's hearing aid. Her x-ray is shown in Figure 29–2. The optimal management is:
   A. Ipecac to induce vomiting
   B. Gastroscopy and removal of the foreign body
   C. Removal of the battery under fluoroscopy, using a magnetic-tipped nasogastric tube device
   D. A laxative to speed passage of the battery
   E. Watchful waiting

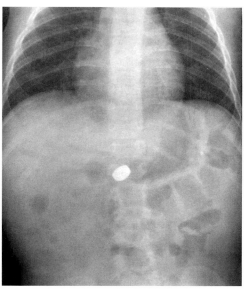

Figure 29–2. *Button battery in stomach.*

ANSWERS AND DISCUSSION

1. **E** Watchful waiting is the optimal management of this child. In general, once a foreign body reaches the stomach, it will traverse the rest of the gastrointestinal (GI) tract and be expelled in the feces. Retrieval of the foreign body by gastroscopy (**A**) or fluoroscopic maneuvers (**B**) is usually not necessary. (If the parents are locked out of somewhere, they might call a locksmith! The key, in fact, seems to be unlocking the pylorus.) The metaclopramide (**C**) will cause gastric contraction and may propel the foreign body into the duodenum, but stimulation of peristalsis is not necessary. White bread (**D**) will be digested from saliva and gastric juice; it does not form a protective coating on the key.

2. **E** The 3-inch broom bristle is the most likely to cause problems. In general, gastrointestinal foreign bodies, once they reach the stomach, will traverse the GI tract and be expelled in the feces. Even the open safety pins (**C**) usually pass without harm. In a remarkable series of 1250 children from Paris with gastrointestinal foreign bodies, complications, usually duodenal perforation, occurred in only 16 (1.3%). Long, rigid, pointed objects (like a 3-inch broom bristle) may perforate the bowel at anatomic points of angulation or fixation (eg, the C-loop of the duodenum). Occasional catastrophies are reported from erosion into the retroperitoneum. Coins (**A** and **B**) from any country usually stick at the esophageal inlet of a 2-year-old, just below the cricopharyngeus muscle, and require extraction. Once they hit the stomach, however, coins should pass through the rest of the GI tract without risk. A 1.5 inch lead from a pencil (**D**) should have less trouble rounding the duodenal C-loop than the 3-inch broom bristle. The lead would not cause lead poisoning since it is graphite.

3. **E** Watchful waiting is the management of button batteries in the stomach, like that for any other foreign body beyond the esophagus. If the battery is lodged in the esophagus, however, extraction is an emergency because of the risk of potentially fatal erosions into the mediastinum. The mechanism of injury is either from alkali leaching out of the battery case or, more likely, by the generation of hydroxyl ions from the tissues as a result of hydrolysis from the electrical cur-

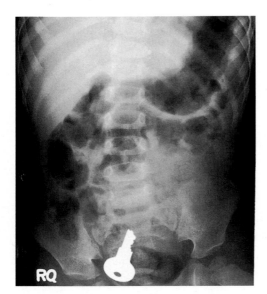

Figure 29–3. *Abdominal film, supine view, taken 3 days after Figure 29–1, showing key in lower intestine, probably sigmoid colon. On following morning, the key passed in child's stool.*

rent of an intact, active cell. The battery will do no harm as long as it keeps moving through the GI tract. Perforation has been reported in a child who had a battery lodged in a Meckel's diverticulum. Ipecac (**A**) is contraindicated, as the battery might move back up into the esophagus during vomiting. The other maneuvers, gastroscopy (**B**) and the magnetic "fishing tube" (**C**), are unnecessary. Laxatives (**D**) have no documented benefit.

FOLLOW-UP   The child is treated as an outpatient. The mother is instructed to return if the boy develops abdominal pain, vomiting, or any problem that worries her. She should call the pediatrician when the key appears in her son's stool or in 3 days if the key fails to appear. After 3 days, the key has not appeared. The pediatrician, who is becoming worried that the foreign body is not moving through the GI tract, repeats the abdominal film (Figure 29–3). The key passes on the fourth day.

BIBLIOGRAPHY

Grosfeld JL, Eng K. Right iliac artery-duodenal fistula in infancy: massive hemorrhage due to "whisk-broom" bristle perforation. *Ann Surg.* 1972;176:761–764.

Kosloske AM. Foreign bodies in children. In: Buntain WL, ed. *Management of Pediatric Trauma.* Philadelphia: Saunders; 1995:459–477.

Litovitz TL. Button battery ingestions: a review of 56 cases. *JAMA.* 1983;249:2495–2500.

Pellerin D, Fortier-Beaulieu M, Gueguen J. The fate of swallowed foreign bodies: experience of 1250 instances of sub-diaphragmatic foreign bodies in children. *Prog Pediatr Radiol.* 1969;2:286–302.

JAUNDICE IN A BABY ON PARENTERAL NUTRITION

HISTORY   A 3-month-old, former 29-week gestational age girl developed severe necrotizing enterocolitis in the first week of life. She underwent extensive small bowel resection and ostomy placement. Total parenteral nutrition (TPN) was initiated at 10 days of life. She recovered well from her operation and NEC and underwent successful stoma closure at 2 months of age. She retained 54 cm of small intestine at the conclusion of this operation. Since then, she has been able to tolerate a gradually increasing fraction of enteral feeding. Currently, she is receiving 20% of her caloric needs and multivitamins by gut and 80% by the parenteral route.

EXAMINATION   The baby's weight is 3.2 kg, and she appears well except for visible jaundice. Her vital signs are normal. Her heart and lung examination is unremarkable. Her abdomen displays a well-healed transverse incision. The liver edge is 2.5 cm below the costal margin and a bit firm. The spleen is palpable at the left costal margin.

LABORATORY   Hemoglobin 9.8, hematocrit 29, white blood cell count 12.2, with 61% neutrophils and 4% bands. INR is 1.8. Electrolytes are normal. Total bilirubin is 9.4 with a direct fraction of 7.9. Alkaline phospatase is 242, aspartate transaminase (AST) is 145, alanine transaminase (ALT) is 130, gamma-glutamyl transpeptidase (GGT) is 204. Abdominal x-ray reveals no abnormalities except for hepatomegaly.
   Please answer all questions before proceeding to discussion section.

✓ QUESTIONS

1. The differential diagnosis includes:
   A. Extrahepatic biliary atresia
   B. Neonatal giant cell hepatitis

   C. Alpha 1 antitrypsin deficiency
   D. All of the above
   E. None of the above

2. The most likely diagnosis is:
   A. Hepatitis C infection
   B. Hepatitis B infection
   C. Alagille syndrome
   D. Total parenteral nutrition (TPN) associated cholestasis
   E. Rh incompatibility

3. Contributing factors to the elevated INR are likely to include:
   A. Systemic vitamin K deficiency
   B. Inadequate synthetic function of the liver
   C. Both
   D. Neither

4. Proven treatment options to alleviate cholestasis due to parenteral nutrition include:
   A. Administration of phenobarbitol
   B. Administration of ursodeoxycholic acid
   C. Provision of partial enteral feeding
   D. All of the above
   E. None of the above

5. Risk factors for parenteral nutrition associated cholestasis include:
   A. Prematurity
   B. Episodes of sepsis
   C. Length of time on TPN
   D. All of the above
   E. None of the above

6. The natural history of parenteral nutrition cholestasis in the infant who continues on TPN is:
   A. Stablilization of cholestasis
   B. Development of chronic liver disease that usually responds to steroids
   C. Cirrhosis and death
   D. Development of severe portal hypertension with maintenance of hepatic synthetic function
   E. Increased risk of hepatoblastoma

7. The cause of parenteral nutrition cholestasis is:
   A. Due to the lipid infusion
   B. Due to the lack of stimulation of gut hormones
   C. Related to overgrowth of intestinal bacteria
   D. Portal vein thrombosis
   E. Unknown

ANSWERS AND DISCUSSION

1. **D** This baby very likely has parenteral nutrition associated cholestasis. Nevertheless, the development of direct hyperbilirubinemia in an infant raises a number of diagnostic possibilities. Care must be

taken to distinguish direct from indirect hyperbilirubinemia, which is likely to be caused by hemolytic disorders. All of the disorders listed can elevate the serum level of direct bilirubin. Extrahepatic biliary atresia is unusual in premature infants and very uncommonly seen in patients on parenteral nutrition. Nevertheless, it should be considered if the stools are acholic and the bilirubin is still rising after cessation of TPN. Neonatal giant cell hepatitis can cause a rising direct bilirubin. Liver biopsy may be required for diagnosis. Alpha 1 antitrypsin deficiency may be diagnosed by a serum test.

2. **D**

3. **C** This patient has evidence of significant cholestasis. This may affect blood coagulation in two ways. First, cholestasis causes significant fat malabsorbtion, including malabsorbtion of fat-soluble vitamins. This problem may be further compounded because a significant portion of this patient's distal ileum was removed. Vitamin K may be absorbed poorly. If it is not supplied parenterally, it should be given in its water-soluble form.

   Parenteral nutrition cholestasis causes hepatic fibrosis and ultimately cirrhosis. Liver synthetic function may be markedly impaired. This includes production of clotting factors.

4. **E** While all of the listed measures are frequently done, none of them are of proven efficacy. Phenobarbitol is thought to promote bile flow and is used to treat other forms of cholestasis. When its use was carefully studied in patients with TPN cholestasis, patients given phenobarbitol actually fared worse than controls. Ursodeoxycholic acid is an exogenous bile acid found in the bile of bears. It promotes increased bile flow and has been used in patients with TPN cholestasis. While pilot studies show some promise, its efficacy remains to be proven. Partial enteral feeding has never been shown to alleviate cholestasis. Rather, several studies report progression of cholestasis in patients receiving partial eneteral feeding in addition to TPN. The only proven method to alleviate parenteral nutrition cholestasis is to discontinue TPN and provide all calories enterally. Nevertheless, provision of partial enteral feeding may promote growth of the gut mucosa and reduce the risk of sepsis. Thus, it should be encouraged.

5. **D** Multiple retrospective reviews of patients with TPN cholestasis attempted to determine why some infants on TPN develop rapidly progressive liver failure while others do not. The answer to this question remains unknown. A consensus of the literature, however, does clearly state that a greater degree of prematurity and increased length of time on TPN are risk factors for cholestasis. Sepsis can cause cholestasis independent of TPN. Episodes of sepsis in a patient on TPN clearly have a synergistic negative effect and markedly accelerate the liver damage.

6. **C** If TPN cannot be discontinued, TPN cholestasis is a progressive, unrelenting disease leading to cirrhosis and death. Parenteral nutrition-associated liver failure is a major indication for liver transplantation in the pediatric population. Care of these patients is complex, as many of them have short gut syndrome and are candidates for small bowel transplantation as well. Steroids (**B**) have no role in the treatment of this disorder. Many of these patients develop severe

portal hypertension (**D**), but this is not independent of marked impairment of hepatic synthetic function. There have been a few anecdotal reports of hepatoblastoma occurring in a patient who had received TPN during infancy. A true relationship has not been proven.

7. **E** Despite two decades of research, the cause of TPN cholestasis remains unknown. Lipid infusion (**A**) does not appear to be the culprit. Total parenteral nutrition cholestasis was reported before lipids came into clinical use. Gut hormone levels (**B**) may be somewhat altered in the fasting state but administration of these hormones has not alleviated cholestasis. Intestinal bacteria (**C**) may have a role in cholestasis, but a variety of antibacterial protocols have had no effect on TPN cholestasis. Portal vein thrombosis (**E**) may be a consequence of cirrhosis but is not directly related to TPN.

BIBLIOGRAPHY

Drowngowski RA, Coran AG. An analysis of factors contributing to the development of total parenteral nutrition-induced cholestasis. *J Parenteral Enteral Nutr.* 1989;13:586–589.

Ginn-Pease ME, Pantalos D, King DR. TPN-associated hyperbilirubinemia: a common problem in newborn surgical patients. *J Pediatr Surg.* 1985; 20(4):436–439.

Hoffman AF. Defective biliary secretion during total parenteral nutrition: probably mechanisms and possible solutions. *J Pediatr Gastroenterol Nutr.* 1995;20:376–390.

Kelly DA. Liver complications of pediatric parenteral nutrition-epidemiology. *Nutrition.* 1998;14:153–157.

Moss RL, Amii L. New approaches to the understanding and etiology of parenteral nutrition associated cholestasis. *Semin Pediatr Surg.* 1999;8:140–147.

Moss RL, Das JB, Ansari G. Hepatobiliary dysfunction during total parenteral nutrition is caused by infusate, not route of administration. *J Pediatr Surg.* 1993;28(3):391–397.

Moss RL, Das JB, Raffensperger JG. Necrotizing enterocolitis and total parenteral nutrition associated cholestasis. *Nutrition.* 1996;12:340–343.

Moss RL, Das JB, Raffensperger JG. Total parenteral nutrition-associated cholestasis: clinical and histopathologic correlation. *J Pediatr Surg.* 1993;28(10):1270–1275.

SUDDEN CARDIAC ARREST IN A POSTOPERATIVE INFANT

HISTORY A 37-weeks' gestation infant male undergoes an uncomplicated repair of esophageal atresia and distal tracheoesophageal fistula. Because of difficulty in obtaining peripheral venous access, a percutaneous central line is placed through the left subclavian vein into the right atrium. The infant was extubated in the operating room and returned to the neonatal intensive care unit where he remained stable for the next 4 days on nasal cannula oxygen. On the fifth postoperative day, there was a transient rise in both the pulse and respiratory rates, and a chest x-ray demonstrated an enlarged cardiac silhouette (Figure 31–1).

Twenty minutes later, the infant suddenly developed bradycardia despite oxygen saturation levels in the nineties. Shortly thereafter, the infant was blue and pulseless. Aggressive resuscitative measures, including endotracheal intubation, mechanical ventilation, administration of inotropic drugs, and bilateral needle thoracostomy, were unsuccessful. The infant was pronounced dead, and a postmortem examination was ordered.

✓ QUESTIONS

1. The possible causes of sudden death in this infant are:
   A. Previously unrecognized congenital heart disease
   B. Fatal cardiac arrhythmia from an associated electrolyte abnormality
   C. Delayed pericardial tamponade complicating central venous line insertion
   D. Air embolism through the central line in the presence of an interatrial communication
   E. All of the above

The principal finding at autopsy was that of a tense pericardial effusion containing approximately 20 mL of straw-colored fluid surround-

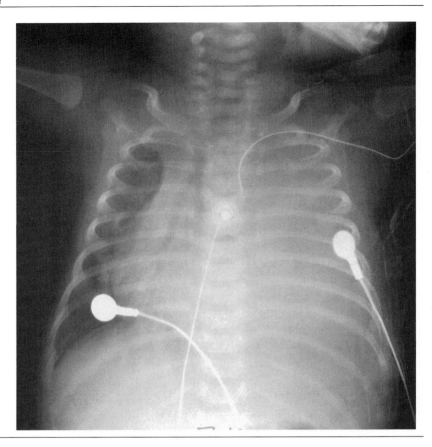

Figure 31–1. *Chest radiograph of a 6-day-old infant who developed sudden cardiac arrest 5 days following repair of esophageal atresia with tracheoesophageal fistula.*

ing a structurally normal heart. There was a focal area of discoloration on the posterior aspect of the right ventricle, which corresponded histologically to an area of partial thickness myocardial necrosis. Death was attributed to cardiac tamponade from hydropericardium, which was caused by focal myocardial injury from the central venous catheter.

2. Which of the following statements regarding cardiac tamponade are *false?*
   A. Cardiac tamponade may occur on an acute or chronic basis
   B. Excluding patients undergoing open heart surgery, cardiac tamponade occurs most commonly in association with penetrating chest injury
   C. Physiologic compromise results from impaired diastolic filling and decreased stroke volume
   D. Fatality from cardiac tamponade correlates directly with patient age

3. Of the following, which factors may be causally associated with the development of cardiac tamponade?
   A. Placement of a central catheter via cut-down technique
   B. Placement of a semirigid plastic versus silastic catheter
   C. Duration of catheter placement
   D. Nature of catheter infusate

4. The diagnosis of cardiac tamponade:
   A. Is made easily on clinical grounds

B. Is suggested by hypotension and decreased central venous pressure

C. Requires the presence of a myocardial perforation

D. Should be considered in any infant with a central venous catheter who develops sudden cardiopulmonary symptoms without evident cause

5. Treatment of cardiac tamponade:
   A. May involve percutaneous placement of a pigtail catheter
   B. Usually requires thoracotomy or sternotomy in the presence of penetrating trauma
   C. Is often not possible because the patient's clinical presentation is precipitous and fatal
   D. May be facilitated by needle pericardiocentesis
   E. All of the above

ANSWERS AND DISCUSSION

1. **E** Sudden death in an apparently healthy infant is unusual and usually signifies a cardiac event, such as a fatal arrhythmia. Typically, cardiac arrest in the infant is secondary to respiratory failure. In these patients, oxygen desaturation and respiratory difficulties precede the cardiac arrest. This patient clearly experienced a cardiac event in the absence of respiratory failure. Any infant with a central line is at risk for inadvertent introduction of air, which in the presence of an atrial septal defect, could result in a coronary embolus and sudden cardiac death. Cardiac tamponade resulting from myocardial perforation is a rare complication of central venous catheters that may occur early (at the time of catheter insertion) or late, presumably due to catheter migration.

2. **D** Age does not appear to be predictive of mortality from cardiac tamponade. If the tamponade is promptly relieved, patients of any age should recover.

3. **B** Although central venous catheters are used frequently, the development of cardiac tamponade in relation to the catheter appears to be an extremely rare event. The more typical complications of central venous catheters are classified as early (usually related to insertion) and delayed. Early complications include hemothorax, pneumothorax, and catheter malposition, while late complications include catheter-associated sepsis or thrombosis, catheter tip migration, and catheter fracture and embolization. In the rare instances that cardiac tamponade does develop, it is usually the result of myocardial perforation by either the catheter or guidewire (percutaneous insertion) at the time of catheter placement. The stiffness of the catheter itself helps determine the risk of cardiac perforation. Most of the catheters in use are either silastic or polyurethane and are less likely to damage the heart than some of the earlier and stiffer polyethylene catheters. Although placement of the catheter at or above the atriocaval junction (confirmed by fluoroscopy at the time of insertion) should minimize the risk of catheter perforation. Cardiac perforation and tamponade weeks to months after appro-

priate catheter placement does occur. Migration of the catheter tip against the wall of the atrium and continuous mechanical trauma may result in focal myocardial necrosis and perforation causing tamponade.

4. **D** Except in cases of penetrating chest injury, where the clinical suspicion of tamponade is very high, the diagnosis is infrequently based on the classic clinical triad of hypotension, central venous pressure elevation, and muffled heart tones (Beck's triad). In instances where the symptomatic presentation is not "sudden death," a chest x-ray showing an enlarged cardiac silhouette or a suspicious position of the catheter tip may suggest the diagnosis. Cardiac ultrasound will usually be confirmatory. Frequently, however, the diagnosis will only be made at autopsy. Most, but not all, cases of cardiac tamponade will have a demonstrable cardiac perforation. Those with a perforation will have blood or infusate in the pericardial sac, while cases of mechanical myocardial injury without perforation will manifest serous inflammatory fluid or "hydropericardium."

5. **E** Treatment of cardiac tamponade requires pericardial decompression, and if perforation exists, suture cardiorrhaphy. Needle pericardiocentesis may be diagnostic and temporizing, but it does not obviate the need for sternotomy or thoracotomy and pericardial exploration. Although fluoroscopically controlled placement of a pigtail catheter is standard treatment for "nontraumatic" pericardial effusions, it is also not definitive if the possibility of cardiac injury exists.

BIBLIOGRAPHY

Collier PE, Blocker SH, Graff DM, et al. Cardiac tamponade from central venous catheters. *Am J Surg.* 1998;176:212–214.

Fioravanti J, Buzzard CJ, Harris JP. Pericardial effusion and tamponade as a result of percutaneous silastic catheter use. *Neonatal Netw.* 1998; 17:39–42.

Parsa MH. Complications of central venous catheter insertion. *Crit Care Med.* 1992;20:443–444.

van Engelenburg KCA, Festen C. Cardiac tamponade: a rare but life-threatening complication of central venous catheters in children. *J Pediatr Surg.* 1998;33:1822–1824.

Wirrell EC, Pelausa EO, Allen AC, et al. Massive pericardial effusion as a cause for sudden deterioration of a very low birthweight infant. *Am J Perinatol.* 1993;10:419–423.

A 5-YEAR-OLD GIRL WITH PUBIC HAIR AND ACNE

HISTORY   A 5-year-old girl has developed pubic hair. Her family first noticed oily skin and acne about 6 months ago. The child has been healthy and active without complaints. She has seen a pediatric endocrinologist.

EXAMINATION   She is a healthy appearing girl in no apparent distress. She is a bit large for her age (in the 95th percentile for height and weight). Her vital signs are normal. She has mild facial acne. Her heart and lungs are normal. Her abdomen is soft and nondistended with a vague fullness in the left upper quadrant. There is no tenderness. She has marked clitoromegaly and the presence of pubic hair. This is shown in Figure 32–1 (see also color plate).

LABORATORY   Hemoglobin 10.8, hematocrit 34, white blood cell count 7.9. Sodium 140, potassium 4.2, chloride 102, bicarbonate 25. Blood, urea, nitrogen (BUN) 4; creatinine 0.5; 17 hydroxyprogesterone 1739 (normal up to 120); androstenedione 6.2 (normal 0.1 to 0.4); dehydroepiandrosterone sulfate (DHEAS) 23,545 (upper limit of normal 650); testosterone 90 (normal < 11).
  Please answer all questions before proceeding to discussion section.

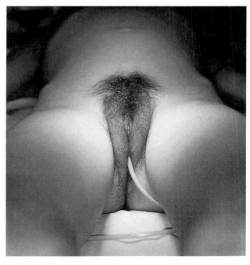

Figure 32–1. *The appearance of this 5-year-old girl with marked clitoromegaly and pubic hair. (See also color plate.)*

✓ QUESTIONS

1. Based on the history and physical appearance of the child only, which is *not* included in the differential diagnosis?
   A. Estrogen-producing ovarian tumor
   B. Adrenocortical carcinoma
   C. Adrenocortical adenoma
   D. 21-hyroxylase deficiency
   E. 11-hydroxylase deficiency

159

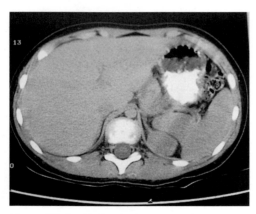

Figure 32–2. *Abdominal computed tomography (CT) scan of a 5-year-old girl with virilization.*

2. An abdominal computed tomography (CT) scan reveals a left adrenal mass (Figure 32–2). The remainder of the abdominal and chest CT scan reveals no other abnormalities. The appropriate management is:
   A. Surgical resection
   B. Obtain serum cortisol and renin studies
   C. Begin treatment with mitotane and follow hormone levels
   D. Treat with three courses of mitotane followed by surgical resection
   E. A CT scan guided needle biopsy of the mass

3. The most accurate way to tell if an adrenal tumor is benign or malignant is
   A. Histologic appearance on hemotoxylin and eosin (H&E) stain
   B. Presence or absence of microscopic vascular invasion
   C. Presence or absence of microvesicular inclusion bodies on electron microscopy
   D. Biologic behavior over time following resection
   E. Presence or absence of a mutation in chromosome 11

4. Survival after resection of an adrenocortical carcinoma is:
   A. Nearly 100%
   B. Poor
   C. Predicted by the value of the preoperative 17 ketosteroid levels
   D. Improved by chemotherapy
   E. Primarily dependent on whether or not the tumor invaded surrounding structures

5. Hyperaldosteronism in children is usually caused by:
   A. Benign adrenal adenoma
   B. Malignant adrenal tumor
   C. Renin-producing tumor of the pancreas
   D. Bilateral adrenal hyperfunction
   E. Wilms' tumor

ANSWERS AND DISCUSSION

1. **A** This child has evidence of virilization. She has pubic hair and clitoromegaly in the absence of breast development. Estrogen-producing tumors can produce pubic hair and enlargement of the genitals in females, but it is also associated with breast development. The differential diagnosis of virilization in young girls includes tumors that produce virilizing hormones and metabolic disorders called "congenital adrenal hyperplasia." The most common virilizing tumors in females are adrenocortical tumors: either adenoma or carcinoma. Ovarian tumors can produce testosterone, but this is quite rare. Congenital adrenal hyperplasia is a group of metabolic disorders where steroid metabolism is interrupted. Due to enzyme defects in the metabolic pathway to create cortisol, intermediates with virilizing effects may accumulate. 21-Hydroxylase deficiency is the most common disorder. 11-Hydroxylase deficiency can produce similar symptoms, but these children typically have hypertension. Female infants with these metabolic disorders typically have abnormal geni-

talia at birth. These disorders, however, can present in a variety of manners, and some are not apparent until early childhood.

2. **A** The presence of a solid adrenal mass in association with virilization and the noted laboratory findings are evidence of a virilizing adrenal tumor. The proper treatment of these tumors is surgical resection. Whether benign or malignant, virilizing adrenal tumors show little response to chemotherapy. Mitotane is an adrenolytic drug that has been used to treat metastatic adrenocortical carcinoma with limited success. Biopsy of the lesion is not indicated because it should be resected regardless of histologic appearance.

3. **D** Adrenal adenomas and adrenocortical carcinomas can appear very similar histologically. In fact, there are no absolute histologic criteria that separate a benign from a malignant adrenal tumor. While overall tumor size and microscopic vascular invasion are useful factors, they are by no means definitive. The only way to be certain that an adrenal tumor is benign is to observe over time that it does not recur following resection. All patients who have had an adrenal tumor resected should be followed closely with serial serum hormone levels as well as abdominal imaging. There are no known features on electron microscopy that predict biologic behavior of adrenal tumors. Adrenal tumors are not known to be related to abnormalities of chromosome 11.

4. **B** Adrenocortical carcinoma is an aggressive tumor, and survival is poor following resection. There is no known effective chemotherapy to treat disseminated or metastatic disease. Treatment of recurrent adrenocortical carcinoma includes aggressive reresection. There are a few long-term survivors reported who have undergone multiple repeat resections of adrenal carcinoma. Preoperative hormone levels do not predict whether or not a tumor is malignant and, when a tumor is malignant, do not predict survival. Invasion of surrounding structures at the time of resection is a poor prognostic sign. Even when the tumors are not grossly invasive, however, outcome is poor.

5. **D** Primary hyperaldosteronism is quite rare in children. This disorder is most commonly caused by bilateral adrenal hyperfunction with or without hyperplasia. In exceptional cases, it may be caused by an adrenocortical adenoma. This is in contrast to the adult experience where adrenal adenomas account for 90% of cases of hyperaldosteronism.

Features of hyperaldosteronism include hypertension, antidiuretic hormone-resistant polyuria, polydypsia, muscle weakness, headaches, and parasthesias within the limbs. Patients usually have hypokalemia and alkalosis. Hyperaldosteronism is not associated with Wilms' tumor.

BIBLIOGRAPHY

Driver CP, Birch J, Gough DC, Bruce J. Adrenal cortical tumors in childhood. *Pediatr Hematol Oncol.* 1998;15:527–532.

Fonkalsrud EW, Dunn J. Adrenal glands. In: O'neill JA, Rowe MI, Grosfeld JL, et al. eds. *Pediatric Surgery.* 5th ed. St. Louis: Mosby-Yearbook; 1998:1555–1573.

Mayer SK, Oligny LL, Deal C, et al. Childhood adrenocortical tumors: case series and reevaluation of prognosis—a 24-year experience. *J Pediatr Surg.* 1997;32:911–915.

Ribeiro RC, Sandrini R. Adrenocortical carcinoma in children: clinical aspects and prognosis. *J Pediatr Surg.* 1993;28:841–843.

Sandrini R, Ribeiro RC, DeLacerda L. Childhood adrenocortical tumors. *J Clin Endocrinol Metab.* 1997;82:2027–2031.

Street ME, Weber A, Camacho-Hubner C, Perry LA. Girls with virilisation in childhood: a diagnostic protocol for investigation. *J Clin Pathol.* 1997;50:379–383.

Teinturier C, Pauchard MS, Brugieres L, et al. Clinical and prognostic aspects of adrenocortical neoplasms in childhood. *Med Pediatr Oncol.* 1999;32:106–111.

Wolthers OD, Cameron FJ, Scheimberg I, et al. Androgen secreting adrenocortical tumours. *Arch Dis Child.* 1999;80:46–50.

A 3-YEAR-OLD GIRL WHO SUDDENLY VOMITS BLOOD

HISTORY A 3-year-old girl is brought to the emergency room after she vomits blood at home. She has no prior history of gastrointestinal disease and is in good general health. She takes no medications and has no history of bleeding or easy bruising. Her only prior hospitalization was for antibiotic treatment of neonatal omphalitis.

EXAMINATION In the emergency room, she appears pale and sweaty. Heart rate is 160 beats per minute, blood pressure 85/55, and respirations 30 per minute. Her sclerae are clear, and her abdomen is soft, with no hepatosplenomegaly, ascites, or prominent periumbilical vasculature. You place bilateral antecubital vein intravenous lines, and draw blood for complete blood count, cross match, and a coagulogram. Two 20 mL/kg boluses of Ringer's lactate are infused. During this resuscitation, she has another emesis of fresh blood.

Please answer all questions before proceeding to discussion section.

✓ QUESTIONS

1. The most likely cause of upper gastrointestinal bleeding in this patient is:
   A. Esophageal varices from extrahepatic portal vein thrombosis
   B. Esophageal varices from parenchymal liver disease
   C. Esophageal varices from hepatic vein obstruction (Budd-Chiari syndrome)
   D. Bleeding duodenal ulcer
   E. Swallowed blood from nasopharyngeal hemorrhage

2. After resuscitation with crystalloid and blood, the patient's condition stabilizes. Her coagulation panel is normal. The next procedure should be:
   A. Placement of a nasogastric tube and iced normal saline lavage

    B. Placement of a Sengstaken-Blakemore tube, and inflation of both esophageal and gastric balloons

    C. Upper gastrointestinal endoscopy

    D. Mesenteric angiography

3. Endoscopy demonstrates large esophageal varices running the distal one third of the esophagus, above the gastroesophageal (GE) junction (Figure 33–1; see also color plate). One varix is actively bleeding. The stomach is full of fresh blood and clot, and although the view is limited, there is no evidence of gastritis or ulceration. The next most appropriate intervention would be:

    A. Emergency interposition of mesocaval shunt

    B. Vasopressin infusion at 0.4 U/min

    C. Intravariceal endoscopic sclerotherapy

    D. Transjugular intrahepatic portosystemic shunt (TIPS) procedure

4. The mortality associated with a first variceal hemorrhage is related to the etiology of the portal hypertension:

    A. True

    B. False

5. Regarding portosystemic shunts, which of the following statements are *false*?

    A. The liver tolerates a portosystemic shunt better in patients with extrahepatic portal hypertension than in those with cirrhosis

    B. Children in whom variceal bleeding cannot be controlled by sclerotherapy should be considered for shunt therapy

    C. Nonselective shunts are associated with a higher incidence of encephalopathy than are selective shunts

    D. Portosystemic shunt procedures are contraindicated in patients with chronic liver disease for whom liver transplantation is a therapeutic option

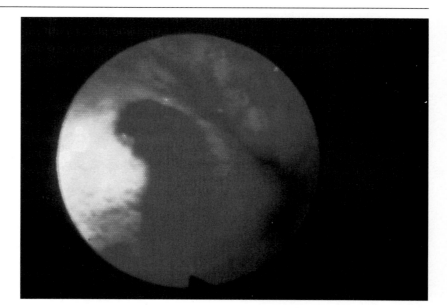

Figure 33–1. *Endoscopic appearance of an actively bleeding esophageal varix. (See also color plate.)*

ANSWERS AND DISCUSSION

1. **A** Brisk upper gastrointestinal bleeding occurring in a previously healthy child, particularly one with a history of neonatal umbilical vein cannulation or omphalitis, is usually caused by esophageal variceal bleeding from extrahepatic portal vein thrombosis and portal hypertension. A useful means of classifying portal hypertension by etiology is to consider the point of venous obstruction anatomically. Extrahepatic obstruction (usually with partial recanalization and development of collateral channels called "cavernomatous transformation") implies vascular obstruction with preservation of normal hepatic function. Intrahepatic obstruction may be pre- or postsinusoidal. Presinusoidal obstruction occurs with congenital hepatic fibrosis and schistosomiasis; in both instances, liver function is well preserved. Postsinusoidal obstruction, on the other hand, is associated with parenchymal liver disease and is the form of portal hypertension seen in association with cirrhosis from any number of causes. Suprahepatic obstruction (hepatic veins or vena cava), a rare cause of portal hypertension, may be seen in association with intraluminal webs and causes the Budd-Chiari syndrome with portal hypertension, destructive hepatic parenchymal disease, and intractable ascites. In the presence of bleeding esophageal varices, the underlying liver function is an important predictor of mortality from first hemorrhage, and liver function must be carefully considered in establishing a treatment algorithm.

2. **C** Upper gastrointestinal endoscopy is the most diagnostically accurate means of assessing the esophagus, stomach, and duodenum in the patient with recent or active hemorrhage, and it should be the first test undertaken once the patient has been stabilized. Not only does endoscopy provide diagnostic and prognostic information, it offers an opportunity to initiate treatment (in the form of injection sclerotherapy or banding) immediately. Although nasogastric tube placement and room temperature saline lavage (iced saline should be avoided since it may exacerbate mucosal injury in the presence of diffuse gastritis) may confirm an upper gastrointestinal bleeding site in a patient presenting with rectal bleeding, it offers little in this clinical setting, except for clearing of blood to facilitate endoscopy. Balloon tamponade of bleeding varices with a Sengstaken-Blakemore tube is effective in stopping hemorrhage, although the rebleed rate after balloon deflation is high. It is essential that airway protection be maintained while the balloon is in use. Mesenteric cannulation and venous phase imaging is helpful in detailing vascular anatomy for shunt therapy. Selective vasopressin infusion through the superior mesenteric artery offers no therapeutic advantage over systemic venous infusion.

3. **C** Direct endoscopic obliteration of esophageal varices can be accomplished by either intravariceal or paravariceal injection (Figure 33–2; see also color plate), or by esophageal banding. It is indicated as a simultaneous procedure at the time of diagnosis as the source of hemorrhage. Because of the correlation between varix size and bleed potential, it is reasonable to sclerose the largest varices at the initial endoscopy. The value of prophylactic sclerotherapy in children is uncer-

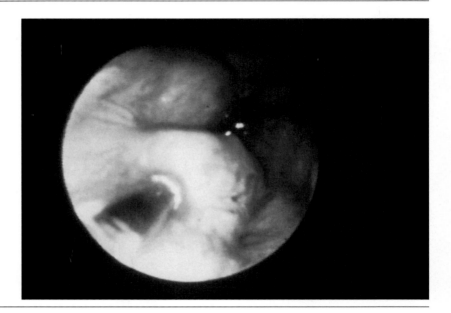

Figure 33–2. *Intravariceal sclerotherapy achieves arrest of hemorrhage. (See also color plate.)*

tain. Complications of sclerotherapy include hemorrhage, esophageal ulceration or stricture, and perforation. Pharmacologic induction of splanchnic vasoconstriction by vasopressin infusion effectively reduces portal blood flow and pressure, and it should be viewed as complementary to sclerotherapy, especially in the presence of active bleeding. The efficacy of sclerotherapy in arresting hemorrhage has made emergency portosystemic shunt operations, for the most part, unnecessary.

4. **A** This is true. An important correlate of mortality after first hemorrhage from esophageal varices is underlying liver function. Therefore, patients with portal hypertension from portal vein thrombosis (PVT) have a mortality rate of less than 5%, in contrast to a 37% mortality rate with first variceal hemorrhage in patients with intrahepatic disease.

5. **D** A decision to opt for portosystemic shunting versus nonshunt therapy for bleeding varices depends on the patient's clinical status, the etiology of the portal hypertension, and the endoscopic and surgical expertise at the institution. The efficacy of endoscopic sclerotherapy has markedly reduced the number of shunt operations performed, although recurrent or intractable hemorrhage, access to endoscopic expertise, and the development of esophageal complications related to repeated sclerosis are all factors that might lead to the consideration of a shunt alternative. Shunt options include nonselective shunts, selective (selective distal splenorenal) shunts, and percutaneous, transjugular intrahepatic portosystemic shunt (TIPS). Nonselective shunts include the end-to-side and side-to-side portacaval shunt, central and distal splenorenal shunts, and mesocaval shunts (end-to-side and interposition). These shunts provide direct portal or mesenteric flow decompression into the systemic circulation and, depending on vascular resistance of the liver, can lead to flow reversal in the portal vein and increased risk of encephalopathy. Selective shunts partition the portal circulation into two compo-

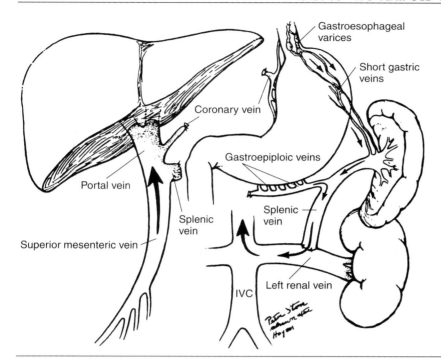

Figure 33–3. *Anatomy of a selective distal splenorenal shunt. Portal inflow to the liver is partitioned, while gastroesophageal varices are decompressed through short gastric veins via a distal splenorenal shunt into the systemic circulation. (From O'Neill JA, Rowe MI, Grosfeld JL, et al. eds. Pediatric Surgery. 5th ed. St. Louis: Mosby-Yearbook; 1998.)*

nents: prograde portal flow to the liver that is uninterrupted, and selective decompression of esophageal varices through short gastrics into the splenic vein, which is anastomosed to the left renal vein. Selective distal splenorenal shunts are, therefore, the shunt procedure of choice for children with portal hypertension, especially those likely to require liver transplantation (Figure 33–3). There is limited experience with TIPS in children, although it has been used successfully as a bridge to transplant in some children with bleeding varices awaiting transplantation. Its efficacy as a definitive procedure is not proven as patency follow-up is short. Patients with intrahepatic liver disease and portal hypertension, who fail sclerotherapy and are candidates for transplantation, should be considered for TIPS or either an interposition mesocaval shunt (which can be ligated at the time of transplant) or a selective distal splenorenal shunt, neither of which appear to increase the technical difficulty of the subsequent transplant operation.

BIBLIOGRAPHY

Altman RP. Portal hypertension. In: O'Neill JA, Rowe MI, Grosfeld JL, et al. eds. *Pediatric Surgery.* 5th ed. St. Louis: Mosby-Yearbook; 1998:1513–1526.

Fonkalsrud EW. Treatment of variceal hemorrhage in children. *Surg Clin North Am.* 1990;70:475–487.

Maksoud JG, Goncalves MEP. Treatment of portal hypertension in children. *World J Surg.* 1994;18:251–258.

A 14-MONTH-OLD BOY WITH AN EMPTY LEFT SCROTUM

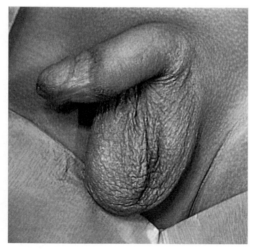

Figure 34–1. *Appearance of the groin of a 14-month-old child with an empty left hemiscrotum.*

HISTORY   A 14-month-old boy is referred to you because his pediatrician could not feel the boy's left testicle. He is an otherwise healthy boy born at term with no significant medical history. He voids normally and has no history of genitourinary problems.

EXAMINATION   The boy appears healthy. Vital signs are normal. He has no dysmorphic features. His heart, lung, and abdominal examination is normal. His right testis resides in the scrotum and has a normal size, shape, and consistency. The left scrotum is empty (Figure 34–1).

LABORATORY   Urinalysis is normal.

Please answer all questions before proceeding to the discussion section.

✓ QUESTIONS

1. Your next diagnostic maneuver should be to:
   A. Obtain an abdominal ultrasound
   B. Obtain a magnetic resonance imaging (MRI) scan of the abdomen and pelvis
   C. Attempt to find the left testis in the groin and manipulate it into the scrotum
   D. Obtain a technetium scan to determine whether or not there is flow to the right testis
   E. All of the above

2. The criteria for the diagnosis of a retractile testis is:
   A. The testis can be brought fully to the bottom of the scrotum without difficulty
   B. The testis remains in the scrotum after manipulation without immediate retraction
   C. The testis is normal in size

168

    D. There is a history that the testis resides spontaneously in the scrotum some of the time

    E. All of the above

HOSPITAL COURSE   You are able to palpate the testis in the left inguinal canal above the level of the inguinal ring. Despite your attempts at manipulation, the testis will not reach the scrotum.

  3. Appropriate management options at this time include:

    A. Diagnostic laparoscopy

    B. Left orchiopexy via a groin approach

    C. Observation until the child is 3 years old with orchiopexy if the testis does not descend spontaneously

    D. Administration of intramuscular testosterone

    E. B or C

  4. Which of the following is true regarding the impact of unilateral undescended testis on testicular function and fertility?

    A. Experimental and clinical studies reveal that the histology of the undescended testis is normal at birth and deteriorates over time

    B. Babies born with unilateral cryptorchidism lack the normal postnatal rise in plasma luteinizing hormone (LH) and testosterone

    C. Paternity rates in unilateral cryptorchidism corrected at puberty are no different than those of the general population

    D. All of the above

    E. None of the above

  5. Which of the following is true about the relationship between undescended testis and malignancy?

    A. Occurrence of malignancy in an undescended testis is rare

    B. Testicular cancer will occur in undescended testes with 300 times greater frequency than in normal testes

    C. Orchiopexy reduces but does not eliminate the risk of cancer

    D. Most testicular tumors occurring in childhood are due to cryptorchidism

    E. All of the above

HOSPITAL COURSE _(CONT.)_   You operate on this patient, doing an orchipexy via a groin approach. You find a normal-appearing testis and bring it into the scrotum with little difficulty. The patient goes home 2 hours after operation and has no further problems.

    Please answer all questions before proceeding to discussion section.

  6. Management of a patient with a unilateral empty scrotum who does _not_ have a palpable testis may include:

    A. Diagnostic laparoscopy

    B. Groin exploration

    C. Administration of human chorionic gonadotropin followed by measurement of serum testosterone levels

    D. A technetium flow study

    E. A or B

7. Undescended testis is associated with which of the following anomalies?
   A. Agenesis of the abdominal wall musculature (prune-belly syndrome)
   B. Gastroschisis
   C. Myelomeningocele
   D. Microcephaly
   E. All of the above

ANSWERS AND DISCUSSION

1. **C** The most common cause of an empty scrotum in childhood is a retractile testis. A retractile testis resides outside of the scrotum due to hyperactivity of the cremaster muscle. The cremaster muscle runs along the spermatic cord, and its contraction elevates the testicle out of the scrotum. This muscle functions to regulate the temperature of the testis and protect it from external trauma. The cremaster muscle retracts in response to low temperature or stimulation of the genitofemoral nerve at the inner thigh. On physical examination, the retractile testis can be gently milked into the scrotum and will stay in the scrotum without continued traction.

   Most authorities believe that a retractile testis is a descended testis and that intervention is not required. Therefore, operation is not recommended. We have followed many such children at yearly intervals and found that virtually all of them will have testes that reside normally in the scrotum by the time of puberty.

   Abdominal ultrasound (**A**) has no role in the management of palpable undescended testes and is probably of little value even when the testis is not palpable. An MRI (**B**) might be useful is identifying nonpalpable testes but would add little to the management of this patient. A technetium scan is useful for determining whether or not acute testicular torsion is occurring. It will not be helpful in the diagnosis of undescended testis (cryptorchidism).

2. **E** **A** through **D** summarize the strict criteria for the diagnosis of a retractile testis. If all of these criteria are met, the testis is not undescended.

3. **B** A unilateral undescended testis should be surgically repositioned in the scrotum sometime between 6 months and 2 years of age (Figure 34–2). Timing of operation is based on experimental studies that suggest that damage to the undescended testis may begin occurring as early as 6 months. Significant histologic injury does not appear to occur prior to age 2, however. Orchipexy at age 6 months can be challenging, and the complication rate may be increased in all but the most experienced hands. There appears to be no harm in waiting until the child is 1 or 2 depending on the experience of the surgeon.

   Diagnostic laparoscopy (**A**) is very useful in the management of a nonpalpable testis. (It allows the surgeon to determine whether or not the) testis is present and whether it is intra- or extra-abdominal. See answer 6.

   Intramuscular testosterone (**D**) has no role in the treatment of cryptorchidism. Some centers have recommended a trial of intramuscular human chorionic gonadotropin (hCG) in an attempt to

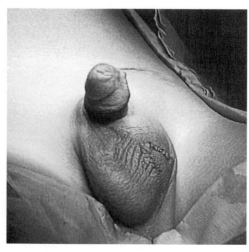

Figure 34–2. *Immediate postoperative appearance following left orchiopexy.*

cause testicular descent hormonally. This treatment is based on the premise that undescended testis is caused by a failure of the hypo-thalamic-pituitary-gonadal axis. The results in a number of studies have been mixed at best. In a prospective double-blind study, hCG was found to be no more effective than placebo. Many investigators believe the hCG can relax the cremaster muscle in cases of retractile testis. They argue that hCG is only "successful" in patients who have retractile rather than true undescended testis. These patients, of course, do not require operaton anyway.

4. **D** All of the statements are true. Both pathologic studies from hu-mans and experimental animal studies have shown that an unde-scended testis may be normal at birth, then it undergoes progressive histologic changes over time. This includes abnormalities in both the Leydig and Sertoli cells. Babies born with undescended testis have an abnormal androgen profile and lack the physiologic increase in LH and testosterone seen after birth. It is not known whether this ab-normality is the primary event causing cryptorchidism or whether it is secondary.

    Despite these histologic and biochemical findings, epidemiologic studies of men treated for cryptorchidism 20 to 30 years ago do not show a difference in paternity rates compared to the general popula-tion. In contrast, men born with bilateral cryptorchidism have a well-documented decrease in fertility.

5. **A** All investigators agree that the incidence of malignancy in unde-scended testes is higher than that for normal testes. The relative risk was once thought to be 50 times that of normal testes but it is prob-ably closer to five to ten times. Nevertheless, the incidence of testicu-lar cancer in the population is about 0.0021%. Even a 100-fold in-crease would only increase the risk to 0.2%. There are no conclusive data to suggest that orchiopexy reduces the risk of malignancy. One can argue that placement of the testicle in the scrotum will facilitate easier diagnosis of a malignancy if it occurs. Most testicular tumors in childhood occur in normal testes. The most common age range for cancer to occur in an undescended testis is 20 to 40 years.

6. **E** Management of unilateral nonpalpable testis is controversial. Diagnostic laparoscopy is safe and extremely effective in determining whether or not a testis is present or in the abdomen. The surgeon will be presented with three possible findings: (1) a testis will be found in the abdomen confirming a high undescended testis (Figure 34–3; see also color plate), (2) a blind ending vas and vessels may be found confirming testicular agenesis or antenatal torsion, or (3) a vas and vessels may be seen exiting the external ring suggesting the presence of the testis in the canal (Figure 34–4; see also color plate).

    The management of each of these three scenarios is different. In the first case, presence of a high intra-abdominal testis, there are sev-eral options. One may attempt orchiopexy via the groin if the testis is very close to the internal ring and the surgeon believes it can be brought down. One can proceed to ligate the spermatic vessels and do an orchiopexy based on the blood supply adjacent to the vas def-erens (Fowler-Stevens orchiopexy). Finally, one can ligate the sper-matic vessels laparoscopically in hopes that the vessels along the vas will hypertrophy for a later Fowler-Stevens approach.

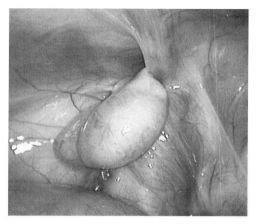

Figure 34–3. *Laparoscopic appearance of a left intra-abdominal testis. The testis is just in-side the internal ring. This child underwent immediate orchiopexy via a groin approach and the testis was successfully mobilized into the scrotum. (See also color plate.)*

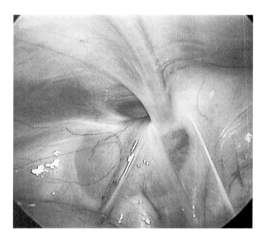

Figure 34–4. *Laparoscopic appearance of a vas and vessels exiting an open internal in-guinal ring suggesting the presence of a testi-cle within the inguinal canal. (See also color plate.)*

In the second case, absent testis, no further intervention is indicated, and the patient is spared a groin exploration and retroperitoneal dissection. In the third case, the surgeon knows the vas and vessels exit the internal ring and should proceed with a groin exploration under the same anesthetic. Usually, a normal testis is found, occasionally an atrophic testis is found in the inguinal canal.

Diagnostic administration of hCG is indicated only in cases of bilateral cryptorchidism to determine if the patient has any functioning testicular tissue. A technetium flow study has no role for reasons already stated.

7. **E** Undecended testis is associated with these and many other anomalies. The vast majority of patients with cryptorchidism, however, are otherwise healthy children.

BIBLIOGRAPHY

deMuinck Keizer-Schrama SM, Hazebroek FW, Matroos AW, et al. Double-blind placebo-controlled study of luteinizing-hormone-releasing-hormone nasal spray in treatment of undescended testes. *Lancet.* 1986; 1:876–880.

Huff DS, Hadziselimovic F, Snyder HM, et al. Histologic maldevelopment of unilaterally cryptorchid testes and their descended partners. *Eur J Pediatr.* 1993;152:5111–5114.

Hutson JM. Undescended testis, torsion, and varicocele. In: O'Neill JA, Rowe MI, Grosfeld JL, eds., *Pediatric Surgery,* 5th ed. St. Louis: Mosby-Year Book; 1998:1087–1099.

Wilson-Storey D, McGenity K, Dickson JAS. Orchiopexy: the younger the better? *J R Coll Surg (Edinb).* 1990;35:362.

A 2-YEAR-OLD BOY
WITH BLOODY STOOLS

HISTORY   A 2-year-old boy is brought to the emergency department after passing two large maroon-colored stools. He has had no abdominal pain. While waiting to see the physician, he passes a third large bloody stool. He is brought directly into a resuscitation room for assessment.

EXAMINATION   He is pale, cool, and restless. His vital signs are temperature 36.1°C (axillary), pulse 160 and weak, blood pressure 80/40, and respirations 36. His weight is 10 kg. His abdomen is scaphoid and soft, and he has dark and fresh blood with clots present in his diaper.
   Please answer all questions before proceeding to discussion section.

✓ QUESTIONS

1. Over the next 10 minutes, his treatment would consist of all of the following *except:*
   A. Placement of a wide bore antecubital intravenous line and a 200 mL warm normal saline bolus
   B. Nasogastric tube placement and aspiration of stomach contents
   C. Blood sent for complete blood count, crossmatch, and coagulation studies
   D. Two radiographic views of the abdomen

2. The differential diagnosis of bleeding in this child includes:
   A. Bleeding esophageal varices
   B. Intussusception
   C. Meckel's diverticulum
   D. Colonic polyp
   E. All of the above

3. After administration of 40 mL/kg of crystalloid, his heart rate is down to 130, and his peripheral perfusion has improved. His naso-

gastric tube drainage is clear, and he is alert and warm. Which of the following diagnostic tests is most likely to reveal the source of bleeding?
A. Mesenteric angiography
B. ^{99m}Technetium scan
C. Flexible esophagogastroduodenoscopy (EGD)
D. Colonoscopy
E. Tagged red cell scan

4. Which of the following statements regarding Meckel's diverticula is *false?*
A. Meckel's diverticula are true diverticula
B. Diverticulitis, mimicking appendicitis, is the commonest presentation
C. Heterotopic gastric tissue is found in approximately 75% of symptomatic patients
D. A Littre's hernia is an inguinal hernia sac containing a Meckel's diverticulum

5. Surgical treatment of Meckel's diverticula:
A. Usually occurs before age 5 years
B. May be accomplished laparoscopically
C. Consists of either diverticulectomy or small bowel resection
D. May not be indicated if found incidentally in asymptomatic patients
E. All of the above

ANSWERS AND DISCUSSION

1. **D** This child is in hypovolemic shock from gastrointestinal bleeding. The initial management should include rapid restoration of intravascular volume with crystalloid and, if necessary, blood. Coagulation studies should be performed. A nasogastric tube should be passed to see whether or not there is fresh blood in the stomach, signifying an upper gastrointestinal source of hemorrhage. Plain abdominal films are of no use in the investigation of gastrointestinal bleeding.

2. **E** The most common cause of lower gastrointestinal bleeding in a 2-year-old child is a colonic (juvenile) polyp (usually a small volume of bleeding), followed by a Meckel's diverticulum (usually a larger volume of bleeding). Intussusception is a common cause of rectal bleeding but is usually associated with abdominal pain and distention. Midgut volvulus with ischemic bowel can cause rectal bleeding and is usually associated with bilious vomiting and abdominal pain. Upper gastrointestinal sources, if brisk, can also present with rectal bleeding and may include peptic ulcer disease and esophageal varices caused by occult portal hypertension from extrahepatic portal vein thrombosis.

3. **B** Investigation of the cause of gastrointestinal bleeding should take place only after hemodynamic stability has been restored. The placement of a nasogastric tube and observation of nonbloody gastric drainage means that a source of bleeding above the ligament of

Treitz is unlikely and that the source is in the small bowel or colon. Given the child's age and the character and rate of hemorrhage, the most likely source is an ileal ulcer caused by unbuffered acid secretion from a Meckel's diverticulum. Although upper and lower endoscopy are often performed first to exclude esophagogastroduodenal and colonic sources of hemorrhage, the test that is most likely to identify bleeding caused by a Meckel's diverticulum is a [99m]Technetium scan (Figure 35–1).

The basic premise of this test is the detection of heterotopic gastric mucosa, which is present in approximately three quarters of all Meckel's diverticula. Gastric mucosal-type surface mucous cells take up pertechnetate ion (carrying the 99m isotope) and secrete it into the bowel lumen. The accuracy of nuclear scanning may be enhanced by the coincident administration of pentagastrin, histamine blockers (for example, ranitidine), and glucagon. Pentagastrin stimulates gastric uptake of pertechnetate, and ranitidine inhibits luminal secretion, so that the radiotracer becomes concentrated within the gastric-type epithelial cells. Glucagon inhibits intestinal peristalsis and thereby reduces the washout of the secreted tracer from the lumen of the diverticulum. [99m]Technetium scintigraphy is reported to have a sensitivity of 85%, a specificity of 95%, and an accuracy of 90%. A negative test should be repeated if the diagnosis is suspected. False-positive tests may be due to intestinal duplications, ulcers, inflammatory bowel disease, bowel obstruction, and occasionally, neoplasms.

Mesenteric angiography is invasive and should be reserved for rapid bleeding (> 1 mL/min) when endoscopy and Meckel's scanning is negative. Tagged red blood cell scintigraphy involves labeling and then reinfusing the patient's own blood. It also requires active bleeding at the time of study to be positive, but at rates lower than those necessary for angiography (~ 0.5 mL/min).

4. **B** Symptoms of Meckel's diverticula are usually caused by heterotopic mucosa (gastrointestinal bleeding) or by persistent vitelline remant fixation to the anterior abdominal wall (leading to intestinal obstruction). In children, inflammation caused by diverticulitis is the least common symptomatic presentation of a Meckel's diverticulum (Figure 35–2).

Meckel's diverticula are "true" diverticula and, therefore, contain all layers of the bowel wall. They are located on the antemesenteric border of the ileum within 100 cm of the ileocecal junction. Their developmental blood supply is from the paired vitelline arteries, which take origin from the aorta. While the left vitelline artery involutes, the right vitelline artery persists as the superior mesenteric artery. The blood supply to a Meckel's diverticulum, therefore, is an end artery coming off the aorta, which explains the propensity for occasional massive hemorrhage.

5. **E** Approximately one half of all children with symptomatic Meckel's diverticula present before age 2, while 80% present by age 5. Abdominal exploration is carried out through a right lower quadrant incision, and the diverticulum is located by tracing the ileum proximal to the ileocecal junction. In instances of continued active bleeding, the bowel downstream of the diverticulum is filled with blood. Once the diverticulum has been located, a decision between

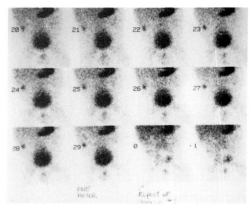

Figure 35–1. *Meckel's scan showing uptake of pertechnetate in the stomach as well as in the kidneys with bladder excretion. There is a persistent "hot spot" in the right lower quadrant consistent with a Meckel's diverticulum with ectopic gastric mucosa.*

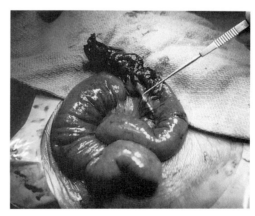

Figure 35–2. *Perforated Meckel's diverticulitis. Note the prominent vitelline artery leading to the tip of the diverticulum.*

diverticulectomy versus small bowel resection must be made. Very broad-based diverticula are less amenable to diverticulectomy due to the potential for luminal encroachment, despite transverse closure of the long axis of the diverticular base. The bleeding site of actively or recently bleeding diverticula should be sought. In most instances, the area of ulceration will be located on the mesenteric border of the ileum, opposite the mouth of the diverticulum, and it is easily oversewn. In addition, the feeding vitelline artery should also be isolated and ligated as it crosses the surface of the ileum. Appendectomy should also be performed. Symptomatic Meckel's diverticula are also very amenable to laparoscopic evaluation and resection with an endoscopic stapler.

The management of incidentally identified, asymptomatic Meckel's diverticula is somewhat controversial, since the lifetime probability of complication is difficult to assess. The best estimate of such a lifetime risk is approximately 5%. Three factors have been identified in retrospective studies as predictive of complications leading to surgical treatment: age less than 40 years, the presence of heterotopic mucosa, and diverticular length greater than 2 cm. Certainly any child with an incidentally discovered Meckel's diverticulum should have it excised, as should all patients with vitelline remnant attachment to the anterior abdominal wall or a history of unexplained abdominal pain.

Older patients discovered to have an incidental, asymptomatic Meckel's diverticulum in whom resection may pose significant infection risk (for example, during vascular prosthetic reconstruction), should not undergo diverticulectomy. Similarly, a Meckel's diverticulum identified during gastroschisis closure should be left because of the risk of suture line breakdown.

BIBLIOGRAPHY

Amoury RA, Snyder CL. Meckel's diverticulum. In: O'Neill JA, Rowe MI, Grosfeld JL, et al. eds. *Pediatric Surgery.* 5th ed. St. Louis: Mosby-Year Book; 1998:1173–1184.

Cullen JJ, Kelly KA. Current management of Meckel's diverticulum. *Adv Surg.* 1996;29:207–214.

St-Vil D, Brandt ML, Panic S, et al. Meckel's diverticulum in children: a 20 year review. *J Pediatr Surg.* 1991;26:1289–1292.

A 7-WEEK-OLD GIRL WITH JAUNDICE

HISTORY You are asked to see a 7-week-old baby girl born at term who was hospitalized for the first few days of life due to hyperbilirubinemia. Her pediatrician is concerned because she still appears visibily jaundiced.

Her mother reports that the infant is thriving. She is feeding very well and has had excellent weight gain. Her mother had an uneventful pregnancy and delivery. The baby passed "normal" meconium stool at 8 hours of life. The baby is now passing two to three light yellow stools per day.

EXAMINATION The baby appears jaundiced but otherwise very healthy and vigorous. Length and weight are in the 75th percentile for age. Vital signs are normal. Her abdomen is slightly distended with a liver edge palpable 4 cm below the right costal margin. The spleen tip is palpable at the left costal margin.

LABORATORY Hemoglobin 10.3, hematocrit 32, white blood cell count 12.2 with 61% neutrophils and 4% bands. INR is 1.8. Electrolytes are normal. Total bilirubin is 9.4 with a direct fraction of 5.6. Alkaline phosphatase is 242, aspartate transaminase (AST) is 145, alanine transaminase (ALT) is 130, gamma-glutamyl transpeptidase (GGT) is 204. Abdominal x-ray reveals no abnormalities except for hepatomegaly.

Please answer all questions before proceeding to discussion section.

✓ QUESTIONS

1. The differential diagnosis includes:
   A. Congenital cytomegalovirus infection
   B. Neonatal giant cell hepatitis
   C. Alpha-1 antitrypsin deficiency

   D. All of the above
   E. None of the above

2. The most likely diagnosis is:
   A. Hepatitis C infection
   B. Neonatal giant cell hepatitis
   C. Alagille syndrome
   D. Extrahepatic biliary atresia
   E. Hemolytic disease due to red blood cell incompatibility

3. Appropriate initial investigative tests may include:
   A. Hepato-iminodiacetic acid (HIDA) scan
   B. Examination of the stools
   C. Abdominal ultrasound
   D. Percutaneous liver biopsy
   E. All of the above

4. All of the above tests have been done, and the diagnosis remains inconclusive. The baby is now almost 8 weeks old, and the bilirubin level is slightly higher. You operate on the baby and obtain a cholangiogram shown in Figure 36–1. You should now:
   A. Close the abdomen, and tell the family that the baby has neonatal giant cell hepatitis
   B. Do an open liver biopsy from both lobes, close the abdomen, and direct the family to the liver transplant team because the baby has uncorrectable biliary atresia
   C. Do an anastomosis between the gallbladder and the porta hepatis
   D. Do an anastomosis between the duodenum and the porta hepatis
   E. Do an anastomosis between a Roux-en-Y loop of jejunum and the porta hepatis

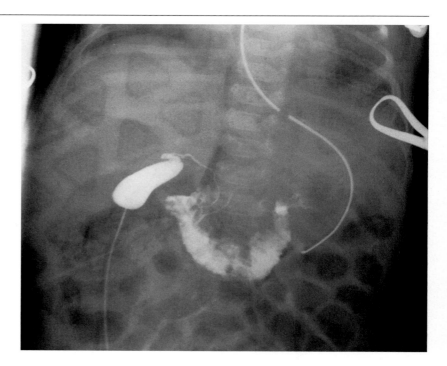

Figure 36–1. *Operative cholangiogram in a 3-month-old infant with direct hyperbilirubinemia.*

5. A liver biopsy taken at the time of the operation shows bridging fibrosis (Figure 36–2; see also color plate). Which of the following is true?
   A. This is a poor prognostic sign, but babies with this degree of liver disease may do quite well
   B. Prognosis is more dependent on the operative findings and surgical result than on liver histology
   C. You have done the wrong operation, and the baby should be referred for liver transplantation immediately
   D. The baby is likely to require transplantation within the next 6 weeks
   E. There is a 50% chance of 10-year survival without further intervention

6. The most common complication after portoenterostomy is:
   A. Anastomotic stricture
   B. Ischemic necrosis of a portion of the liver
   C. Cholangitis
   D. Small bowel obstruction
   E. Biliary-cutaneous fistula formation

7. Important prognostic factors following portoenterostomy include:
   A. Age at operation
   B. Whether or not bile drainage is established
   C. Histologic severity of preoperative liver damage
   D. Presence or absence of jaundice 8 weeks following operation
   E. All of the above

ANSWERS AND DISCUSSION

1. **D** This baby has direct hyperbilirubinemia. This is defined as hyperbilirubinemia with the conjugated fraction making up greater than 50% of the total. The most common cause of jaundice in the newborn period is due to the accelerated breakdown of red blood cells and causes unconjugated hyperbilirubinemia. This probably accounted for the jaundice in this baby just after birth; however, jaun-

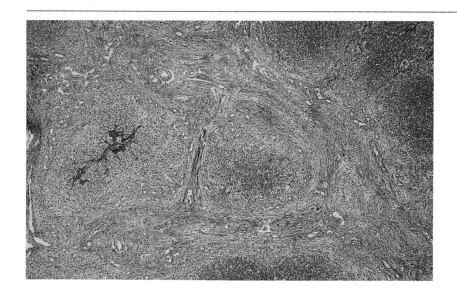

Figure 36–2. *This is the histologic appearance of a liver biopsy taken from a 12-week-old baby with extrahepatic biliary atresia. It is shown at × 15 magnification and has been stained with trichrome. Collagen (fibrous tissue) appears blue. Portal triads are surrounded by fibrosis, and trails of fibrous tissue "bridging" to other parts of the liver are seen. Nodule formation suggests that the patient is progressing from bridging fibrosis to cirrhosis. (See also color plate.)*

dice that persists longer than 4 weeks and juandice due to conjugated bilirubin are pathologic.

The differential diagnosis is broad. It includes congenital TORCH infections (*to*xoplasma, *r*ubella, *c*ytomegalovirus, *h*erpes virus), neonatal giant cell hepatitis, alpha-1 antitrypsin deficiency, extrahepatic atresia, Alagille syndrome, and other less common disorders.

2. **D** In a baby who is healthy and thriving, yet has a markedly elevated serum direct bilirubin, biliary atresia is the most likely diagnosis. Most babies with congenital infections have failure to thrive. Babies with congenital disorders, such as Alagille syndrome, have other stigmata of the syndrome (eg, abnormal vertebrae, ocular abnomalities). Babies with infectious hepatitis tend to have markedly elevated transaminase levels.

While the differential diagnosis of direct hyperbilirubinemia is broad, biliary atresia is the only disorder requiring prompt intervention. Therefore, the diagnosis of "biliary atresia" or "not biliary atresia" is somewhat urgent. One should not necessarily await the results of a lengthy and extensive work-up when biliary atresia is strongly suspected. Invasive tests may be necessary to rule biliary atresia in or out. If it is ruled out, the work-up may proceed in a more stepwise and slower paced manner.

3. **E** The evaluation of conjugated hyperbilirubinemia involves a combination of clinical examination, noninvasive laboratory tests, sonographic and nuclear medicine imaging, and when necessary, invasive diagnostic tests, including percutaneous liver biopsy, operative cholangiography, or both. In all cases, the diagnosis must be expeditious, since the age of the infant at operation for biliary atresia is closely related to outcome.

Examination of the stools is easy and inexpensive. If the stools are green, biliary atresia is extremely unlikely. On the other hand, clay colored or acholic stools are strongly suggestive of biliary atresia. Light yellow stools are a suspicious but nonspecific finding. Serum biochemistry profiles, including total and conjugated bilirubin, transaminases, GGT, and alkaline phospatase, may reflect changes more consistent with biliary obstruction than hepatocellular inflammation but are just as often nonspecific. Serum screening for metabolic disease (alpha-1 anti-trypsin deficiency and cystic fibrosis) and hepatitis (A, B, C, TORCH) is essential to the work-up, yet the results often take days to weeks to return. Abdominal ultrasound is useful for excluding other causes of extrahepatic biliary obstruction (eg, choledochal cyst), and if a fasting study fails to demonstrate a gallbladder, the diagnosis of biliary atresia is quite likely.

Nuclear scintigraphy (HIDA scan) is an essential diagnostic test. Administration of phenobarbital prior to the procedure optimizes hepatocellular uptake of radionucleide through cytochrome p450 enzyme induction. In this test, a radionucleotide is given intravenously that is taken up by the liver and excreted in the bile. If the isotope is seen in the liver and later in the bile duct and intestine, bile duct patency is confirmed, and biliary atresia is ruled out. A HIDA scan such as this rules out biliary atresia with virtually 100% certainty. In contrast, a HIDA scan showing uptake by the liver without excretion for 48 hours is suspicious for biliary atresia (Figure 36–3).

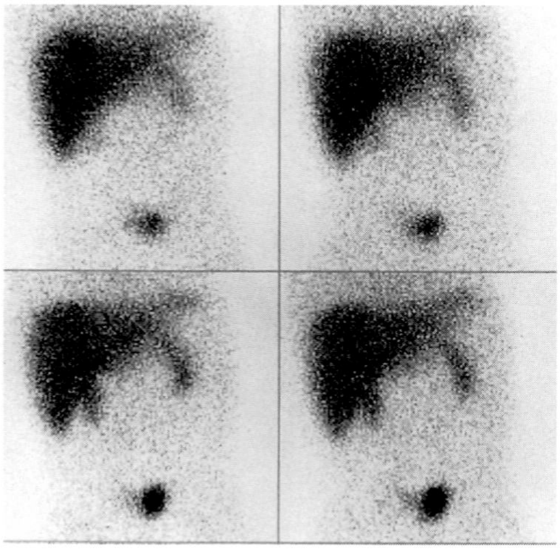

Figure 36–3. *This image is taken from a hepato-iminodiacetic acid (HIDA) scan 12 hours after injection. A dense hepatic shadow is seen. Both kidneys are visualized, as is the bladder. The isotope is taken up secondarily by the kidneys and excreted in the urine. There is no isotope seen in the region of the gallbladder or in the intestine. When this finding persists over 48 hours, the study is consistent with, but not readily diagnostic of, biliary atresia.*

Percutaneous liver biopsy demonstrating cholestasis, bile duct proliferation, and minimal inflammation in the hepatic lobules is virtually diagnostic of extrahepatic biliary obstruction and mandates abdominal exploration. On the other hand, it is not essential that percutaneous liver biopsy be done in all cases prior to laparotomy and cholangiography. Demonstration of an atretic extrahepatic biliary tree by cholangiography performed through the gallbladder or by endoscopic retrograde cholangiopancreatography (ERCP) (infrequent in infants) confirms the diagnosis of biliary atresia and must be done prior to proceeding with portoenterostomy (see following).

4. **E** This operative cholangiogram was done by placing a tube directly in the gallbladder and injecting contrast. It shows a patent gallbladder and a very small common bile duct with flow of contrast into the duodenum. The second small duct to the left of the common bile duct is the pancreatic duct. The common hepatic ducts and intrahepatic ducts are not seen. This suggests that the patient has biliary atresia. The surgeon, however, must be extremely cautious to be certain that the contrast does not flow into the proximal biliary tree simply because the distal tree provided a path of least resistance. Therefore, when confronted with this finding, the surgeon should clamp the common bile duct atraumatically and repeat the contrast injection to be certain the proximal tree is not patent. This was done in this case. Figure 36–4 shows a diagram of this patient's portal anatomy.

This patient has biliary atresia. About 20% of patients with biliary atresia have a patent common bile duct and a cholangiogram similar to Figure 36–1. In the remaining cases, the cholangiogram would show only the gallbladder or would be impossible to do because the gallbladder would have no lumen.

The treatment for biliary atresia is the Kasai hepatic portoenterostomy. The condition is "correctable," and liver transplantation is reserved for cases in which this operation fails (see later). A Kasai procedure involves excision of all prevascular ductal and fibrous tissue in the porta hepatis up to the undersurface of the liver. An anastomosis is then done between a Roux-en-Y loop of jejunum and the portal plate (Figure 36–5).

Some authors reported using the gallbladder, when patent, for anastomosis to the portal plate (**C**). This technique is fraught with late complications and has been abandoned in favor of the Kasai procedure. The duodenum cannot be used for anastomosis for two reasons. First, a tension-free anastomosis is difficult. Second, a Roux-en-Y loop free of the fecal stream is important to decrease the risk of bacterial cholangitis.

5. **A** At the time of portoenterostomy, a liver biopsy should always be done. This is an important prognostic factor that determines prognosis following operation. Cirrhosis is an ominous finding, with most patients requiring liver transplantation within 6 months or less. Fibrosis, on the other hand, portends a mixed prognosis. As a group, these patients clearly do not do as well as those without fibrosis. Many of these patients, however, will be free of jaundice for 5 to 10 years following Kasai portoenterostomy.

In general, portoenterostomy will provide long-term biliary drainage with good liver function in about one third of patients. The

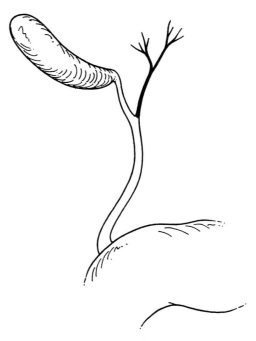

Figure 36–4. *Diagram of the patient's anatomy depicted in the cholangiogram (Figure 36–1). The gallbladder and common bile duct are patent, but the common hepatic duct is atretic. (From Raffensperger JG, ed. Swenson's Pediatric Surgery. 5th ed. Norwalk, CT: Appleton & Lange, 1990: Figure 76–1B.)*

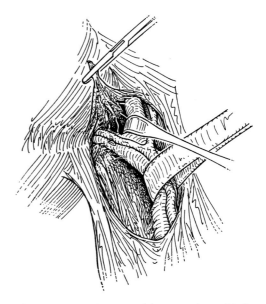

Figure 36–5. *Diagram of the porta hepatitis in biliary atresia. The forceps is holding the fibrous remnants of the extrahepatic biliary system. The vessel loop is around the hepatic artery and portal vein. The fibrous tissue will be resected from the hilum of the liver, and an anastomosis will be done here. (From Raffensperger JG, ed. Swenson's Pediatric Surgery. 5th ed. Norwalk, CT: Appleton & Lange, 1990: Figure 76–6C.)*

remainder will deteriorate and require transplantation. Even among the two thirds of patients who will require a liver transplant, many of them are palliated for years by portoenterostomy. The success of liver transplantation is greater in older patients than in infants, and donor availability is markedly better. Therefore, pediatric surgeons around the world agree that portoenterostomy is the initial treatment of choice for biliary atresia.

Liver transplantation is recommended for three groups of patients: (1) those who never obtain bile drainage following portoenterostomy, (2) those who develop growth delay and stigmata of liver failure in the face of poor bile drainage, and (3) those with good bile drainage but severe disabling sequelae of liver disease.

6. **C** Cholangitis is the most common complication after portoenterostomy. The reported incidence is 40% to 60%, and the pathogenesis is not clear. Presumed enterobiliary reflux has induced surgeons to try placing an antireflux valve in the Roux-en-Y jejunal loop in an effort to decrease the occurrence of cholangitis. This has not been proven to be effective.

Cholangitis is manifested by fever and progressive jaundice. It is treated with intravenous antibiotics. Repeated episodes of cholangitis will accelerate the liver's deterioration and correlates with a poor prognosis.

7. **E** All of the prognostic factors are important. Age at operation appears to be the most important predictive factor for long-term outcome. In a Japanese review, 10-year survival for patients diagnosed prior to age 60 days was 68% and for patients diagnosed after age 91 days was 15%.

BIBLIOGRAPHY

Bates MD, Bucuvalas JC, Alonso MH, et al. Biliary atresia: pathogenesis and treatment. *Semin Liver Dis.* 1998;18:281–293.

Matsuo S, Suita S, Kubota M, et al. Long-term results and clinical problems after portoenterostomy in patients with biliary atresia. *Eur J Pediatr Surg.* 1998;8:142–145.

Ohi R. Surgical treatment of biliary atresia in the liver transplantation era. *Surg Today.* 1998;28:1229–1232.

Ohi R, Masaki N. The jaundiced infant: biliary atresia and other obstructions. In: O'Neill JA, Rowe MI, Grosfeld JL, eds. *Pediatric Surgery.* 5th ed. St. Louis: Mosby-Year Book; 1998.

Okazaki T, Kobayashi H, Yamataka A, et al. Long-term postsurgical outcome of biliary atresia. *J Pediatr Surg.* 1999;34:312–315.

Ryckman FC, Alonso MH, Bucuvalas JC, et al. Biliary atresia—surgical management and treatment options as they relate to outcome. *Liver Transpl Surg.* 1998;4(5 Suppl 1):S24–S33.

A 2-YEAR-OLD BOY WITH FEVER AND DROOLING

HISTORY   You are asked to evaluate a 2-year-old boy with a 24-hour history of high fever and difficulty in swallowing. He appeared to complain of a sore throat 2 days ago and developed a fever yesterday. His mother reports his temperature was 104°F 2 hours ago.

EXAMINATION   The child is very fussy and appears toxic. Temperature 39.5°C, heart rate 180, blood pressure 100/60, respiratory rate 28. The child is sitting up and drooling slightly. He refuses to take his bottle. His tympanic membranes are moderately erythematous. He is not eager to allow you to look in his mouth, but his tonsils appear normal. His pharynx is red and bulging. He is breathing rapidly but without stridor or respiratory distress. His cry is normal. Lung fields are clear to auscultation. His heart and abdominal examination is normal.

LABORATORY   Hemoglobin 11.4, hematocrit 38, white blood cell count 19.5 with 79% polymorphonuclear leukocytes and 12% bands.
    Please answer all questions before proceeding to discussion section.

✓ QUESTIONS

1. The most likely diagnosis is:
    A. Epiglottitis
    B. Croup
    C. Retropharyngeal abscess
    D. Pharyngitis with penicillin-resistant *Streptococcus pneumoniae*
    E. Otitis media

2. The most appropriate study to confirm the diagnosis is:
    A. Ultrasound
    B. Computed tomography (CT) scan
    C. Magnetic resonance imaging (MRI) under general anesthesia

D. Blood culture
E. No further investigation is needed

3. Treatment options for this condition include:
   A. A trial of oral antibiotic therapy
   B. Intravenous antibiotics
   C. Surgical incision and drainage via the mouth
   D. Surgical incision and drainage via an anterior cervical incision
   E. B and C

4. With respect to the peripharyngeal space:
   A. It extends from the base of the skull in a superior direction to the hyoid bone in the inferior direction
   B. It communicates with the retropharyngeal space
   C. Infection may spread to this space from the salivary glands, tongue, or teeth
   D. Abscesses of this space may be drained by the intraoral route
   E. All of the above

ANSWERS AND DISCUSSION

1. **C** A toxic-appearing child with a high fever and a bulging pharynx has a retropharyngeal abscess until proven otherwise. Epiglottitis is an acute bacterial infection of the supraglottic structures, most commonly caused by *Haemophilus influenzae* type B. It presents with severe stridor and impending airway obstruction. If epiglottitis is suspected, a lateral radiograph of the neck can be done to confirm the diagnosis. Croup is a viral infection that presents with low-grade fever, hoarseness, rhinorrhea, and a characteristic barking cough. Pharyngitis with resistant pneumococcus is a possibility but would be unlikely to cause the child to appear so toxic and certainly would not cause a bulging mass in the pharynx. Furthermore, pharyngitis tends to occur in conjunction with tonsillitis, where the tonsils appear normal in most cases of retropharyngeal abscess. Otitis media does not cause this constellation of signs and symptoms.

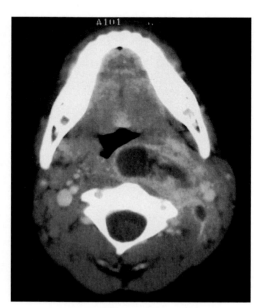

Figure 37–1. *Computed tomography scan of the neck in a patient with retropharyngeal abscess. The pus appears as a low-density mass with ring enhancement between the vertebral column and the pharynx.*

2. **B** In children, the retropharyngeal space is home of two large chains of lymph nodes. These nodes are prominent in children and recess by adulthood. Supparative infection in this nodal chain results in an accumulation of pus between the pharynx and the prevertebral fascia. The most effective way to evaluate this area is by means of CT scan of the neck with intravenous contrast. This study nicely shows the pathology and delineates the anatomy necessary for surgical drainage. Ultrasound examination of the retropharyngeal space is difficult and less reliable. An MRI is less useful and requires general anesthesia. Blood cultures may be helpful in identifying the infective organisms, but they will not reveal the source of the infection.

   Figure 37–1 shows a CT scan of the neck in a patient with a retropharyngeal abscess.

3. **E** Retropharyngeal infections can take the form of cellulitis or true abscesses. If the patient is not in respiratory distress and does not appear profoundly septic, a trial of intravenous antibiotics is reasonable. Unless there is considerable improvement over 24 to 36 hours,

surgical drainage is appropriate. The most effective and expeditious way to drain a retropharyngeal abscess is via the intraoral route. Great care should be taken during intubation to avoid rupture of the abscess and spillage of purulent material into the unprotected airway. After intubation, the endotracheal tube is retracted laterally, and the abscess is directly incised and drained.

This area cannot be directly accessed through a cervical incision. Drainage via this route is less effective, requires placement of a drain across the carotid sheath, and leaves a scar on the patient's neck. Oral antibiotics are never appropriate for infections of this severity.

Figure 37–2 (see also color plate) shows the appearance of the abscess viewed through the mouth at operation. The abscess has just been incised, and pus can be seen draining out of the bulging mass. One should make every effort to avoid spillage of pus into the airway.

4. **E** All of the statements are true regarding the peripharyngeal space. This space communicates with the retropharyngeal space, and infection can spread from one to the other.

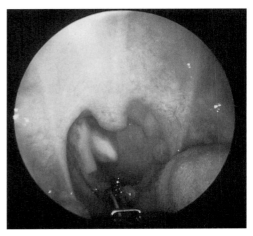

Figure 37–2. *Transoral drainage of a retropharyngeal abscess. (See also color plate.)*

BIBLIOGRAPHY

Boucher C, Dorion D, Fisch C. Retropharyngeal abscesses: a clinical and radiologic correlation. *J Otolaryngol.* 1999;28(3):134–137.

Gaglani MJ, Edwards MS. Clinical indicators of childhood retropharyngeal abscess. *Am J Emerg Med.* 1995;13(3):333–336.

Lalakea MI, Messner AH. Retropharyngeal abscess management in children: current practices. *Otolaryngol Head Neck Surg.* 1999;121(4):398–405.

A FOREIGN BODY IN THE ESOPHAGUS IN A 5-YEAR-OLD GIRL

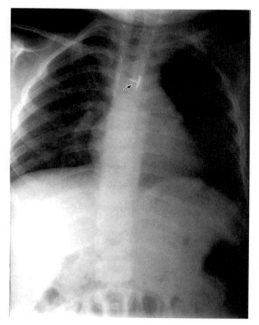

Figure 38–1. *Chest x-ray, frontal view, showing thumbtack (arrow) in upper mediastinum. Without lateral view, one cannot be certain whether it is in trachea, esophagus, or elsewhere.*

HISTORY   This 5-year-old girl swallowed a thumbtack late one afternoon. There was no pain, vomiting, or excessive salivation. She told her mother what had happened and was brought to the hospital. X-rays were obtained (Figures 38–1 and 38–2), and she was transferred to a center for pediatric surgical treatment.

EXAMINATION   She is a well-developed, well-nourished, quiet girl in no respiratory distress. Pulse is 96 per minute, blood pressure 90 systolic, temperature 37°C (orally). Eyes and ears are unremarkable. The pharynx is normal with no evidence of bleeding or inflammation. The neck is supple without masses. The trachea is in the midline. There is no subcutaneous emphysema. Lungs are clear to percussion and auscultation. No cardiac murmur is audible. The abdomen is soft without masses. The remainder of the physical examination is within normal limits.

LABORATORY   Hemoglobin 12.6 gm%, hematocrit 35%, white blood cell count 7200/mm³. Urinalysis is within normal limits. Repeat chest x-rays identical to Figures 38–1 and 38–2 were obtained.
    Please answer all questions before proceeding to discussion section.

✓ QUESTIONS

   1. Appropriate management of this patient would be:
      A. Prompt esophagoscopy
      B. Esophagoscopy if the tack is stationary for 24 to 36 hours
      C. Removal of the tack by dislodgement with a Foley catheter
      D. Immediate ingestion of white bread and milk

HOSPITAL COURSE   The patient has not eaten for several hours. Esophagoscopy is performed under general anesthesia. Figure 38–3 shows the foreign body removed (very gently) from the junction of the upper and middle thirds of the esophagus. There is no bleeding or inflammation at the site. She is discharged a few hours later.

2. The most common esophageal foreign bodies in children are:
   A. Coins
   B. Tacks
   C. Toys
   D. Raw vegetable particles
   E. Meat particles

3. The method of choice for removal of meat particles impacted in the esophagus is:
   A. Esophagoscopy
   B. Extraction with Foley catheter (under fluoroscopy)
   C. Extraction with Fogarty catheter (under fluoroscopy)
   D. Instillation of a dilute solution of papain
   E. Instillation of a dilute solution of hydrochloric acid

ANSWERS AND DISCUSSION

1. **A** Prompt esophagoscopy is the best management for this patient with a sharply pointed foreign body lodged in the upper esophagus. The fact that the tack has not moved on repeat roentgenogram suggests that its tip may be embedded in the esophagus with the potential for perforation. As long as it remains in the esophagus, it can be reached and withdrawn. Delay for 24 to 36 hours (**B**) would have no advantage. Foley catheters (**C**) have been used for removal of rounded, smooth objects, such as coins, from the esophagus. The technique consists of passage of the catheter tip beyond the foreign body, inflation of the balloon with contrast material, and retrograde dislodgement of the foreign body under fluoroscopic control. The method described in **C**, however, is incorrect because the technique is not appropriate for a sharply pointed object, which may perforate the esophagus or the balloon during manipulation. A few experts have condemned the Foley catheter technique because the airway is not protected during the crucial moment when the coin pops out of the esophagus. The coin could drop back into the glottis, producing respiratory arrest. In the hands of a skilled practitioner, however, with proper positioning and with resuscitation equipment close at hand (including pediatric laryngoscope, endotracheal tubes, suction, oxygen, Ambu ventilation bag, and Magill forceps), such a catastrophe is unlikely. Dietary oddities, such as bread and milk (**D**), have no value and should not be given, particularly if general anesthesia is contemplated.

2. **A** Coins are by far the most common esophageal foreign body. Swallowed foreign bodies are usually radiopaque and, thus, easier to identify than airway foreign bodies. The film should include the neck, since foreign bodies may lodge in the pharynx or proximal esophagus. Because the normal resting esophagus is flattened in the anterior-posterior direction, radiographic orientation of a swal-

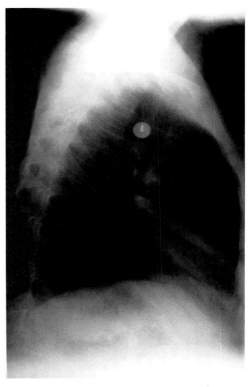

Figure 38–2. *Chest x-ray, lateral view, locates the tack in esophagus, behind the tracheal air column, and anterior to the vertebral column.*

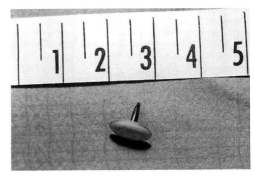

Figure 38–3. *Thumbtack removed from esophagus of patient shown in Figures 38–1 and 38–2.*

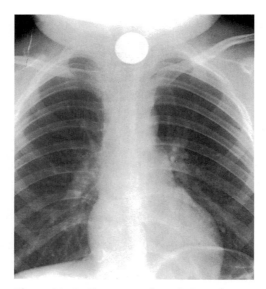

Figure 38–4. *Chest x-ray, frontal view, showing coin in proximal esophagus.*

lowed coin is characteristically flat in the frontal view (Figure 38–4), and on edge in the lateral view (Figure 38–5). The esophagus has four sites of anatomical narrowing: the cricopharyngeus, the thoracic inlet, the aortic arch, and the diaphragmatic hiatus. Most coins lodge between the cricopharyngeus and thoracic inlet. They are not visible on examination of the posterior pharynx but come into view as soon as the esophagoscope slides through the cricopharyngeus. The coin in Figures 38–4 and 38–5 (which was actually *two* pennies!) is in the typical location.

3. **A** Esophagoscopy is the treatment of choice for removal of an impacted meat particle. The meat may be grasped under direct vision with a forceps and removed or nudged distally into the stomach. Foley catheters (**B**) are used for removal of radiopaque objects, such as coins. A meat particle would not be visible under the fluoroscope. Fogarty catheters (**C**) are useful for bronchoscopic extraction of airway foreign bodies and might be used as an adjunct to esophagoscopy. Use of a papain solution (**D**) is a controversial technique; both success and (rarely) esophageal perforation have been reported. Hydrochloric acid (**E**) is not an option. The esophagus might dissolve along with the meat particle. (Swallowing acid, however, generally injures the stomach, whereas alkali typically injures the esophagus.)

BIBLIOGRAPHY

Campbell JB, Quattromani FL, Foley LC. Foley catheter removal of blunt esophageal foreign bodies: experience with 100 consecutive children. *Pediatr Radiol.* 1983;13:116–118.

Kosloske AM. Foreign bodies in children. In: Buntain WL, ed. *Management of Pediatric Trauma.* Philadelphia: Saunders; 1995:459–477.

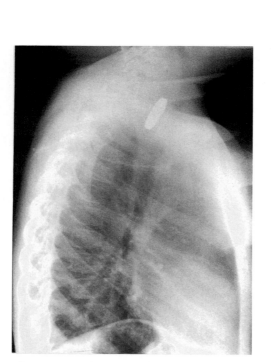

Figure 38–5. *Chest x-ray, lateral view. The coin is on edge because of normal esophageal flattening in the anterior-posterior diameter.*

A 6-MONTH-OLD INFANT WHO TURNED BLUE AND STOPPED BREATHING

HISTORY A 6-month-old male infant is brought to the emergency room after an episode in which he turned blue and stopped breathing. The episode occured about 30 minutes after a meal of rice cereal and formula. His mother gave him cardiopulmonary resuscitation (CPR) while his father drove them to the emergency room. Past history is significant; he was a term infant with esophageal atresia and tracheoesophageal fistula (TEF) who made an uncomplicated recovery after repair and was discharged at 2 weeks of age. He had a peculiar, "barky" cough but otherwise did well until 3 months of age, when he required a 3-day readmission for pneumonia. At 5 months of age, following a feeding, he experienced a cyanotic episode that resolved spontaneously. He was seen by his pediatrician, who recommended an antireflux medication. A second cyanotic episode occurred 1 week later, unrelated to feedings. The present (third) episode is much worse than the others, but by the time they reach the emergency room, the infant is breathing again; in fact, he is crying lustily.

EXAMINATION The patient is a well-developed male infant who stops crying when his mother holds him. He is breathing without difficulty, although circumoral cyanosis is noted. Blood pressure is 78/58, pulse 136, respirations 40/min, temperature 37.0°C. Weight is 6.1 kg. The trachea is in the midline. He has a well-healed right thoracotomy scar. Breath sounds are equal. A few rhonchi are audible throughout the chest. No heart murmur is heard. The abdomen is soft, without masses or hernias. The remainder of his examination is unremarkable.

LABORATORY Hemoglobin 13 gm%, hematocrit 39%, white blood cell count 11.0. Chest x-ray shows a normal heart and lungs. The oxygen saturation is 92% on room air.

Please answer all questions before proceeding to discussion section.

✓ QUESTIONS

1. Management should include all of the following *except:*
   A. Hospital admission with monitoring
   B. Endotracheal intubation for 24 to 48 hours
   C. Barium swallow
   D. Bronchoscopy
   E. A 24-hour pH probe

2. The diagnosis of tracheomalacia in an infant is optimally established by:
   A. Rigid bronchoscopy with the patient under neuromuscular blockade
   B. Rigid bronchoscopy with the patient breathing spontaneously
   C. Flexible fiberoptic bronchoscopy with the patient breathing spontaneously
   D. Videofluoroscopy
   E. Dynamic computed tomography (CT) scan

3. The surgical management of severe tracheomalacia is:
   A. Median sternotomy, segmental tracheal resection, and anastomosis
   B. Right thoracotomy, segmental esophageal resection, and anastomosis
   C. Right thoracotomy, suspension of anterior aortic arch from sternum
   D. Left thoracotomy, suspension of anterior aortic arch from sternum
   E. Left thoracotomy, suspension of distal trachea from sternum

4. Stridor is noted in a 4-week-old premature infant who is ready for discharge from the neonatal "growers" unit. She spent the first 2 weeks of life in the neonatal intensive care unit for respiratory distress syndrome. She was intubated a total of 6 days, including one reintubation when the endotracheal (ET) tube became dislodged. Her stridor persists in spite of inhalation treatments with a bronchodilator. The differential diagnosis includes all of the following *except:*
   A. Subglottic stenosis
   B. Type IV branchial cleft cyst
   C. H-type TEF
   D. Vascular ring
   E. Gastroesophageal reflux

5. Which *one* of the following is considered the diagnostic procedure of choice for infants and children with stridor?
   A. Neck and airway films
   B. Airway videofluoroscopy
   C. Barium esophagram
   D. Fiberoptic laryngoscopy
   E. Operative laryngoscopy and bronchoscopy

6. The type of vascular ring that most commonly causes significant symptoms is:
   A. Double aortic arch
   B. Right-sided arch with ligamentum arteriosum (Neuhauser's anomaly)
   C. Anomalous innominate artery
   D. Anomalous left common carotid artery
   E. Anomalous right subclavian artery

ANSWERS AND DISCUSSION

1. B The infant does not need prophylactic endotracheal intubation as long as he is monitored (**A**) in hospital. Barium swallow (**C**) or, alternatively, esophagoscopy will rule out (or rule in) esophageal stricture at the anastomosis or posterior esophageal compression from a vascular ring. Either of these abnormalities could trigger an episode of cyanosis from aspiration. Bronchoscopy (**D**) is crucial to several diagnoses, including tracheomalacia, vascular ring, and recurrent TEF. (A missed, double TEF is also possible, although ideally this diagnosis would have been made at an earlier tracheobronchoscopy just prior to repair.) The 24-hour pH probe (**E**) is the acid test (pun, sorry!) for gastroesophageal reflux, which may also produce a "near-miss" cyanotic episode.

2. B The essential study for diagnosis of tracheomalacia is (**B**) rigid bronchoscopy with the patient breathing spontaneously. The diagnosis cannot be made if the patient is receiving positive pressure ventilation, as would be the case with (**A**) neuromuscular blockade. Flexible bronchoscopy (**C**) may carry significant risk in infants with tracheal abnormalities because the flexible fiberscope has no channel for ventilation. If the infant should become hypoxic during the procedure, ventilation cannot be restored by slipping the bronchoscope beyond the segment of tracheomalacia, as can be done with the rigid bronchoscope. Further, the view through the rigid telescope, which employs the Hopkins rod-lens system, is unsurpassed. Radiologists recommend (**D**) cinefluoroscopy of the airway or (**E**) dynamic CT scan for diagnosis of tracheomalacia, but the essential diagnostic study remains direct visualization of the defect at bronchoscopy. Virtually all infants with esophageal atresia or TEF have a mild degree of tracheomalacia, which accounts for the signature "barky" cough. No treatment is necessary for mild tracheomalacia, and the child usually outgrows the peculiar cough. A few infants, however, have tracheomalacia so severe that life-threatening episodes ("dying spells") occur. For them, operation is life saving.

3. D The procedure of choice is aortopexy (ie, suspension of the anterior arch from the sternum). The approach by left thoracotomy is technically easier than from the right side (**C**). Since the aortic arch is located anterior to the distal trachea, it is anatomically impossible to suspend the trachea (**E**) from the sternum at this level (T4). The adventitia between the aorta and the trachea should *not* be dissected in order to allow the trachea to move forward with the aorta. Intraoperative bronchoscopy is recommended. Tracheal resection

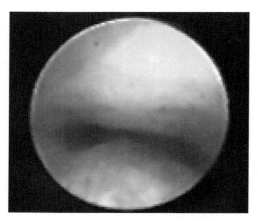

Figure 39–1. *Bronchoscopic photograph showing severe tracheomalacia. (See also color plate.)*

(**A**) would carry greater risk than aortopexy, and esophageal resection (**B**) would not correct the problem.

4. **B** Branchial cleft cyst is not in this differential diagnosis. (Type IV doesn't exist.) All of the other conditions may produce stridor. Subglottic stenosis (**A**) may develop after endotracheal intubation, although it usually follows prolonged or traumatic intubation, which was not the case here. The stenosis occurs at the level of the cricoid, the narrowest point of the neonatal airway. H-type TEF (**C**) is typically diagnosed in the first month of life following pneumonia from aspiration. Vascular ring (**D**) also usually presents in the first month. Cyanosis and dysphagia, the classic symptoms, worsen as the infant grows and the vascular ring tightens. Gastroesophageal reflux (**E**), a common problem among premature infants, may likewise produce stridor. The differential diagnosis of stridor in a 4-week-old infant goes on forever and includes many other choices not listed (eg, micrognathia, vocal cord paralysis, laryngomalacia, tracheomalacia, laryngeal web or cleft, subglottic hemangioma, laryngotracheal infection, and others).

5. **E** Operative laryngoscopy and bronchoscopy is the study of choice for sorting out this large differential (see answer 4). The other studies are good for identification of one or another of the conditions, but they are not definitive.

6. **A** Double aortic arch accounts for 50% of all the vascular rings that cause clinical problems. The anomalous right subclavian artery (**E**) occurs more often, but it is usually asymptomatic. Neuhauser's anomaly (**B**) accounts for approximately 15% of symptomatic patients. The other, less common variants (**C** and **D**) produce respiratory symptoms by anterior compression of the trachea, but they are incomplete rings and have no effect on swallowing.

HOSPITAL COURSE Bronchoscopy is performed, showing severe tracheomalacia above the carina (Figure 39–1; see also color plate) at the level of the repaired TEF. Esophagoscopy shows no anastomotic stricture or esophageal deformity. The 24-hour pH probe shows mild gastroesophageal reflux. On the third hospital day, aortoplexy is performed via a left thoracotomy. Bronchoscopy following the procedure shows a patent trachea (Figure 39–2; see also color plate). The infant makes an uncomplicated recovery. He is discharged on antireflux medications. The "dying spells" never recur.

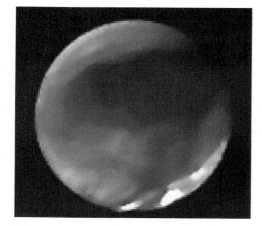

Figure 39–2. *Bronchoscopic photograph after aortopexy. (See also color plate.)*

BIBLIOGRAPHY

Azizkhan RG, Caty MG. Subglottic airway. In: Oldham KT, Colombani PM, Foglia RP, eds. *Surgery of Infants and Children: Scientific Principles and Practice.* Philadelphia: Lippincott-Raven; 1997:897–913.

Benjamin B, Cohen D, Glasson M. Tracheomalacia in association with congenital tracheoesophageal fistula. *Surgery.* 1976;79:504–508.

Filler RM, Forte V. Lesions of the larynx and trachea. In: O'Neill JA Jr, Rowe MI, Grosfeld JL, et al. eds. *Pediatric Surgery.* 5th ed. St. Louis: Mosby-Year Book; 1998:863–872.

Filler RM, Rossello PJ, Lebowitz RL. Life-threatening anoxic spells caused by tracheal compression after repair of esophageal atresia: correction by surgery. *J Pediatr Surg.* 1976;11:739–748.

Othersen HB Jr, Filler RM. Tracheomalacia. In: Othersen HB Jr, ed. *The Pediatric Airway.* Philadelphia: Saunders; 1991:97–106.

Tunkel DE, Yueh B. Otolaryngologic disorders. In: Oldham KT, Colombani PM, Foglia RP, eds. *Surgery of Infants and Children: Scientific Principles and Practice.* Philadelphia: Lippincott-Raven; 1997:825–834.

A 13-YEAR-OLD BOY
WITH A SUNKEN CHEST

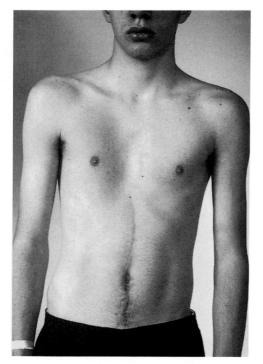

Figure 40–1. *Teenage boy with moderately severe and slightly asymmetric pectus excavatum deformity.*

HISTORY   A 13-year-old boy is referred for evaluation of a deformed anterior chest wall (Figure 40–1). The deformity has been present from birth, but it has become more prominent coincident with his pubertal growth spurt. A systems review indicates that the boy has periodic twinges of anterior chest wall pain and a decreased tolerance for strenuous exercise compared with his peer group. He also reports feeling increasingly self-conscious about the appearance of his chest, and refuses to take off his shirt in the company of friends. The boy is accompanied by his mother who is concerned that his self-consciousness is leading to social withdrawal and isolation.

EXAMINATION   The boy is tall and lean and is noted to have hypermobile joints but no dysmorphic features. His anterior chest wall, which demonstrates a funnel deformity, is nontender. His cardiac impulse is laterally displaced, and he has a grade II/VI systolic ejection click and murmur. His lungs are clear.
    Please answer all questions before proceeding to discussion section.

✔ QUESTIONS

1. Which of the following statements regarding the presentation and diagnosis of pectus excavatum is true?
   A. The diagnosis becomes evident during the first year of life in 90% of patients
   B. Girls are affected three times as frequently as boys
   C. Marfan syndrome is present in 25% of patients with pectus excavatum
   D. There is a strong correlation between symptoms and severity of deformity

2. Preoperative evaluation of patients with pectus excavatum:
   A. Is unnecessary if the patient is asymptomatic
   B. Should include pulmonary function tests and noninvasive cardiovascular function tests in patients
   C. Is unlikely to be predictive of a physiologic necessity for operation
   D. All of the above

3. Operative correction of the deformity should not be performed unless:
   A. The patient is symptomatic
   B. The asymptomatic patient is highly motivated to have corrective surgery to improve cosmesis
   C. The surgeon is certain that the deformity will progress without intervention
   D. Mitral valve prolapse has been excluded by preoperative echocardiography

4. Surgical correction of pectus excavatum:
   A. Usually involves subperichondrial excision of deformed costal cartilages
   B. Is usually accomplished through a transverse or curvilinear inframammary incision with or without metal strut sternal fixation
   C. Is amenable to minimally invasive surgical techniques
   D. All of the above

5. Pectus excavatum may recur after surgical correction:
   A. True
   B. False

ANSWERS AND DISCUSSION

1. **A** Pectus excavatum, which is the most common anterior chest wall deformity, is most often present at birth or becomes apparent within the first year of life. It is more common, by a ratio of 3:1, in male patients than female patients. The cause of the deformity is unknown, but the observation that pectus excavatum can occur after surgical correction of congenital diaphragmatic hernia lends credence to the theory that muscular traction on the sternum by the diaphragm leads to the deformity. Musculoskeletal abnormalities, most commonly scoliosis, have been noted in approximately 20% of patients with pectus excavatum. Marfan syndrome occurs infrequently (< 1% of patients), but it should be considered if marfanoid features are noted, since plans for pectus surgery might be influenced by the diagnosis of previously unrecognized aortic disease. The vast majority of patients with pectus excavatum do not have symptoms. The correlation between symptoms, such as cartilage or precordial pain, exertional dyspnea, and palpitations, and the severity of deformity is quite poor; however, their presence should prompt a diagnostic work-up, including pulmonary function testing and echocardiography. Pulmonary function testing is usually normal. However, mild restrictive lung defects and decreased voluntary minute ventilation have been reported in pectus patients.

2. **D** The decision to investigate a patient with pectus excavatum is determined mainly by the presence or absence of symptoms. The vast majority of patients who seek consultation for surgical correction have no physical symptoms but rather a desire for cosmetic alteration. The few patients who have symptoms, such as chest pain, dyspnea, or palpitations, should undergo pulmonary function testing, looking for a restrictive lung defect. A patient with a murmur or cardiac symptoms, such as chest pain or palpitations, should undergo echocardiography to look for evidence of mitral valve prolapse or cardiac chamber compression or displacement. Even among patients with symptoms, the likelihood that preoperative testing will identify a significant cardiopulmonary abnormality is quite low.

   Despite efforts to demonstrate a physiologic benefit to pectus excavatum repair, pre- and postoperative pulmonary function evaluations have, for the most part, failed to demonstrate any significant change in either vital capacity, total lung capacity, or maximal voluntary ventilation. In fact, a number of studies have actually demonstrated a functional decrease in these parameters soon after surgery that may reflect a decrease in chest wall compliance. It has been observed that exercise tolerance determined by total exercise time and maximal oxygen consumption may increase after pectus repair coincident with a decrease in heart rate at a given level of work. The observation has led to the hypothesis that improvement in exercise capacity and work efficiency is due to improved stroke volume, perhaps related to cardiac chamber decompression. Cardiac function studies (cardiac catheterization and radionuclide angiography) provide some support for this hypothesis.

3. **B** Only a small percentage of patients referred for consideration of repair of pectus excavatum have true symptoms. The vast majority of patients have no symptoms but request repair to improve cosmesis, and it is essential that these patients have reasonable expectations of what the operation can and cannot accomplish. It is very difficult to project, at an early age, how a given deformity will progress with time, which is the reason most surgeons recommend delaying correction until early adolescence. Patients with pectus excavatum who have a coincident cardiac murmur should undergo echocardiography, since some of these patients may have Marfan syndrome and associated aortic root pathology. The coexistence of mitral valve prolapse with pectus excavatum has been reported and in approximately 50% of patients, disappears after surgical correction of the chest wall deformity. This may be the result of ventricular chamber, and hence mitral valve annulus deformity which is correctable by sternal realignment.

4. **D** Surgical correction of pectus excavatum involves excision of deformed costal cartilages with perichondrial preservation, and sternal realignment with or without temporary metal strut support. The operation is usually done through either a transverse or curvilinear inframammary incision, except in Marfan patients, in whom a vertical incision (in anticipation of the eventual need for sternotomy and aortic valvular reconstruction) should be used. Sternal realignment is accomplished by making a wedge osteotomy through the anterior sternal cortex and then cracking the posterior cortex by forced anterior angulation. Sutures placed in the anterior sternum to close the

osteotomy usually suffice in maintaining the sternal correction, although some surgeons choose to reinforce this with a retrosternal strut. One innovation to the surgical treatment of pectus excavatum has been the development of a minimally invasive technique that permits placement of a metal bar behind the sternum. This bar rests on the parasternal chest wall and forcibly maintains the sternum in a position of correction. The bar remains in place for a recommended 2-year period to allow structural remodeling of the anterior chest wall and is then removed.

5. **A** The phenomenon of acceleration of deformity coincident with the pubertal growth spurt is well recognized and may even occur after surgical correction. It is, therefore, important to inform the patient of this possibility prior to operation.

BIBLIOGRAPHY

Cahill JL, Lees GM, Robertson HT. A summary of preoperative and postoperative cardiorespiratory performance in patients undergoing pectus excavatum and carinatum repair. *J Pediatr Surg.* 1984;19:430–433.

Shamberger RC. Congenital chest wall deformities. In: O'Neill JA, Rowe MI, Grosfeld JL, et al. eds. *Pediatric Surgery.* 5th ed. St. Louis: Mosby-Year Book; 1998.

Shamberger RC, Welch KJ. Cardiopulmonary function in pectus excavatum. *Surg Gynecol Obstet.* 1988;166:383–389.

AN INFANT BOY
WITH A TENSE MASS
IN THE GROIN

HISTORY This 8-week-old premature infant boy comes to the emergancy room with an incarcerated left inguinal hernia. A lump in the left groin has been noted intermittently for the past week. On the morning of admission, the infant is irritable and refuses his feeding. The inguinal area is swollen and seems tender. The family doctor is unable to reduce the hernia in his office.

He was a premature infant who weighed 1400 g at birth. He was born to a 16-year-old gravida I, para I mother whose pregnancy was complicated by a urinary tract infection just prior to delivery at 30 weeks' gestation. Presentation was breech. Apgar scores were not known. He required transfer to a neonatal intensive care unit because of increasing respiratory distress. He received 30% to 40% oxygen but required endotracheal intubation becuase of apnea and bradycardia. After 3 days, he was extubated.

Subsequent occasional spells of apnea/bradycardia resolved with minimal stimulation. At 3 weeks of age, he was transferred back to a nursery near home. A clubfoot on the left foot was treated with casts, which were changed weekly. He made good progress and was discharged home at 6 weeks of age. At discharge the testes were palpable in the upper scrotum, but no inguinal hernia was noted.

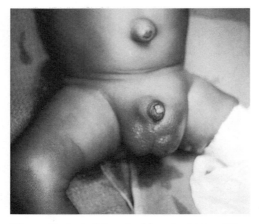

Figure 41-1. *Left inguinal hernia. Note pitting edema of left side of scrotum. Umbilical hernia is also present. Cast on left leg is for correction of talipes equinovarus (clubfoot).*

EXAMINATION He is an irritable but active male infant. Pulse is 168/min, temperature is 37°C rectally, respirations 36/min, blood pressure is 80/50. Weight is 6 lbs, 1 oz, height is 47 cm, and head circumference is 35 cm. His head appears large, with flattening in both temporal areas. The fontanelles are normal. There are no neck masses. The chest is clear to auscultation and percussion. No cardiac murmur is audible. The abdomen is moderately distended. An umbilical hernia protrudes with a 1.2-cm fascial defect. He is uncircumcised. There is a large, tense left inguinal hernia with marked scrotal edema (Figure 41-1). Both testes are in the scrotum. The anus is patent. The left leg is enclosed in a cast.

LABORATORY Hematocrit 34%, hemoglobin 11.7 gm%, white blood cell count 10,900/mm^3 with segments 9, bands 2, lymphocytes 83, and monocytes 6. Chest x-ray shows a normal heart and lungs. Urinalysis reveals a pale yellow urine with a specific gravity of 1.012, a pH of 6.0. Testing for protein is negative, as was glucose and acetone. There are no red blood cells and white blood cells are rare.

HOSPITAL COURSE After a few minutes of gentle manipulation (by the attending surgeon), the left inguinal hernia is reduced. The infant is admitted to the hospital. The following day, bilateral inguinal herniorrhaphy is performed under general anesthesia. The umbilical hernia is also repaired. He is monitored postoperatively in the hospital; apneic spells do not occur. Moderate swelling of the left testis and scrotum is noted at discharge the following day. At follow-up 1 week later, the swelling is resolving, and the incisions are healing well.

Please answer all questions before proceeding to discussion section.

✓ QUESTIONS

1. Which of the following is the *most* correct statement regarding pediatric inguinal hernias?
   A. The left side is more frequently affected than the right
   B. The pathogenesis is a congenital weakness of the inguinal floor
   C. In girls, the sac is adherent to the ligament of the ovary
   D. There is an inverse relationship between gestational age and risk of hernia
   E. Elective herniorrhaphy should be deferred until the infant is about 6 months of age

2. The following statements about incarcerated inguinal hernia in the pediatric patient all are accurate *except*:
   A. Incarceration is most frequent in the first year of life
   B. Infarction of incarcerated bowel is a frequent complication
   C. Infarction of the ovary is rare
   D. Testicular atrophy is an occasional complication following incarceration
   E. Inguinal lymphadenopathy may mimic incarcerated hernia

3. Which of the following conditions may be associated with an increased risk of inguinal hernia?
   A. Twinning
   B. Prematurity
   C. Hydrocephalus
   D. A and B
   E. All of the above

4. An irritable, 6-month-old male infant presents with acute onset of right scrotal swelling. There is a firm, ovoid, irreducible mass that extends from the external inguinal ring to the lower portion of the scrotum. He cries whenever the mass is touched. Which of the following is the most accurate maneuver to distinguish incarcerated hernia from acute hydrocele?
   A. Transillumination
   B. Needle aspiration

C. Rectal examination
D. Doppler ultrasound examination of the scrotum
E. Immediate surgical exploration

5. No matter which operative technique is employed, the most important step in the surgical repair of a pediatric inguinal hernia is:
A. High ligation of the sac
B. Complete excision of the sac
C. Reconstruction of the inguinal canal
D. Replacement of the spermatic cord in its anatomic location
E. None of the above

6. Which of the following is the *best* indication for exploration of the (asymptomatic) contralateral side during inguinal herniorraphy in a child?
A. A thickened spermatic cord on the contralateral side
B. A negative herniogram
C. A boy under 2 years of age
D. A girl under 6 years of age
E. A clinical hernia presenting on the left

7. A 12-month-old boy presents with a left inguinal hernia. The consensus for management of the contralateral side (which is normal on examination) is:
A. Exploration
B. No exploration
C. Exploration only if laparoscopy is positive
D. Exploration only if there is a history of prematurity
E. None of the above (ie, there is no consensus)

8. Which of the following statements is true regarding anesthesia for inguinal herniorraphy in an infant?
A. Postoperative monitoring in the hospital is indicated for all premature infants up to 1 year of age
B. Postoperative monitoring in the hospital is indicated for a 9-week-old term infant
C. Apneic spells rarely occur more than 18 hours postanesthesia
D. Infiltration of the herniorraphy incisions with local anesthetic is usually contraindicated in premature infants
E. Spinal or epidural anesthesia is usually contraindicated in premature infants

9. All of the following statements about *umbilical* hernias in infancy and childhood are correct *except*:
A. Umbilical hernias are common in African American children
B. Spontaneous closure of the defect occurs in the majority of children by age 3 or 4 years
C. Strapping the hernia with a velcro waistband does not speed the closure
D. Laparoscopic repair should be performed if the defect persists beyond age 3 or 4 years
E. Incarceration, strangulation, and evisceration are rare indications for repair

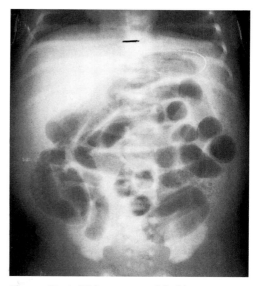

CASE 42

A 2-DAY-OLD GIRL
WITH ABDOMINAL DISTENTION
WHO IS FEEDING POORLY

HISTORY   Your opinion is requested on a 2.3 kg, 2-day-old, 36-week gestational aged girl who is feeding poorly, has not passed stool, and is becoming distended. She has been regurgitating frequently, and her father worries that not much breast milk is staying down.

EXAMINATION   The baby is slightly lethargic. Temperature 37.0°C, pulse 167, blood pressure 80/55, respiratory rate 34. The heart and lungs are normal. The abdomen is moderately distended but soft and nontender to deep palpation with no mass or hepatosplenomegaly. Rectal examination reveals an empty rectal vault.

LABORATORY   An abdominal flat plate is shown in Figure 42–1.
   Please answer all questions before proceeding to discussion section.

Figure 42–1. *Kidney, ureter, bladder (KUB) view of the abdomen.*

✓ QUESTIONS

1. You suspect:
   A. Mechanical obstruction of the small bowel
   B. Functional obstruction of the small bowel
   C. Mechanical obstruction of the large bowel
   D. Functional obstruction of the large bowel
   E. Hypomotility of the large and small bowel

2. A rectal examination demonstrates a patent and normally located anus. There is no presacral mass nor is there an explosion of stool when the examining finger is withdrawn. The mother is not diabetic and did not have gestational diabetes mellitus. Which is true?
   A. Small left colon syndrome is now much less likely
   B. Meconium plug syndrome bears further consideration
   C. Hirschsprung disease is no longer your provisional diagnosis

D. Rectal atresia is eliminated, and there appears to be more small bowel (than colon) loops involved

E. Megacystis-microcolon-intestinal hypoperistalsis syndrome becomes your provisional diagnosis

3. You ask for a contrast enema. Your radiologist asks, "Which contrast?"
   A. Barium
   B. Gastrograffin
   C. Gastrograffin and *N*-acetyl cysteine
   D. Renograffin
   E. Isotonic water soluble

4. The enema is shown in Figure 42–2. The radiologist shows you a small piece of firm green fecal matter that extruded from the rectum during the study. You note:
   A. With surprise, that an initial green plug is typical of meconium ileus
   B. A transition zone in the proximal descending colon and conclude this must be Hirschsprung disease
   C. The baby clearly has meconium plug syndrome but Hirschsprung disease is not excluded from consideration
   D. Neuronal intestinal dysplasia (NID) is often responsible for stool of this quality
   E. That it would be a good time to perform a sweat chloride test (iontophoresis)

5. By the following morning, the patient has not passed any more stool and is still moderately distended. The radiologist calls you after reviewing the baby's abdominal films and tells you they are unchanged. You ask the radiologist:
   A. To repeat the study and use 60 mL of 20% *N*-acetyl cysteine per liter of contrast
   B. To send the patient back to the neonatal intensive care unit to prepare for operation
   C. Not to do any further enemas for now, fearing perforation

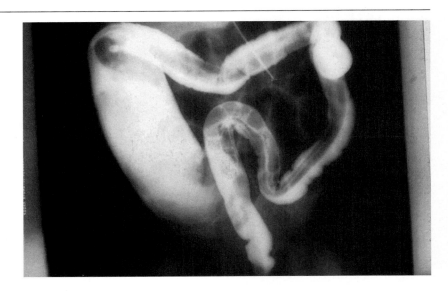

Figure 42–2. *Contrast enema.*

D. To take films looking for anomalies of the vertebral column and radial limbs

E. To save some stool for culture and sensitivity (C+S)

6. With the second enema, the colon entirely clears, the colon caliber (when unobstructed) is near normal, and the child begins to stool spontaneously the next day with progressively diminishing abdominal distention. You do all *but*:
A. Tell the parents you need to biopsy their daughter's rectum
B. Perform serology for cystic fibrosis and, perhaps, iontophoresis in a month's time
C. Diagnose small left colon syndrome and suggest glucose tolerance testing
D. Point out that an immature myenteric nervous system may be responsible for these symptoms
E. Counsel the parents that lifelong problems are unlikely

ANSWERS AND DISCUSSION

1. **D** The presence of multiple dilated loops of bowel suggests a distal obstruction. The absence of markedly dilated loops and the slowly progressive history make ileal atresia less likely. Statistically, the most common congenital cause of colon obstruction is Hirschsprung disease, a functional blockage caused by failure of the involved segment to relax. Hypomotility of the premature typically occurs in younger, smaller neonates.

2. **B** Less than half of babies with small left colon syndrome are born to diabetic mothers, therefore, the data given do not drastically reduce this possibility. Hirschsprung disease (HD) is still the most likely diagnosis, but failure to pass stool explosively means it would have to be segmental disease extending above the examining finger—the sigmoid colon or higher. True—there is not rectal atresia—but with the exception of Dravidian Indians from Tamilnadu in the South of India, this is an exceptionally rare problem to begin with and was never high on the list. Also, on a plain film in a neonate, one can guess at but not positively distinguish between large bowel and small. Hirschsprung disease behaves similarly to megacystis-microcolon-intestinal hypoperistalsis syndrome and is much more common. Meconium plug syndrome is a common cause of neonatal large bowel obstruction.

3. **E** Barium is the best medium to visualize details of the bowel wall and to remain cohesive for enteroclysis, but when given preoperatively—potentially pushed above an obstruction—using it risks retention, desiccation, or leakage, or a combination of these, at the time of operation. Gastrograffin is thinner, does not provide as stark contrast, and is so hypertonic (~1500 mOsm) that children have intravascularly dehydrated from the fluid shifts that take place when it is used in the bowel lumen. Renograffin is an intravascular contrast solution. Gastrograffin diluted to serum iso-osmolality (280 mOsm) or another agent of similar osmolality is optimal. This trades-off the stark contrast of barium for the benefits of water soluble contrast, which include solubilizing meconium, reabsorption if not excreted, and minimal toxicity with intraoperative spill.

4. **C** The x-ray and physical findings are diagnostic of meconium plug syndrome (MP). The contrast in Figure 42–2 outlines the long thick plug of meconium from the rectum to the midtransverse colon. There is a marked increase in caliber proximal to this point (transition zone). Meconium plug syndrome occurs when thick, viscid meconium becomes impacted in the left colon and acts as an obstruction.

   The contrast enema may be therapeutic. The water soluble agent will loosen the thick plug of meconium from the bowel wall and allow it to pass. Meconium plug syndrome is associated with Hirschsprung disease in about 20% to 30% of cases (see following). Meconium ileus causes obstruction of the ileum, not the left colon. Furthermore, the initial "meconium plug" associated with meconium ileus is gray not green as the secretions are so viscid that bile does not penetrate to the most distal luminal contents. Iontophoresis is not useful until after 48 hours of life because of early serum changes affecting electrolyte balance. In fact, even with pilocarpine it is difficult to generate the 0.05 g of sweat required to prove a chloride level > 60 mEq/L that is diagnostic. Most practitioners prefer serologic genetic testing during the first few weeks of life, which is about 85% sensitive. The stool associated with NID is similar to that of HD—anywhere from normal to claylike, depending on the length of the diseased segment.

5. **A** The study with water soluble contrast has been partially therapeutic. A repeat study or studies will probably complete colon evacuation. While not mandatory, adding *N*-acetyl cysteine to the irrigation solution may help to solubilize stool concretions. No operation (other than a rectal biopsy, which requires no preparation) is indicated. There is no suggestion of VACTERL syndrome or spina bifida occulta, therefore, spine and extremity films are not indicated. In a nontoxic neonate, stool C+S is of no value.

6. **C** The extruded plug is shown in Figure 42–3. The return of the colon to normal caliber, the "plug of meconium," and the rapid return to a normal stooling pattern are consistent with MP syndrome. This is a poorly understood entity thought to be caused by an immature myenteric nervous system. As this system matures (days to weeks), one expects stooling to become normal. Meconium plug syndrome is usually not indicative of an underlying disorder. Most babies have normal gastrointestinal function after passage of the plug. Hirschsprung disease, however, is associated in 20% to 30% of cases, and cystic fibrosis is found in a few percent of cases. Therefore, suction rectal biopsy to rule out Hirschsprung disease and testing for cystic fibrosis are mandatory.

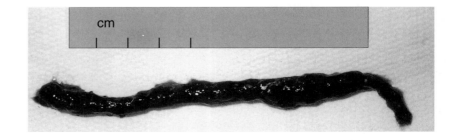

Figure 42–3. *Meconium plug following evacuation. Most babies have normal bowel function following passage of the plug.*

BIBLIOGRAPHY

Berdon WE, Slovis TL, Campbell JB, Baker DH, Haller JO. Neonatal small left colon syndrome: its relationship to aganglionosis and meconium plug syndrome. *Radiology.* 1977;125:457–462.

Hussain SM, Meradji M, Robben SG, Hop WC. Plain film diagnosis in meconium plug syndrome, meconium ileus and neonatal Hirschsprung's disease: a scoring system. *Pediatr Radiol.* 1991;21:556–559.

A NEWBORN WITH RESPIRATORY DISTRESS

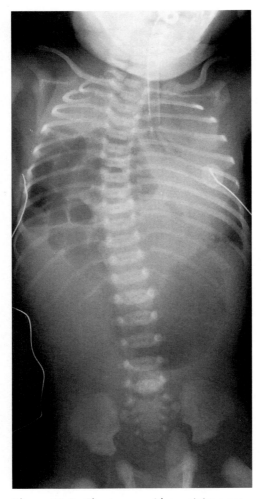

Figure 43–1. *Chest x-ray with suspicious pattern in right hemithorax.*

HISTORY   A neonatologist from an outside institution calls you to request the transfer of a 2.7-kg, 36-week gestational aged, neonate at 6 hours of life with persistent, worsening cyanosis. The baby's Apgar scores were 3 and 5 at 1 and 5 minutes, respectively. The baby was resuscitated with bag mask ventilation and intubated with some difficulty in the delivery room.

EXAMINATION   The referring doctor tells you that the baby is blue and pale. Peripheral perfusion is poor with a capillary refill time of 3.5 seconds. The heart tones are difficult to hear. Breath sounds are normal.

LABORATORY   The chest x-ray is shown in Figure 43–1.
   Please answer all questions before proceeding to discussion section.

✓ QUESTIONS

1. Your differential diangosis does *not* include:
   A. Defect in the pleuroperitoneal membrane
   B. Congenital cystic adenomatoid malformation (CCAM)
   C. Congenital diaphragmatic hernia (CDH)
   D. Right lower lobe collapse
   E. Right diaphragm eventration

2. You accept transfer and do all *but*:
   A. Recommend immediate placement of a nasogastric or orogastric tube
   B. Recommend placement of intravenous lines and expeditious fluid delivery
   C. Recommend intubation before trying more conservative measures

   D. Mobilize your main operating room staff for rapid hernia repair
   E. Suggest the pH be checked and, if abnormal, have it corrected during transfer

3. When you confirm this is a right-sided diaphragmatic hernia, you collaborate with the neonatologists to:
   A. Use conventional ventilation, keeping mean airway pressure as low as possible
   B. Use high pressures and average frequency ventilation
   C. Start tolazoline
   D. Start high-frequency ventilation
   E. Prepare the nitrous oxide delivery system

4. Using optimal ventilation including 100% F_{IO_2}, the child's mean airway pressure is 32 torr and his preductal P_{O_2} is 60. You note:
   A. With surprise that right-sided hernias are less common than left and usually do better than this
   B. This is a good case for partial liquid ventilation
   C. His oxygenation index (OI) is less than 50, therefore, he does not meet extracorporeal membrane oxygenation (ECMO) criteria
   D. He should be excluded from ECMO because of the risk of intraventricular hemorrhage (IVH) with systemic anticoagulation in a premature infant
   E. His OI is over 40, unless he rapidly improves, he will be a candidate for ECMO

5. The baby improves markedly. Two days later, he is on conventional ventilation with a peak inspiratory pressure of 22 mmHg, a ventilatory rate of 40, and and F_{IO_2} of 40%. Your plan for the CDH is to:
   A. Prepare to fix it through the abdomen
   B. Prepare to fix it through the right chest
   C. Discuss surgery with the parents, obtain informed consent, and warn them of a 20% association with chromosomal abnormalities
   D. Plan to perform a fundoplication at the time of surgery because so many of these children will have gastroesophagel reflux (GER)
   E. Order various radiologic investigations

6. A curious medical student asks you the difference between a Morgagni and Bochdalek hernia. You say many things, but you do *not* say:
   A. Morgagni herniae are about one-quarter as common as Bochdalek ones
   B. Both arise when the four diaphragm anlage do not fuse by the tenth week of gestation
   C. A Bochdalek hernia tends to be posterolateral and is caused by a persistent pleuroperitoneal canal
   D. A Morgagni hernia tends to be central and anterior and is caused by an inadequate transverse septum
   E. The latter occurs in 1:2000 pregnancies and in 1:5000 live births

7. Concerning the repair of a Bochdalek defect, the following is untrue:
   A. If small, it can be closed primarily with nondissolving sutures; if large, with thin (1 mm) Goretex

    B. The recurrence rate is markedly increased when prosthetic material is used
    C. If a peritoneal sac is found in the chest, it should be excised
    D. The associated malrotation must be fixed with a Ladd's procedure
    E. Two thirds of children will have GER; one third will require fundoplication

8. Associated syndromes include all of the following but:
    A. Beckwith-Wiedemann syndrome
    B. Fryn syndrome
    C. Pentralogy of Cantrell
    D. Trisomy 9, 13, and 18
    E. Currarino's triad

ANSWERS AND DISCUSSION

1. **D** There is a space occupying lesion in the right chest. This is almost certainly caused by bowel passing through a congenital diaphragmatic hernia. A congenital cystic adenomatoid malformation can cause bubbles of gas in the chest as the cysts fill with air. The abdominal gas pattern, however, should be normal. A right lower lobe collapse would pull the mediastinum right and not cause atelectasis of the upper hemithorax.

2. **D** If congenital diaphragmatic hernia is in the differential diagnosis, it is wise to avoid triggers of persistent fetal circulation (PFC), which include acidosis, hypoxemia, hypothermia, and dehydration. Persistent fetal circulation occurs when hypoxia induces severe pulmonary hypertension. This high pulmonary pressure causes anatomic right-to-left shunting at the foramen ovale and ductus arteriosus. Breathing is currently imperiled and transfer necessary—the safest measure to ensure an airway is rapid intubation. It would be premature to consider thoracotomy or laparotomy. Efforts should concentrate on stabilization, transfer, and evaluation. The principles of transfer are to keep the child warm, hydrated, and decompressed, which applies to most neonatal transfers.

3. **A** The goals of ventilation for the baby with a diaphragmatic hernia include maintaining arterial oxygenation and CO_2 levels in a range that will not exacerbate pulmonary hypertension and minimizing peak and mean airway pressures to reduce the effect of barotrauma, which can cause a pneumothorax and injure the pulmonary parenchyma. Conventional ventilation is the first-line strategy. Both peak and mean airway pressures should be kept as low as possible. Tolazaline is an alpha-receptor blocker that causes vasodilation. While it dilates the pulmonary arterial bed, it similarly dilates the systemic circulation. Thus, any reduction in pulmonary pressure is offset by systemic hypotension. High-frequency ventilation is an extremely useful modality in diaphragmatic hernia. It may allow effective ventilation with less barotrauma. It is generally introduced when conventional ventilation at "reasonably safe" settings has failed. Nitric (not nitrous) oxide is a selective pulmonary vasodilator that

may be useful. Research evidence has not yet shown a benefit in patients with a diaphragmatic hernia.

4. **E** The ratio of left-to-right CDH is 10:1, but new experience with antenatal ultrasounds suggest they are equally morbid. Perfluorocarbon partial liquid ventilation, when used with oxygen in a standard ventilator, is still experimental but has anecdotally produced some impressive results. Extracorporeal membrane oxygenation (ECMO) *inclusion* criteria include:

- An alveolar–arterial oxygen difference of greater than 610 for 10 hours
- An OI over 40 on several consecutive arterial blood gases over 30 minutes
- A PaO_2 < 50 torr for 4 hours
- Severe barotrauma
- Acute deterioration with 2 hours of PaO_2 < 40 torr or pH < 7.15
- Two hours of ventilation index (MAP × ventilator rate) > 1000 and $PaCO_2$ > 40 torr post-CDH repair
- Failure of nitric oxide
- Reversible cardiopulmonary failure

ECMO *exclusion* criteria include:

- Grade II intraventricular hemorrhage
- Weight < 2 kg (relative)
- Age < 32 weeks postconception because of the risk of IVH (relative)
- Severe chromosomal abnormalities (conveniently left vague)
- Cyanotic congenital heart disease (unless used as a bridge to surgery)
- Uncontrolled bleeding
- Irreversible cardiopulmonary damage

The most commonly used indicator, the OI, is a product of mean airway pressure and FIO_2 divided by the best *postductal* PO_2, which is the blood circulated to all but the head and upper extremities.

5. **A** For several years, it has been accepted practice to wait for at least 1 to 2 days of stable behavior before surgical repair of CDH in children who are initially unstable. The stress of general anesthesia and repair can exacerbate the baby's pulmonary hypertension. Furthermore, most surgeons believe the repair transiently worsens pulmonary function. The chance of chromosomal anomalies is much lower than 20% in the live born infant with CDH. It is true that many patients will have GER, but most surgeons will wait to treat those babies unresponsive to medical therapy (about 30%).

6. **A** Morgagni herniae represent only 2% to 5% of all CDHs. The diaphragm is formed by the fusion of four anlage: two lateral pleuroperitoneal membranes that grow toward the midline where they meet esophageal mesenchyme in the posterior midline growing forward toward the anterior midline where it meets muscles of the body wall. **E** emphasizes the "hidden mortality" of CDH in which almost one half the affected fetuses are spontaneously aborted or stillborn.

7. **D** Small to moderate diaphragmatic hernias may be simply closed with sutures after mobilization of the posterior rim from retroperitoneal attachments. Prosthetic material is necessary to close large defects. In these cases, the hernia recurrence rate is significant. It is not unreasonable to perform a Ladd's procedure (most patients will have malrotation), but many believe the adhesions resulting from intestinal manipulation during repair will prevent subsequent volvulus. While many children with CDH have gastroesophageal reflux, most can be managed medically.

8. **E** Only Fryn syndrome is commonly associated with CDH, with the others listed occasionally associated with CDH. Currarino's triad refers to anal narrowing, presacral mass, and a spinal anomaly often involving the meninges.

BIBLIOGRAPHY

Harrison MR, Bjordal RI, Langmark F, Knutrud OJ. Congenital diaphragmatic hernia: the hidden mortality. *J Pediatr Surg.* 1978;13:227–230.

Lally KP. Extracorporeal membrane oxygenation in patients with congenital diaphragmatic hernia. *Semin Pediatr Surg.* 1996;5:249–255.

Langer JC. Congenital diaphragmatic hernia. *Chest Surg Clin North Am.* 1998;8:295–314.

Thebaud B, Mercier JC, Dinh-Xuan AT. Congenital diaphragmatic hernia: a cause of persistent pulmonary hypertension of the newborn which lacks an effective therapy. *Biol Neonate.* 1998;74:323–326.

The Congenital Diaphragmatic Hernia Study Group. Does extracorporeal membrane oxygenation improve survival in neonates with congenital diaphragmatic hernia? *J Pediatr Surg.* 1999;34:720–724.

A 3-YEAR-OLD BOY WITH A PROLAPSED RECTUM

HISTORY You are called by an anxious physician from the emergency room about a 3-year-old boy with a 4-cm long bulbous protrusion of rectal mucosa through the anus. This occurred about 3 hours ago while the child was sitting on the toilet. The child's parents are hysterical, but the child appears comfortable and does not complain of pain.

EXAMINATION Vital signs are temperature 37.0°C, heart rate 92, blood pressure 110/57, respiratory rate 20. The heart and lungs are normal. The abdomen is flat, soft, nondistended, and nontender to deep palpation in all quadrants. You do not feel any masses or hepatosplenomegaly. Protruding from the rectum is a 4-cm length of mucosa that appears edematous and a bit purple but viable.

Please answer all questions before proceeding to discussion section.

✓ QUESTIONS

1. Which of the following are associated with rectal prolapse?
   A. Diarrhea
   B. Straining at stool
   C. Constipation
   D. Spontaneous reduction
   E. All of the above

2. What is the most important *first* step in management of this child?
   A. Abdominal computed tomography (CT) scan with intravenous and oral contrast
   B. Abdominal ultrasound
   C. Intravenous fluid administration and broad-spectrum antibiotics
   D. Attempt at manual reduction
   E. Barium enema

3. Management should include screening for which of the following disease(s)?
   A. Inflammatory bowel disease
   B. Cystic fibrosis
   C. Prostatic rhabdomyosarcoma
   D. Familial polyposis coli
   E. A and B

4. The natural history of rectal prolapse is:
   A. Spontaneous resolution in the majority of cases
   B. Recurrence leading to incarceration and need for emergency operation in 20%
   C. Encopresis and chronic fecal incontinence in 30%
   D. Up to one third of patients will be diagnosed with a serious underlying disorder
   E. None of the above

5. Successful surgical options include:
   A. Posterior sagittal incision with resection of the coccyx and suspension of the rectum to the sacrum
   B. Placement of a circumferential circlage wire or suture to narrow the anal opening
   C. Injecting hypertonic saline or 5% phenol into the perianal tissues as a sclerosant
   D. Placement of full thickness sutures through the rectum and sacrum suspending the sacrum
   E. All of the above

ANSWERS AND DISCUSSION

1. **E** Rectal prolapse is a relatively common disorder that occurs in early childhood. It is associated with protracted straining at stool or long periods of time sitting on the toilet. The vast majority of children with rectal prolapse have a history of abnormal defecation. This history varies from frequent diarrhea to prolonged constipation with straining at stool. These events lead to stretching of the suspensory ligaments of the pelvis and the pelvic peritoneum.

   The suspensory ligaments of the pelvis are muscular. If prolapse can be prevented, these structures will regain their normal tone, and the problem will not recur. Thus, in most cases, the treatment of rectal prolapse consists of treatment of the underlying disorder.

   Rarely, a sigmoid intussusception may present as rectal prolapse. Placement of the examining finger through the anus, next to the prolapse, allows the examiner to differentiate between this and rectal prolapse.

2. **D** In almost all cases, the prolapsed rectum can be gently reduced inside the anus by the physician. This is accomplished by means of gentle circumferential pressure to reduce the edema followed by reduction of the tissue through the anus. The longer the prolapse is untreated, the greater the degree of bowel edema and the more difficult it is to reduce. Abdominal imaging has no role in the treatment of this disorder. Barium enema will not help reduce the prolapse. If barium enema is done after reduction, it is invariably normal. Unless

the patient is in shock or the bowel is ischemic, intravenous fluids and antibiotics are not necessary. Prompt reduction without delay is the cornerstone of management.

3. **B** Rectal prolapse may be a presenting sign of cystic fibrosis. One review found that one fifth of children with cystic fibrosis have rectal prolapse at some time during childhood. The reason for this is not entirely clear but is probably related to abnormally thick mucus in the rectum. Most authors believe that all children with rectal prolapse should be tested for cystic fibrosis.

There is no direct association between rectal prolapse and inflammatory bowel disease. Prostatic rhabdomyosarcoma presents in this age group but causes a pelvic mass, obstipation, or both rather than prolapse. Familial polyposis does not cause prolapse.

4. **A** Most cases of rectal prolapse are successfully treated by addressing the underlying stooling disorder. Acute ischemia or necrosis of the prolapsed segment is very rare. Most children go on to have normal bowel function. Encopresis or fecal incontinence are not expected. Except for the few patients with cystic fibrosis, patients with rectal prolapse are otherwise healthy children.

5. **E** There are a large number of accepted procedures for the treatment of rectal prolapse. This is because all of them are moderately effective, yet none is clearly superior. The basis for **A** and **D** is surgical suspension of the rectum to fixed bony structures. **B** relies on a suture to prevent prolapse long enough for the pelvic sling to return to normal strength and tone. **C** depends on formation of sclerosing scar between the rectum and perirectal tissue.

BIBLIOGRAPHY

Altemeier WA, Culbertson WR, Schowengerdt C, et al. Nineteen years experience with the one stage perineal repair of rectal prolapse. *Ann Surg.* 1971;173:993–1006.

Ashcraft KW, Garred JL, Holder TM. Rectal prolapse—17 year experience with posterior repair and suspension. *J Pediatr Surg.* 1990;25:992–995.

Ashcraft KW, Holder TM. Acquired anorectal disorders. In: Ashcraft KW, ed. *Pediatric Surgery.* 2nd ed. Philadelphia: WB Saunders; 1993:410–415.

Pearl RH, Ein SH, Churchill B. Posterior sagittal anorectoplasty for pediatric recurrent rectal prolapse. *J Pediatr Surg.* 1989;24:1100–1102.

Shwachman H, Redmond A, Khaw K-T. Studies in cystic fibrosis: report of 130 patients diagnosed under 3 months of age over a 20 year period. *Pediatrics.* 1970;46:335–343.

A NEWBORN WITH ABDOMINAL DISTENTION AND GREEN VOMITING

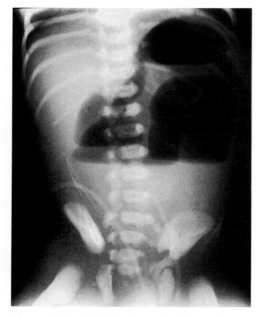

Figure 45–1. *Upright abdominal film of a newborn with bilious vomiting.*

HISTORY   A neonatologist calls you to see a 10-hour-old, term, 3-kg boy who is mildly distended and vomiting bile after feeding attempts. He has not passed stool, his anus is perforate, and a nasogastric tube has been passed, and it has drained 45 mL of bilious fluid.

EXAMINATION   He does not appear toxic. His pulse is 120, and mean arterial pressure (MAP) is 45 mmHg. His heart and lungs are normal. His abdomen is markedly distended with some large bowel loops visible through the abdominal wall. His abdomen is not tender, and you do not feel a mass.

LABORATORY   An upright view of the abdomen is shown in Figure 45–1.
   Please answer all questions before proceeding to discussion section.

✓ QUESTIONS

1. Your provisional diagnosis would be:
   A. Jejunal atresia
   B. Ileal atresia
   C. Meconium ileus
   D. Meconium cyst
   E. Hirschsprung disease

2. Which radiology sign is incorrectly matched?
   A. Ground glass appearance: meconium ileus
   B. Calcifications: meconium ileus, meconium cyst, antenatal volvulus, neuroblastoma
   C. Inverted J sign: septic ileus

   D. Question mark sign: long segment Hirschsprung disease
   E. Pneumatosis intestinalis: bowel ischemia of any origin, baro-
      trauma, benign

3. Of the following, which would be *least* useful?
   A. Complete blood count (CBC)
   B. Electrolytes
   C. Glucose
   D. C-reactive protein (CRP)

4. If offered one investigation prior to an operation, which would you
choose?
   A. Abdominal ultrasound
   B. Abdominal computed tomography (CT) scan
   C. Barium enema
   D. Water soluble contrast enema
   E. Upper gastrointestinal (GI) series

5. Which of the following should be done prior to operation?
   A. Placement of nasogastric tube
   B. Administration of antibiotics
   C. Restoration of normal intravascular volume
   D. Normalization of serum electrolytes
   E. All of the above

6. You find an atretic proximal jejunum that is markedly dilated con-
nected by a fibrous cord to much smaller distal bowel (Figure 45–2;
see also color plate). You would classify this lesion as an atresia type:
   A. I
   B. II
   C. IIIa
   D. IIIb
   E. Cannot classify from information given

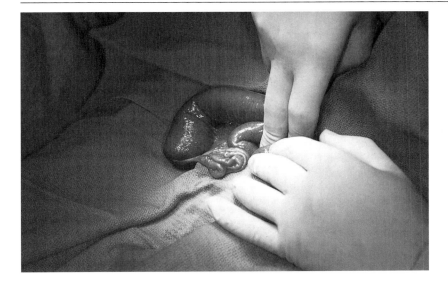

Figure 45–2. *Operative findings showing dilated proximal bowel and contracted distal
bowel connected by a fibrous cord. A considerable caliber discrepancy between proximal
and distal bowel is typical of jejunal atresia.
(See also color plate.)*

7. Assuming there is a 5:1 caliber discrepancy, which of the following would be your preferred anastamosis?
   A. Tapered end-to-back
   B. Bishop-Koop
   C. Santulli with removal of bulbous proximal tip
   D. Side-to-side
   E. No anastamosis: proximal stoma until dilated bowel recovers

8. If you found proximal jejunal atresia and multiple (> 15) distal atresias, what would be your preferred operative strategy?
   A. Resect each atresia, and reanastamose whatever is left
   B. Resect long atresia segments, and enteroplasty short segments
   C. Close the abdomen, and give the parents the bad news
   D. Resect the proximal bulb, taper, and pass a feeding tube from the nose through the entire length of small bowel any way you can
   E. Bring out a proximal stoma, and investigate the distal bowel subsequently without sacrificing it

9. Who described the first animal model of jejunoileal atresia, and how does it differ from duodenal atresia?
   A. Ladd: later event in gestation
   B. Gross: problem of vascularization
   C. Barnard: not a problem of recanalization
   D. Hirschsprung: windsock deformity less common
   E. Todani: passage of distal gas is not possible in a complete atresia

10. Of the following, the most common site and type of small bowel atresia is:
    A. Duodenum, III
    B. Ileum, II
    C. Jejunum, III
    D. Jejunum, IV
    E. Colon, IIIb

11. Key principles of operative repair for jejunal atresia include all but:
    A. Measure length of remaining bowel and include in operative report
    B. Using air, liquid, or a catheter, rule out distal obstruction(s)
    C. Avoid bringing out a proximal jejunal stoma whenever possible
    D. Avoid keeping a neonate's abdomen open longer than 1 hour: hypothermia may cause irreversible bleeding
    E. Excise thickened and dilated bulb, taper proximally, fishmouth distally, confirm distal bowel patency, end-to-oblique anastomosis, and closure of mesenteric defect

12. Predictors that a case of short bowel syndrome will be problematic include all but:
    A. Less than 50 cm of small bowel
    B. Loss of the ileocecal valve
    C. Total parenteral nutrition (TPN) cholestasis
    D. No remaining ileum
    E. No remaining colon

13. Jejunoileal atresia:
    A. Type IIIb is associated with prematurity and low birth weight
    B. Is usually associated with maternal polyhydramnios

C. Types I, II, and III are associated with normal gut length
D. Tends to be distal in the jejunum or proximal in the ileum
E. Has a 30% association with chromosomal abnormalities

ANSWERS AND DISCUSSION

1. **A** The absence of stool and relatively mild abdominal distention coupled with bilious vomiting suggest a high mechanical bowel obstruction. All the other possibilities are more distal and should be associated with greater abdominal distention and more loops on radiologic examination. The upright abdominal x-ray in Figure 45–1 shows a few dilated loops of bowel with air fluid levels and no distal gas. These findings are diagnostic of jejunal atresia.

2. **C** Uncomplicated meconium ileus presents with viscid chyme that is fairly homogeneous (ground glass) and traps bubbles rather than layering (soap bubbles). Complicated meconium ileus may involve free air, a pseudocyst of meconium from a large contained, but not healed, perforation, or calcifications that are the abdomen's response to an old perforation. For this reason, calcifications may also be seen in antenatal volvulus. Microcalcifications are a classical sign of neuroblastoma—albeit uncommon at birth. The inverted J sign describes one loop of bowel with more fluid accumulated in the distal limb (from peristalsis) and more air in the proximal limb, findings consistent with bowel that continues to peristalsis against a mechanical obstruction. For this reason, it is not usually found in sepsis, where an ileus pattern is much more common. Narrow, foreshortened colon that has lost typical haustrations and some of the sigmoid curvature may be observed following contrast enema in long segment Hirschsprung disease. In this configuration, it roughly resembles a question mark (?) when contrast enema is performed. Pneumatosis intestinalis may be caused by any of the etiologies listed, depending on the clinical setting.

3. **D** This patient has an obvious partial or complete bowel obstruction. All causes may elevate the CRP (acute phase reactant), therefore, it is not useful in differentiating among them. It is more important to stabilize the patient expeditiously and then operate.

4. **D** This patient is likely to have jejunal atresia and, at the time of operation, it will be necessary to verify that there are not multiple atresias. If a preoperative enema (isosmotic water-soluble contrast is the safest in a preoperative abdomen) is normal, only the small bowel will have to be investigated during the operation. If this has not been performed, it may be necessary to enlarge the incision so that the entire colon may be visualized. These advantages—potentially smaller incision and less operative time—are not worth the risks of delay and hypothermia and so should be balanced against the child's stability and optimal time of operation. From the information given, this obstruction is likely a high one, and the enema is not likely to show the cause of it. An upper gastrointestinal series is not necessary. The plain films are diagnostic of complete jejunal obstruction.

5. E The cardinal goal in the management of this patient will be resuscitation, evaluation, and then operation. A nasogastric tube, antibiotics, cross-match, blood work, informed consent, appropriate intravenous lines, rehydration, ionic hemostasis, and warming all need to be performed or arranged. Unlike the child with volvulus, the preoperative phase for jejunoileal atresia should be thorough and complete.

6. E The following classification was proposed by Bland in 1889 with modifications in the 1960s and 1970s to include types IIIB and IV:
  I. Membrane with (windsock) or without central perforation (21%)
  II. Fibrous cord connecting proximal and distal (25%)
  IIIa. Absent segment with mesenteric defect (24%)
  IIIb. Absent segment with mesenteric defect and vascular supply to distal small bowel arising from collateral branches of the right colic artery (apple peel or Christmas tree deformity) (8%)
  IV. Multiple atresias (23%)

The information given so far explicity neglects the results gleaned from running the entire bowel, a *treacherous oversight*. For that reason, there is insufficient data to know if it is only a type II or possibly a type IV (although admittedly, most II vascular configurations are associated with just one atresia).

7. A A functional end-to-end anastamosis (transverse division proximal, oblique division distal) is synonymous with end-to-oblique or end-to-back and is extremely similar to end-to-end after the distal end is fishmouthed (slit in the antimesenteric midline to increase lumen caliber). The key is tapering the proximal segment. This usually involves removing the bulbous tip too, depending on the length of bowel that will remain. Proximal jejunal atresias demonstrate some of the most marked caliber discrepancies of any bowel anastamoses. The child's proclivity to TPN-induced liver failure and long-term outcome may well depend on the early and efficient functioning of this anastamosis. An end-to-vented-side anastamosis (Bishop-Koop) is one way of rationalizing caliber discrepanicies. Usually these are 7:1 or greater and are often seen with meconium ileus. A short 2- to 5-cm chimney connects the distal bowel to the skin that serves to apply constant pressure toward distal stool migration with a pop-off function out the stoma until the distal bowel is sufficiently dilated. A vented side-to-end anastamosis (Santulli) is mentioned only to be condemned. This arrangement encourages rapid stool egress to skin level through the proximal limb without exerting significant distending pressure on the distal, small-caliber bowel. A stoma this high is disastrous and should rarely be performed.

8. D There is no absolutely right answer to this question, and the situation is a dreaded one, often not apparent until one is in the operating room (because the first atresia prevents radiologic appreciation of the subsequent ones). In type IV atresias, it is reasonable to entertain the idea of multiple anastamoses—as many as five or seven sometimes. But when they are in excess of ten (sometimes there may be 20 or 30), one must either excise segments or use another strategy. Some of the type I atresias can be enteroplastied and all type II or III must be excised. But if type I atresias are numerous, another strategy is to force a small (4 to 6 Fr) silicone catheter from the nose through the stomach and small bowel and down into the cecum (assuming it is beyond the atresias) or out through an appendicostomy to the abdominal wall. In this way, the lumen will be stented. It is far from an uncomplicated procedure but remains one of a few viable options.

9. **C** It is important to emphasize the different theories of duodenal atresia (aberrant recanalization, Tandler 1900) in contrast to jejunoileal atresia (vascular accident, Louw 1952), which is thought to occur later in pregnancy. The South African surgeon famous for the first heart transplant, Barnard, also created the first animal model for jejunoileal atresia by ligating the vascular arcades of fetal dogs. Todani is known for modification of the Altmeier classification of choledochal cysts.

10. **C** Relative to live births, classical teaching is that jejunoileal atresia occurs in ~1:500 cases, duodenal atresia in ~1:5000 cases, and colonic atresia in 1:20,000 cases, although these numbers vary considerably from series to series. In a large series from South Africa and Indiana, type III(a and b) atresias are most common. Jejunal lesions may be more common than ileal ones.

11. **D** While this rule may be true of small for gestational age premature infants with perforated necrotizing enterocolitis who are operated on emergently, it is not true for jejunoileal atresia in infants who are usually healthy otherwise and normal-sized for dates. In these children, appropriate measures before operation (plastic skin barrier, exothermic gel pad, warm air fan, complete rehydration) are taken to ensure sufficient operative time for more complicated procedures, if necessary.

12. **B** While the classical teaching is that an ileocecal valve is worth 25 to 50 cm of small bowel—by virtue of slowing gastrointestinal transit that permits increased absorption—this fact has not been borne out in at least one series. Term neonates have about 200 cm of small bowel and do very well if only the ileocecal valve is lost. In the other circumstances, there is significant short gut syndrome, which is proportional to the loss of short bowel and, to a lesser extent, colon.

13. **A** Apple peel atresia (type IIIb) is associated with low birth weight and prematurity. The reason is not clear. The more distal the atresia, the more gut there is available to absorb fluid; therefore, the lower the chance of polyhdramnios, which is estimated at 24% for jejunoileal atresias. Type III atresias are associated with a loss of intestinal length. Atresias tend to be high and low—proximal in the jejunum and distal in the ileum. Duodenal atresias, but not jejunoileal atresia, has a 30% association with trisomy 21.

BIBLIOGRAPHY

Dalla-Vecchia LK, Grosfeld JL, et al. Intestinal atresia and stenosis: a 25-year experience with 277 cases. *Arch Surg.* 1998;133(5):490–496.

Dillon PW, Cilley RE. Newborn surgical emergencies: gastrointestinal anomalies, abdominal wall defects. *Pediatr Clin North Am.* 1993; 40:1289–1314.

Kimble RM, Harding JE, Kolbe A. Does gut atresia cause polyhydramnios? *Pediatr Surg Intl.* 1998;13:115–117.

Newborn Surgery. Prem Puri: Butterworth-Heinemann; 1996.

A TERM INFANT WITH EXCESSIVE SALIVATION

HISTORY   A 2700 g, term male infant is born at a rural hospital to a 34-year-old, gravida 4, para 3 mother whose pregnancy was complicated by polyhydramnios. Vaginal delivery is uneventful. Apgars are 8 at 1 minute and 9 at 5 minutes. As he is transported to the hospital nursery, excessive salivation (Figure 46–1; see also color plate) is noted.

EXAMINATION   The patient is a well-developed, active male infant. Pulse 140, temperature 98.2°F, respirations 30/min, blood pressure 78/ 52. He is breathing easily without cyanosis or jaundice. No anomalies of the head, neck, trunk, or extremities are evident. Copious secretions are suctioned from his mouth. Breath sounds are audible on both sides of the chest. No cardiac murmur is heard. The abdomen is soft and without distention. No masses are palpable. Genitalia are normal. A drop of meconium is visible at the anus.

LABORATORY   Hemoglobin 17.0 gm%, hematocrit 60%, white blood cell count 18,000/mm³, differential normal.

HOSPITAL COURSE   A nasogastric tube is inserted but meets an obstruction about 8 cm beyond the nostril. A "babygram" (Figure 46–2) is obtained. He is begun on nasal oxygen, and a pulse oximeter is placed. Oxygen saturation remains between 92% and 98% as long as he is suctioned frequently. The neonatal transport team is called, and the infant is transported to a pediatric surgical center for definitive care.
   Please answer all questions before proceeding to discussion section.

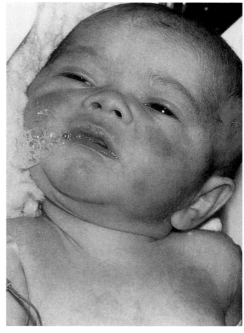

Figure 46–1. *Appearance of a newborn infant with excessive salivation. (See also color plate.)*

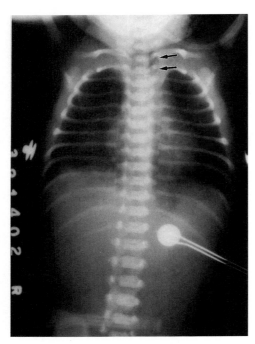

Figure 46–2. *"Babygram" showing an air-filled proximal esophageal pouch (arrows), containing a faintly visible catheter. The abdomen is gasless.*

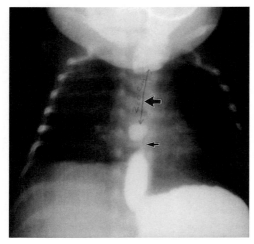

Figure 46–3. *Contrast study showing a 2.0-cm gap (large arrow) between proximal and distal ends of esophagus. An unexpected finding was a narrowed segment (small arrow) of distal esophagus.*

✓ QUESTIONS

1. Gasless abdomen is associated with:
   A. Isolated esophageal atresia
   B. Esophageal atresia with proximal tracheoesophageal fistula (TEF)
   C. Esophageal atresia with distal TEF
   D. A and B
   E. All of the above

2. All of the following statements regarding isolated esophageal atresia are true *except:*
   A. Isolated esophageal atresia is the second most common anatomic variant after proximal atresia with distal TEF
   B. Initial management should be gastrostomy and suction of the upper pouch
   C. Mechanical bouginage to stretch the proximal pouch is essential to permit primary anastomosis of the esophagus in the first weeks of life
   D. Anastomotic complications occur in a higher percentage of cases following repair of isolated esophageal atresia than following repair of other anatomic variants of the anomaly
   E. The risk of aspiration pneumonia is less for isolated atresia than for other anatomic variants

HOSPITAL COURSE *(CONT.)*   After gastrostomy, the infant is treated by suction on the upper pouch and gastrostomy feedings. A contrast study (Figure 46–3) is obtained at 5 weeks of age. Thoracotomy is performed at 6 weeks of age, and end-to-end esophageal anastomosis is completed with minimal tension. The distal esophagus is well developed. An intramural nodule (Figure 46–3, arrow) is removed and proves to be cartilage (ie, a tracheal remnant!). He does well postoperatively. A mild postoperative stricture requires dilation.

3. An infant with esophageal atresia undergoes thoracotomy for possible esophageal anastomosis at 6 weeks of age. In spite of maximal mobilization, the esophageal pouches remain about 2 cm apart. Which of the following procedures is the *best* option?
   A. Circular myotomy of the proximal pouch, end-to-end anastomosis under tension
   B. Segmental jejunal interposition
   C. Colonic interposition
   D. Emergency construction and placement of a reverse gastric tube
   E. Cervical esophagostomy and esophageal replacement (with colon or stomach) 6 to 12 months later

4. Which of the following statements regarding the outcome of esophageal replacement is true?
   A. Isoperistaltic interposition of the colon is superior to antiperistaltic interposition
   B. Retrosternal placement of the colon is superior to retrohilar placement
   C. Interposition of the transverse colon is superior to interposition of right or left colon

D. Anastomotic leak is more common with colonic interposition than with reverse gastric tube
E. Pyloroplasty is usually recommended with colonic interposition

5. All of the following statements regarding pediatric esophageal surgery are true *except:*
A. The diagnosis of proximal TEF or double TEF (associated with esophageal atresia) is best made at the operating table by complete mobilization of the upper pouch
B. Endoscopy is the definitive method for diagnosis of laryngotracheoesophageal cleft
C. H-type TEF is usually repaired via a right cervical incision
D. Gastric transposition is an alternative for esophageal replacement in children
E. Caustic injury to the esophagus has decreased in frequency in the United States during the past 20 to 25 years

6. Figure 46–4 is the barium esophagram at 14 months of age in an infant with repaired esophageal atresia with widely separated pouches. Postoperatively, she had an anastomotic leak, which healed, and a severe stricture, which recurred in spite of multiple dilations. She also had a Nissen fundoplication to correct gastroesophageal reflux. The treatment of choice now is:
A. Colonic interposition
B. Reverse gastric tube
C. Gastric interposition
D. Repeat thoracotomy, resection of stricture, primary anastomosis
E. Surgeon's choice

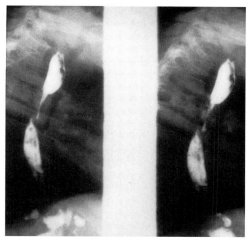

Figure 46–4. *Severe esophageal stricture 1 year following repair of wide-gap esophageal atresia (in a patient different from the one shown in Figures 46–2 and 46–3).*

ANSWERS AND DISCUSSION

1. **D** Air normally enters the gastrointestinal (GI) tract by swallowing. If the infant has esophageal atresia, however, the air must enter via a TEF, which is in continuity with the stomach. Isolated atresia (**A**) and atresia with proximal TEF (**B**) have no such connection; hence, the gasless abdomen.

2. **C** A lesson from history: bouginage of the upper pouch is not essential. Howard and Myers who introduced the technique in Melbourne later abandoned it (even as others jumped on the bandwagon) after their serendipitous discovery that anastomosis was usually possible in about 6 to 10 weeks, whether or not bouginage was carried out. All of the other statements are true. Isolated esophageal atresia comprises 8% to 10% of cases in every series (**A**), second only to the blind upper pouch with distal fistula. Initial management is by gastrostomy (for feeding) and suction of the upper pouch (**B**); the pouches are invariably too far apart to permit anastomosis in the first week. Anastomotic complications (**D**) (leak and stricture) occur in a higher proportion of cases with isolated esophageal atresia because of the wide gap between pouches and the resulting tension on the anastomosis. Most anastomotic complications are a function of the gap. Aspiration pneumonia is less common with isolated atresia (**E**) than with other variants because aspiration of gastric juice is anatomically impossible prior to repair. Aspiration of saliva may oc-

cur, but it is not as injurious to the airways because saliva is much less acidic than gastric juice.

3. **A** Ideally, one never performs an anastomosis under tension. The best choice in this scenario, however, is (**A**) to accept the risk of leak or stricture rather than abandon the esophagus (**B** to **E**). The circular myotomy adds about 1 cm of length to the upper pouch, decreasing the tension slightly. A patch of pleura, pericardium, or azgous vein may be used to buttress the anastomosis, limiting leakage. Myers stated the guiding principle: "One's own oesophagus is the best oesophagus," (ie, "There's no esophagus like an esophago-esophagus"). The surgeon should make every effort to retain the native esophagus without placing the baby in a life-threatening position. The trend in management is to wait for esophageal growth, while maintaining the infant on gastrostomy feedings and suction of the proximal pouch. End-to-end esophageal anastomosis is almost always possible after 6 to 20 weeks. Esophageal replacement by colon (**C**) or by reverse gastric tube (**D**) are standard methods of esophageal substitution, but are options for later, if the native esophagus cannot be salvaged. They are not appropriate emergency operations in a 6-week-old infant. The use of jejunum (**B**) as an esophageal substitute in children is limited by its precarious blood supply.

4. **E** Pyloroplasty is usually recommended in conjunction with colonic interposition in order to overcome gastric stasis and delayed emptying that may occur after the procedure. (Stasis may also occur in the colon graft, which typically becomes elongated and redundant as the child grows.) All of the other statements are false. The colon conduit generally lacks peristalsis and empties by gravity; placement in an isoperistaltic or antiperistaltic (**A**) position makes no difference. Results are similar with retrosternal versus retrohilar (**B**) placement of the graft. Outcomes are similar for colonic interposition (**C**) whether right, left, or transverse colon is used. Anastomotic leak (**D**) complicates the postoperative course of one third to one half of children who undergo either colonic interposition or gastric tube esophagoplasty. Neither technique is clearly superior. The cervical anastomosis is especially vulnerable because of marginal blood supply. An anastomotic leak is usually followed by stricture. The existence of multiple different operations for a single surgical problem usually indicates that none of the operations has worked wonderfully. Gurus in this subject agree that the ideal conduit has yet to be developed.

5. **A** The diagnosis of proximal TEF or double TEF is usually made by a preoperative contrast study of the proximal pouch (performed by a skilled pediatric radiologist) or by preoperative tracheobronchoscopy. Unfortunately, a small proximal fistula can be missed with either technique. Fortunately, however, both are rare, comprising a total of about 2% of esophageal anomalies. At endoscopy, the proximal TEF typically looks like a little mucosal bump on the membranous trachea, which should be gently probed with the tip of a ureteral or Fogarty catheter to identify a fistula. Extensive mobilization of the upper pouch to rule out these rare variants is unnecessary and risks injury of the recurrent laryngeal nerve(s). All of the

other statements are true. Laryngotracheoesophageal cleft (**B**), the most severe variant of TEF, is best diagnosed endoscopically; contrast studies are more hazardous. Most H-type TEFs can be repaired through a low cervical incision (**C**). The right side is preferred to avoid injury to the thoracic duct. Gastric transposition (**D**), a technique used in adults with esophageal carcinoma, is the procedure of choice for esophageal replacement at the Hospital for Sick Children, Great Ormond Street, London. The stomach is mobilized in the abdomen and drawn up to the neck without thoracotomy, using stay sutures, via a tunnel in the posterior mediastinum. In 83 such procedures in children, Spitz reported a 7.2% mortality, 12% leak rate, and 12% stricture rate—outcomes that were superior to those cited for other techniques. Caustic ingestion (**E**), once a major injury leading to esophageal replacement in children, has decreased in the United States following the mandated packaging of caustic agents with child-proof caps. Lye burns of the esophagus still occur, however, usually when a child swallows a caustic substance that was poured out of the original container and left in a cup or bottle by a careless adult.

6. **E** Different pediatric surgeons will select different operations in this situation. Any one of the procedures may correct the problem, but, unfortunately, all carry risks. In a difficult clinical situation, the wise surgeon chooses the operation at which he or she is most experienced. (This author's bias would be [**D**], which has worked in this situation and preserves the esophagus. A few months' delay could be advantageous since the stricture may still be too long to permit primary anastomosis after resection; another centimeter or two of esophageal growth might make the difference between success and failure.)

BIBLIOGRAPHY

Anderson KD, Randolph JG. The gastric tube for esophageal replacement in children. *J Thorac Cardiovasc Surg.* 1973;66:333–342.

Brown AK, Tam PK. Measurement of gap length in esophageal atresia: a simple predictor of outcome. *J Am Coll Surg.* 1996;182:41–45.

Harmon CM, Coran AG. Congenital anomalies of the esophagus. In: O'Neill JA Jr, Rowe MI, Grosfeld JL, et al. eds. *Pediatric Surgery.* 5th ed. St. Louis: Mosby-Year Book; 1998:941–967.

Howard R, Myers NA. Esophageal atresia: a technique elongating the upper pouch. *Surgery.* 1965;58:725–727.

Kosloske AM. Axygous flap technique for reinforcement of esophageal closure. *J Pediatr Surg.* 1990;25:793–794.

Millar AJW, Cywes S. Caustic strictures of the esophagus. In: O'Neill JA Jr, Rowe MI, Grosfeld JL, et al. eds. *Pediatric Surgery.* 5th ed. St. Louis: Mosby-Year Book; 1998:969–979.

Myers NA. Large gap between the segments: international symposium on oesophageal atresia. *Z Kinderchir Suppl.* 1975;17:3–28.

Puri P, Blake N, O'Donnell B, et al. Delayed primary anastomosis following spontaneous growth of esophageal segments in esophageal atresia. *J Pediatr Surg.* 1981;16:180–183.

Spitz L. Esophageal replacement. In: O'Neill JA Jr, Rowe MI, Grosfeld JL, et al. eds. *Pediatric Surgery.* 5th ed. St. Louis: Mosby-Year Book; 1998: 981–995.

AN ABDOMINAL WALL DEFECT IN A NEWBORN

HISTORY   A 3-kg term infant is born by elective cesarean section with a large, antenatally diagnosed omphalocele. The fascial defect is large, approximately 8 cm, the amnion is intact, and the contained viscera include stomach, most of the intestine, liver, and spleen (Figure 47–1; see also color plate). The baby is pink and breathing comfortably on room air.

Please answer all questions before proceeding to discussion section.

✓ QUESTIONS

1. The antenatal evaluation of this infant would have likely included:
   A. Maternal serum alpha-fetoprotein (MSAFP)
   B. Serial ultrasounds

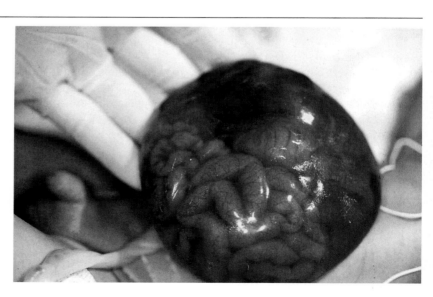

Figure 47–1. *Giant omphalocele with intact amnion containing all hollow and solid viscera. Primary closure was impossible, and placement of a prosthetic silo was necessary to achieve gradual reduction of herniated viscera. (See also color plate.)*

    C. Amniocentesis
    D. Fetal echocardiography
    E. All of the above

2. An antenatal diagnosis of a large omphalocele is considered a contraindication to vaginal delivery:
    A. True
    B. False

3. The frequency of association of other congential malformations with omphalocele is:
    A. Ten percent
    B. Fifty percent
    C. Ninety percent

4. The most common associated cardiovascular malformation is:
    A. Ebstein's anomaly
    B. Ventricular septal defect
    C. Tetralogy of Fallot
    D. Atrial septal defect

5. All of the following feautres help to distinguish omphalocele from gastroschisis *except:*
    A. The location of the umbilical cord relative to the defect
    B. Coexistent intestinal atresia
    C. Coexistent malrotation
    D. Presence of covering amnion

6. Factors precluding primary abdominal wall closure include:
    A. High required ventilator pressures
    B. The presence of associated malformations
    C. Hepatic outflow obstruction
    D. Omphalocele sac rupture

7. The mortality rate is determined by:
    A. Associated malformations
    B. The size of the fascial defect
    C. The tightness of primary abdominal closure
    D. The occurrence of sepsis

ANSWERS AND DISCUSSION

1. **E** Improved prenatal diagnosis has led to an increased awareness of abdominal wall defects, which are often first suspected by an elevated maternal serum alpha-fetoprotein (MSAFP). An elevation of MSAFP to two multiples of the median is 78% predictive of omphalocele. Ultrasonography can detect abdominal wall defects as early as 10 weeks' gestation and can easily distinguish omphalocele from gastroschisis based on the presence of an amniotic covering and the umbilical cord insertion site. Doppler sonography is useful for characterizing herniation of solid viscera, such as liver or spleen. Amniocentesis and karyotyping should be considered in light of the 20% association with major chromosomal malformations (trisomy 13, 18, and 21), for which termination may be a consideration. Fetal

echocardiography should be performed to detect life-threatening cardiac defects.

2. **A** Although small omphaloceles containing only intestine can be safely delivered vaginally, the main risks associated with attempted vaginal delivery of large omphaloceles are dystocia, amnion rupture, and solid viscous (liver, spleen) injury.

3. **B** The reported incidence of anomalies associated with omphalocele ranges from 37% to 81%. Approximately two thirds of these malformations are major (cardiovascular, central nervous system, and genitourinary), while one third are minor (skeletal, gastrointestinal, and genitourinary). Approximately 20% have a chromosomal abnormality (trisomy 13 to 15, 18, and 21) or the Beckwith-Weidemann syndrome (macrosomia, macroglossia, and hypoglycemia).

4. **C** The cardiovascular malformation most commonly associated with omphalocele is tetralogy of Fallot, followed by atrial septal defect.

5. **C** Malrotation, or more commonly, nonrotation (small bowel on the right side, colon on the left) is seen in omphalocele and gastroschisis since the normal process of midgut herniation, rotation, reduction, and fixation is disrupted in both. Omphaloceles are umbilical defects that always have an amniotic covering, while in gastroschisis the bowel is unprotected and the defect lies to the right of the umbilicus. Gastroschisis is more often associated with intestinal injury in the form of atresias, stenoses, and short gut, and it is the condition and length of the intestine and the required duration of parenteral nutrition that is the principal determinant of outcome.

6. **C** Primary abdominal wall (fascia and skin) closure is always the preferred treatment, and it is possible for most smaller omphaloceles that do not contain liver. If a primary closure requires forcible visceral reduction to the extent that respiratory function is impaired, vena caval or hepatic venous return is impeded or mesenteric blood flow is compromised, then attempts at primary closure should be abandoned, and a prosthetic "silo" (with amnion preservation) placed for gradual visceral reduction (Figure 47–2). The baby returns to the nursery and is maintained on parenteral nutrition with nasogastric intestinal decompression. The viscera are reduced gradually by mechanical means until delayed primary abdominal wall closure is possible. Other treatment options for giant omphaloceles not amenable to primary closure include skin flap closure and amnion escharization. Both techniques create large ventral hernias that require eventual secondary closure.

7. **A** The principal determinant of outcome in omphalocele is the presence of associated life-threatening malformations, most commonly cardiovascular, chromosomal, or both.

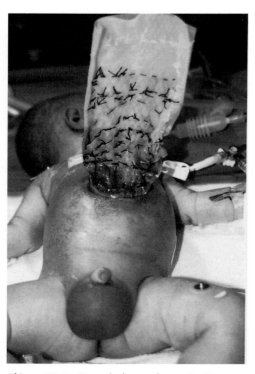

Figure 47–2. *Same baby as shown in Figure 47–1 1 week after placement of an abdominal silo over the intact amnion with twice daily reductions. The viscera have returned to the abdominal compartment, and delayed primary fascial closure is now possible.*

BIBLIOGRAPHY

Cooney DR. Defects of the abdominal wall. In: O'Neill JA, Rowe MI, Grosfeld JL, et al. *Pediatric Surgery.* 5th ed. St. Louis: Mosby-Year Book; 1998.

Grosfeld JL, Weber TR. Congenital abdominal wall defects: gastroschisis and omphalocele. *Curr Probl Surg.* 1982;19:157.

Sermer M, et al. Prenatal diagnosis and management of congenital defects of the anterior abdominal wall. *Am J Obstet Gynecol.* 1987;156:308.

A NEWBORN GIRL
WITH RESPIRATORY DISTRESS

HISTORY A 41-week gestational aged girl is born via cesarean section for failure to progress. The amniotic fluid is stained dark green with thick fluid. Initial Apgar score is 4. The baby is rapidly intubated and ventilated. At the time of intubation, meconium is found in the trachea. With mechanical ventilation and 100% oxygen, the baby's color and perfusion become normal. The infant is stabilized in the neonatal intensive care unit on the following ventilator settings: pressure 24/5, rate 30, F_{IO_2} 0.40. Chest radiograph shows diffuse bilateral airspace disease.

Over the next 12 hours, the infant requires marked increases in ventilatory parameters to maintain adequate oxygenation and ventilation. You are called to evaluate the patient for extracorporeal membrane oxygenation (ECMO). At this time, ventilator settings are pressure 40/5, rate 80, F_{IO_2} 1.0.

EXAMINATION The baby is 4800 g. She is agitated and thrashing about despite having received large doses of morphine. Vital signs are temperature 37.4°C, heart rate 190, blood pressure 80/60. Capillary refill time is 2 seconds in all four extremities. Breath sounds are equal but coarse and squeaky bilaterally. Lung expansion is poor despite the high inspiratory pressure. The heart sounds are distant but normal without murmur. There is moderate total body edema, but the remainder of the examination is otherwise normal.

LABORATORY Oxygen saturation from a pulse oximeter probe on the right index finger is 89%. Arterial blood gas data from the umbilical artery catheter are pH 7.32, P_{CO_2} 34, P_{O_2} 41, oxygen saturation 63%. Electrolytes and complete blood count are normal. A repeat chest radiograph is shown in Figure 48–1.

Please answer all questions before proceeding to discussion section.

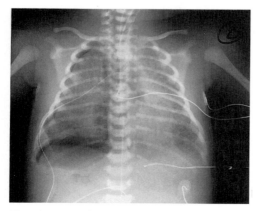

Figure 48–1. *Chest x-ray of newborn with respiratory failure.*

✓ QUESTIONS

1. Why does the oxygen saturation from the pulse oximeter differ markedly from the measured saturation from the arterial blood gas?
   A. The pulse oximeter is inaccurate because the patient has poor peripheral perfusion
   B. The patient has congenital heart disease causing an intracardiac right-to-left shunt
   C. The patient has a right-to-left shunt outside the heart
   D. Oxygen saturation is fluctuating rapidly in this critically ill baby; both values are accurate
   E. Ventilation perfusion mismatch from the aspirated meconium has caused a large intrapulmonary shunt

2. Correct initial management includes:
   A. Placement of a chest tube in the right chest
   B. Cannulation and placement on venovenous ECMO
   C. Cannulation and placement on venoarterial ECMO
   D. Initiation of high-frequency oscillatory ventilation
   E. Delivery of inhaled nitric oxide at 20 ppm

3. Which of the following constitute appropriate reasons to institute ECMO?
   A. An oxygen index (OI = [mean airway pressure × percent FIO_2] / PaO_2) of greater than 40
   B. Severe barotrauma on required ventilator settings
   C. A predicted mortality of 80% using conventional therapy
   D. Cardiac arrest requiring cardiopulmonary resuscitation
   E. All of the above

4. This baby fails to respond to high-frequency ventilation, inotropic support, and nitric oxide therapy. The decision is made to institute venovenous ECMO. Which of the following statements regarding venovenous ECMO compared to venoarterial ECMO is true?
   A. It results in increased survival of patients with respiratory failure and normal cardiac function
   B. Preserving the right carotid artery decreases the risk of ischemic damage to the right side of the brain
   C. It results in better long-term neurologic outcome than venoarterial ECMO
   D. It should not be used when there is echocardiographic evidence of poor ventricular function
   E. Increases in ECMO flow rate will not improve systemic perfusion

5. The baby is placed on ECMO. What is her chance of survival?
   A. Less than 10%
   B. Twenty-five percent
   C. Fifty percent
   D. Seventy-five percent
   E. Greater than 90%

6. ECMO is *least* effective for which of the following conditions?
   A. Sepsis
   B. Meconium aspiration syndrome

C. Respiratory distress syndrome
D. Viral pneumonia
E. Congenital diaphragmatic hernia

7. With respect to the cost of treating patients with ECMO compared to treatment with conventional ventilation, which is true?
A. The ECMO costs 20% more than conventional therapy
B. The costs are roughly equivalent
C. The ECMO costs more because hospital stays are longer
D. The ECMO results in lower hospital charges but higher professional fees

8. Which of the following about ECMO is true?
A. Extracorporeal membrane oxygenation (ECMO) appears to be very effective, but there is no direct evidence that survival is improved
B. Extracorporeal membrane oxygenation (ECMO) improves survival slightly but often at the expense of severe neurologic compromise
C. Extracorporeal membrane oxygenation (ECMO) improves survival without compromising neurologic outcome
D. Extracorporeal membrane oxygenation (ECMO) will likely be replaced by nitric oxide therapy
E. Extracorporeal membrane oxygenation (ECMO) improves outcome in babies with pure pulmonary hypertension, but the results in sepsis and pneumonia are equivocal

ANSWERS AND DISCUSSION

1. **C** The pulmonary arterial bed of neonates differs markedly from that of adults in two important ways. It is very muscular, and it is exquisitely sensitive to oxygen. Hypoxic neonates develop severe pulmonary hypertension resulting in pulmonary arterial pressures that far exceed systemic pressures. This causes right-to-left shunting at the level of the ductus arteriosus. Thus, **C** is the correct answer. Both oxygen saturation measurements are correct. The pulse oximeter on the right arm is measuring oxygen saturation of blood ejected from the left ventricle prior to its dilution with pulmonary arterial (venous) blood at the level of the ductus arteriosus (preductal). The blood gas drawn from the umbilical artery catheter in the aorta is distal to the level of the ductus (postductal); therefore, it has a lower oxygen saturation.

   B and **E** are incorrect. Any form of intracardiac or intrapulmonary shunt would affect all arterial blood equally. Saturation would be equivalent above or below the ductus arteriosus. **A** is incorrect. Modern pulse oximeters function well even in states of moderate hypoperfusion. If the oximeter is accurately tracking the heart rate, it should be accurate.

2. **A** The chest radiograph reveals a right pneumothorax. Barotrauma is extremely common in neonates requiring high levels of ventilatory support. Any clinical deterioration should be evaluated with a repeat chest x-ray. Physical examination is notoriously insensitive for detecting a pneumothorax. Placement of a chest tube will allow expansion of the lung and may result in enough improvement to avoid

high-frequency ventilation or ECMO. In the rush to proceed to ECMO or other complex strategies, it is easy to miss a problem as easily treated as a pneumothorax. Barotrauma can also result in pneumomediastinum and pulmonary interstitial emphysema. While neither of these entities requires specific treatment, they are markers that the current ventilation strategy is injuring the lung. Figure 48–2 shows reexpansion of the right lung following chest tube placement.

3. **E** All of the responses are true. Initially, an OI of greater than 40 was required to meet ECMO criteria. Data suggest that this value should be significantly decreased. In the early years of ECMO use, it was only instituted when the patient was felt to have a greater than 80% chance of mortality by conventional treatment. This criteria has been broadened as well. Since conventional therapy for neonates is constantly improving, rigid criteria for ECMO will never exist. Most centers no longer use rigid criteria but rather use ECMO based on clinical judgment of the treating physicians. In patients requiring CPR, ECMO has been used with 60% survival.

4. **E** Venoarterial (VA) ECMO requires cannulation of the right internal jugular vein and common carotid artery. Blood is removed from the right-sided circulation, oxygenated, and returned to the left. It provides pulmonary and cardiac support. Venovenous (VV) ECMO is accomplished via a double lumen cannula in the right atrium (Figure 48–3). Blood is drained from the atrium and returned to the atrium directed out the tricuspid valve. Venovenous ECMO provides only pulmonary support and does not augment cardiac output. It is appropriate for babies with respiratory failure and a normal heart (most neonates requiring ECMO). Carotid cannulation and ligation is not necessary. Figure 48–4 shows the double lumen venovenous cannula properly positioned with its tip at the base of the heart and inflow directed through the tricuspid valve.

Survival with VV ECMO is equivalent to that with VA. Many patients with profound desaturation have poor cardiac function. This is not a contraindication to VV ECMO. As soon as ECMO is established and oxygenation improves, the heart functions normally. While preservation of the right carotid artery can only be good, statistical analysis of neurologic problems in ECMO patients have failed to show a difference between patients treated with VV or VA ECMO. The long-term implications of carotid ligation are unknown. These data may not exist until the current cohort of ECMO patients reach their seventh and eighth decades.

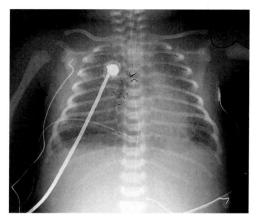

Figure 48–2. *Reexpansion of right lung following chest tube placement.*

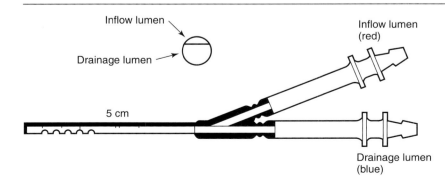

Inflow lumen

Drainage lumen

5 cm

Inflow lumen (red)

Drainage lumen (blue)

Figure 48–3. *Double lumen venovenous ECMO cannula.*

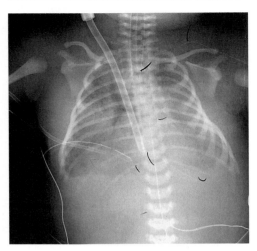

Figure 48–4. *Chest x-ray showing properly positioned double lumen venovenous ECMO catheter. The tip is at the base of the right atrium.*

5. **E** Data from the Extracorporeal Life Support Organization registry reported a 94% survival for neonates with meconium aspiration treated with ECMO. Survival for other diagnoses are respiratory distress syndrome 84%, primary pulmonary hypertension 82%, sepsis or pneumonia 76%, and congenital diaphragmatic hernia 59%.

6. **E** See statistics in answer 5. The treatment of congenital diaphragmatic hernia (CDH) remains a challenge. While complex statistical analysis suggests that ECMO has probably improved survival, the impact has been small. The severe pulmonary hypertension that occurs in these patients is exceedingly difficult to treat. While pulmonary hypoplasia is an important factor, the degree of hypoplasia does not directly correlate with outcome.

7. **B** Data suggest that the daily cost of caring for a patient on ECMO is double that for conventional therapy. The hospital stay in ECMO patients, however, is about half that for similar patients treated conventionally. Thus, the cost is about the same.

8. **C** This controversial question has finally been answered unequivocally. The first trial published by Bartlett and coworkers in 1985 used a "play the winner" strategy that favored randomization toward the therapy with success. In this trial, one patient died on conventional therapy and eleven out of eleven patients treated with ECMO survived. This study was widely criticized for its randomization technique. O'Rourke and associates used a related strategy in 1989. These results were also criticized. One published prospective randomized trial from the United Kingdom has shown without question that ECMO markedly increases survival over conventional therapy.

BIBLIOGRAPHY

Anderson HL, Snedecor SM, Tetsoru Otsu, et al. Multicenter comparison of conventional veonarterial access versus venovenous double lumen catheter access in newborn infants undergoing extracorporeal membrane oxygenation. *J Pediatr Surg.* 1993;28:530–535.

Bartlett RH, Roloff DW, Cornell RG, et al. Extracorporeal circulation in neonatal respiratory failure: a prospective randomized study. *Pediatrics.* 1985;76:479.

Kanto WP, Bunyapen C. Extracorporeal membrane oxygenation: controversies in selection of patients and management. *Clin Perinat.* 1998; 25:123–135.

Lally KP. Extracorporeal membrane oxygenation in patients with congenital diaphragmatic hernia. *Semin Pediatr Surg.* 1996;5:249–255.

O'Rourke PP, Crone R, Vacanti J, et al. Extracorporeal membrane oxygenation and conventional medical therapy in neonates with persistent pulmonary hypertension of the newborn: a prospective randomized study. *Pediatrics.* 1989;84:957.

Pearson GD, Short BL. An economic analysis of extracorporeal membrane oxygenation. *J Inten Care Med.* 1987;2:116.

UK Collaborative ECMO Trial Group. UK collaborative randomized trial of neonatal extracorporeal membrane oxygenation. *Lancet.* 1996;348:75.

IN UTERO DIAGNOSIS OF A FETUS WITH CONGENITAL DIAPHRAGMATIC HERNIA

HISTORY   A 35-year-old primigravid female is referred for a fetal sonogram at 23 weeks' gestation after she is noted by her obstetrician to be large for dates. The ultrasound (Figure 49–1) demonstrates a live fetus with a three vessel umbilical cord and increased amniotic fluid volume. There is an apparent left-sided diaphragmatic hernia with a dilated stomach, intestine, spleen, and liver in the left hemithorax. The fetal heart is displaced into the right hemithorax.

LABORATORY   An amniocentesis and fetal echocardiogram were ordered.

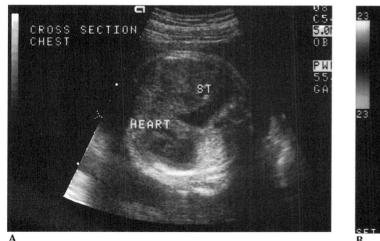
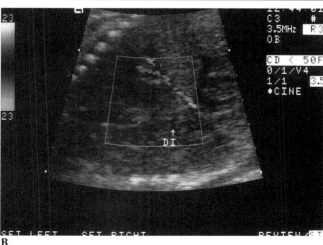

A   B

Figure 49–1. A. *Transverse sonogram through the fetal thorax shows herniation of the fetal stomach (ST) and other viscera with displacement of the heart across midline.* **B.** *A longitudinal Doppler sonogram through the fetal thorax and abdomen shows vascular flow across the diaphragm (DI) into the thorax within the herniated left lobe of fetal liver.*

Please answer all questions before proceeding to discussion section.

✓ QUESTIONS

1. Prenatal diagnosis of a congenital malformation increases the likelihood of survival after birth:
   A. True
   B. False

2. The cause of increased amniotic fluid volume (polyhydramnios) in this pregnancy is:
   A. Increased placental blood flow
   B. Fetal polyuria
   C. Gastric outlet obstruction
   D. None of the above

3. The most common chromosomal abnormality detected in association with congenital diaphragmatic hernia (CDH) diagnosed in utero is:
   A. Trisomy 13
   B. Trisomy 18
   C. Trisomy 21
   D. Deletion of short arm of chromosome 11

4. Fetal echocardiography is extremely accurate in identifying cardiac malformations associated with CDH:
   A. True
   B. False

5. The most common cardiac association of CDH (not including patent ductus arteriosus or patent foramen ovale) is:
   A. Left heart "smallness" or hypoplasia
   B. Atrial septal defect (ASD)
   C. Ventricular septal defect (VSD)
   D. Tetralogy of Fallot

6. Based on the sonographic data given, the expected mortality for this baby at birth with best available postnatal care (including ECMO) would be estimated to be:
   A. Ten percent
   B. Thirty percent
   C. Sixty percent
   D. Ninety percent

7. Fetal tracheal occlusion is a treatment option for high-risk fetal diaphragmatic hernia:
   A. True
   B. False

ANSWERS AND DISCUSSION

1. **B** Intuitively, one might surmise that the diagnosis of a condition prior to birth might improve postnatal outcome. Awareness of the

condition before birth permits planned delivery in specialized centers, and in select circumstances, an opportunity for prenatal intervention, but for the most part, such awareness has little impact on outcome. In fact, survival outcome comparisons between groups of patients with congenital malformations diagnosed prenatally as opposed to postnatally illustrates the concept of the "hidden mortality" of prenatal diagnosis. Infants with one congenital malformation diagnosed prenatally are at risk for other malformations that may contribute to fetal or early neonatal demise; hence, infants that "survive" to be diagnosed postnatally are self-selected to a better outcome. This phenomenon has been observed with a number of congenital malformations for which diagnoses can be made prenatally, including esophageal atresia, cystic hygroma, and CDH.

2. **C** Polyhydramnios occurring in association with CDH is usually the result of gastric outlet obstruction caused by kinking or extrinsic compression of the herniated intrathoracic stomach. This prevents egress of swallowed amniotic fluid and results in amniotic fluid accumulation. Some authors consider the development of polyhydramnios to be reflective of the severity of pulmonary hypoplasia, and, therefore, an unfavorable outcome indicator for CDH.

3. **B** There are a number of genetic associations of CDH, but in most series, the most common is trisomy 18. It is important to perform an amniocentesis or some form of invasive sampling to identify those fetuses who have a life-threatening chromosomal abnormality in addition to CDH, since it will impact a family's decision making. Other genetic conditions associated with CDH include Fryns syndrome, Marfan syndrome, and Beckwith-Weidemann syndrome.

4. **B** Fetal echocardiography has not proven to be particularly reliable in providing accurate anatomic diagnoses of cardiac defects associated with CDH. This can be attributed to a number of factors including sonographer expertise, fetal positioning, and anatomic distortion of the heart due to mediastinal compression.

5. **A** Increasingly, the most frequent cardiac association with CDH is a condition called left heart hypoplasia or "smalless." It has been postulated that in utero mediastinal compression by herniated intrathoracic viscera compresses both the lungs and heart, resulting in "cardiopulmonary hypoplasia." Impaired cardiac function in association with pulmonary hypoplasia and pulmonary hypertension appears to be a particularly lethal combination for the infant with CDH.

6. **C** The mortality rate for isolated CDH diagnosed before 24 weeks' gestation with the best postnatal therapy, including ECMO, has been reported to be 58%. Attempts to identify reliable prenatal predictors of outcome have been, for the most part, unsuccessful, although early gestational diagnosis and herniation of the left lobe of liver into the left hemithorax have proven to be fairly accurate predictors of neonatal mortality despite ECMO support. More recently, echocardiographic measurements of fetal heart size and the ratio of fetal lung area to head circumference have shown promise as reliable predictors of postnatal outcome.

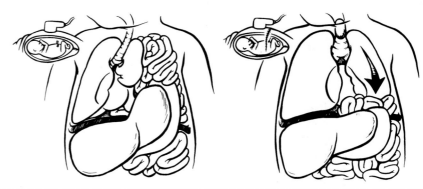

Figure 49–2. *A schematic showing the physiologic effects of fetal tracheal occlusion. Note that the intraluminal tracheal "plug" has resulted in lung growth, mediastinal shift back-to-midline, and a gradual reduction of herniated abdominal viscera.*

7. **A** Fetal tracheal occlusion of "PLUG" (Plug the Lung Until it Grows) (Figure 49–2) is currently being investigated as in utero therapy for cases of antenatally diagnosed CDH deemed, by prognostic criteria, to have a near 0% chance of survival with optimal postnatal care, including ECMO. The physiologic basis for tracheal occlusion as a treatment for high-risk CDH is the observation, in both animal models and human "experiments of nature," that fetal tracheal obstruction results in supraphysiologic lung growth and gradual reduction of the herniated viscera so that at birth, the baby is born without lung hypoplasia or associated pulmonary hypertension (Figures 49–2 and 49–3). The mechanism of accelerated lung growth in the presence of tracheal occlusion is not understood, but it is believed to be mediated by mechanical and hormonal growth stimuli triggered by the prevented egress of fluid from the fetal lungs into the amniotic cavity. Fetal tracheal occlusion has evolved from an open procedure to a minimally invasive one done with 2- to 3-mm instrument ports through the uterine wall (Figure 49–3). Fetal lung growth can be followed sonographically after the procedure, and at cesarean delivery, it is necessary to maintain the fetoplacental circulation while a patent neonatal airway is established.

BIBLIOGRAPHY

Fauza Do, Wilson JM. Congenital diaphragmatic hernia and associated anomalies: their incidence, identification, and impact on prognosis. *J Pediatr Surg.* 1994;29:1113–1117.

Harrison MR, Adzick NS, Estes JM, et al. A prospective study of the outcome of fetuses with congenital diaphragmatic hernia. *JAMA.* 1994; 271:382–384.

Metkus AP, Filly RA, Stringer MD, et al. Sonographic predictors of survival in fetal diaphragmatic hernia. *J Pediatr Surg.* 1996;31:148–151.

Sharland GK, Lockhart SM, Heward AJ, et al. Prognosis in fetal diaphragmatic hernia. *Am J Obstet Gynecol.* 1992;166:9–13.

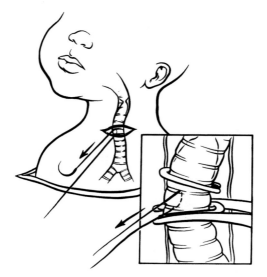

Figure 49–3. *Another technique of tracheal occlusion: the tracheal "clip." The advantage of this procedure is that it can be done without hysterotomy using standard minimally invasive surgical techniques, employing warm saline (rather than CO_2), low pressure insufflation.*

A 7-YEAR-OLD BOY WITH A LAP BELT ABDOMINAL INJURY

HISTORY   A 7-year-old boy is a rear seat, lap belt restrained passenger in a head-on collision at 55 mph. The driver, the boy's father, suffers severe chest and facial injuries, and the driver of the other car is killed instantly. After a 45-minute extrication, the boy is transported by helicopter to a nearby trauma center. He was reported as unconscious for approximately 10 minutes after impact. At the trauma center, he is awake but confused and complains of diffuse abdominal and pelvic pain. He appears to be breathing easily, and his oxygen saturaton is 100% on 50% oxygen by face mask. His vital signs are pulse 110, blood pressure 110/67, respirations 28, temperature 35.1°C. His weight is estimated to be 20 kg. He has two large bore antecubital intravenous (IV) lines that are infusing normal saline at 10 mL/h.

EXAMINATION   The boy is conversant but confused with no externally evident head injury, and his ears are clear. His neck is immoblized by hard collar. The trachea is midline; the clavicles are intact. His lungs are clear; his abdomen is flat. He has a faint bruise and skin abrasion across his lower abdomen between the anterior superior iliac spines (Figure 50–1), with mild, but nonlocalized, abdominal tenderness. His pelvis is tender to compression. The rectal examination is normal. His extremities are normal.

LABORATORY   A chest and three-view cervical spine (anterior-posterior, lateral, odontoid) x-rays are normal. The x-ray of the pelvis demonstrates bilateral iliac wing fractures. Blood work and urinalysis are sent out.

Please answer all questions before proceeding to discussion section.

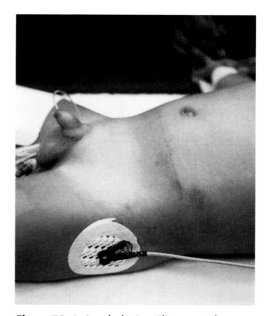

Figure 50–1. *Lap belt sign (iliac crest, lower abdominal wall abrasion, and contusion) in a child involved in a high-speed motor vehicle accident with two point (lap) restraint. In addition to the intra-abdominal injuries shown in Figure 50–2, he also suffered a traction injury to his thoracic spinal cord rendering him paraplegic.*

243

✓ QUESTIONS

1. Your bolus intravenous orders for this patient are:
   A. A 200 mL Ringer's lactate
   B. A 400 mL warmed Ringer's lactate
   C. A 400 mL 5% albumin
   D. No bolus required as patient has stable vital signs

2. What further radiologic investigations should be obtained?
   A. A computed tomography (CT) head (noncontrast); kidney, ureter, bladder (KUB); abdominal ultrasound; lateral thoracolumbar spine x-rays
   B. A CT head (noncontrast), CT abdomen/pelvis (with enteral contrast)
   C. A CT head (noncontrast), CT abdomen/pelvis (IV and enteral contrast), lateral thoracolumbar spine x-rays
   D. A CT head (with IV contrast), CT abdomen/pelvis (IV and enteral contrast)

3. While waiting to go to CT scan, the patient's heart rate is noted to be up to 125, and blood pressure 100/60. You would now order the following IV fluids:
   A. A 400-mL warmed Ringer's lactate bolus
   B. A 200-mL O-negative blood tranfusion over 30 minutes
   C. A 400-mL 5% albumin
   D. A 200-mL warmed Ringer's lactate

HOSPITAL COURSE The head CT scan is normal. The abdominal CT scan shows a scant amount of free fluid and a small retroperitoneal hematoma from the pelvic fracture. There is no injury to liver or spleen. The lumbar spine x-rays show no sign of fracture or dislocation. The child is now alert and verbally appropriate, and repeat abdominal examination demonstrates mild lower abdominal tenderness. The hematocrit is 32, white blood count 15,000, and amylase 110. Urinalysis is normal.

4. All of the following statements regarding diagnosis of blunt traumatic small bowel injuries are true *except:*
   A. A CT scan demonstrating a large quantity of free fluid, in the absence of a solid organ injury, is strongly suggestive of a small bowel injury
   B. Serum amylase level is a reliable indicator of bowel perforation
   C. The accuracy of a *negative* CT scan in predicting the *absence* of a small bowel injury is poor
   D. Peritoneal lavage may be helpful in the evaluation of an unconscious patient with an unreliable physical examination

5. The constellation of injuries associated with lap belt restrained head-on crashes include all of the following *except:*
   A. Liver laceration
   B. Small bowel perforation
   C. Duodenal hematoma
   D. Chance fracture of lumbar spine

6. The correct treatment in this case would be to:
   A. Admit the child to the pediatric intensive care unit for close observation and serial abdominal examinations
   B. Perform diagnostic peritoneal lavage (DPL)
   C. Take the child to the operating room for exploratory laparoscopy
   D. Take the child to the operating room for exploratory laparotomy

7. The delay in operative treatment of small bowel injury attributable to the time required for clinical signs to evolve is associated with an increased complication rate:
   A. True
   B. False

ANSWERS AND DISCUSSION

1. **B** Even though this patient appears hemodynamically stable, his injury mechanism and the presence of a pelvic fracture place him at high risk for the development of hypovolemic shock. He should, therefore, receive 20 mL/kg of warmed resuscitative crystalloid and continued close hemodynamic monitoring.

2. **C** In addition to chest, three-view cervical spine, and pelvic x-rays, all head-injured trauma patients should receive a noncontrast head CT scan. A double contrast (intravenous and enteral) CT scan of the abdomen and pelvis should be done to look for intra-abdominal injury, and in this instance, the injury mechanism and lap belt abdominal wall abrasion mandate that a lumbar spine injury be sought.

3. **A** According to Advanced Trauma Life Support (ATLS) recommendations, resuscitation of traumatic hypovolemic shock involves two boluses (20 mL/kg each) of crystalloid, followed by blood as needed to achieve hemodynamic stability.

4. **B** The diagnosis of small bowel injury in the context of blunt trauma and in the absence of obvious signs of peritonitis is a difficult one. Serum amylase levels are elevated in only about one third of patients with traumatic bowel perforation and may be elevated in the setting of facial trauma (salivary amylase) or mild pancreatic injury. Computed tomography (CT) scans do not reliably diagnose small bowel injury, in fact, in most series of traumatic small bowel perforation, the scan is normal in well over 50% of patients later found to have a small bowel injury. Diagnostic accuracy of a small bowel disruption goes up significantly if the CT scan demonstrates a large amount of free fluid without solid organ (liver or spleen) injury or in the presence of enteral contrast extravasation or free intraperitoneal air. These CT findings are infrequent, however, and the vast majority of patients with small bowel injury will have a normal CT scan on admission. An associated traumatic head injury makes the diagnosis of a small bowel injury more obscure, since the patient's altered level of consciousness creates a situation where physical examination of the abdomen is unreliable for the detection of peritonitis. Diagnostic peritoneal lavage (DPL) has been proposed as a useful diagnostic adjunct in situations where the CT findings or physical examination is equivocal. If intestinal succus, bile, food

fibers, or high amylase levels are discovered, then a small bowel injury should be suspected and a laparotomy performed. Most patients with a small bowel injury, however, have only blood in the lavage fluid, and since most pediatric trauma patients with intraperitoneal blood will not require operation, this is not a distinguishing finding. Diagnostic laparoscopy has been employed successfully and accurately in children with equivocal findings after lap belt injury, and it should now be considered part of the diagnostic armementarium. Since the vast majority of children with blunt abdominal trauma can be managed without operation, it is essential that a high index of suspicion of injury be maintained to identify the occasional child who requires laparotomy. This is particularly true in those patients with injury mechanisms (lap belt injuries, handle bar impalement injuries) known to predispose to small bowel disruption.

5. **A** Seat belt injuries are the result of a collision, usually head-on, with sudden deceleration and flexion of the upper torso about a fulcrum (the lap belt). This injury mechanism may result in a constellation of injuries to the abdominal wall, intestinal viscera and mesentery, retroperitoneum, and lumbar spine known collectively as the "lap belt" syndrome. Often the only visible sign of a lap belt injury is the imprint the belt leaves in the form of a bruise or abrasion on the anterior abdominal wall (seat belt sign). In more severe injuries, the rectus muscle may be partially or even completely transected, making the distinction between abdominal wall and intra-abdominal injuries difficult. Intra-abdominal injuries are most commonly traction avulsion injuries to the small bowel mesentery resulting from the sudden deceleration, and antemesenteric small bowel perforations caused by visceral impingement between seat belt and spine (Figure 50–2). Retroperitoneal structures including the duodenum and kidney are vulnerable to injury, presumably by the same mechanism. The injuries incurred by the lumbar spine result from forced flexion and axial distraction and are potentially the most devastating. The injury may be purely osseous, purely ligamentous, or a combination of the two. A well-recognized spinal injury is a horizontal fracture through the spinous process, lamina, transverse

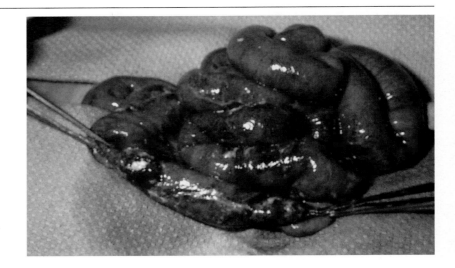

Figure 50–2. *Findings at laparotomy: two antemesenteric perforations in the midileum with multiple regions of seromuscular hemorrhage and contusion. A resection of the areas of perforation was performed.*

process, and pedicles, called a "chance fracture." The stretch tolerance of a child's ligaments and bones is four times that of the spinal cord, and this may lead to normal x-rays in a patient with a spinal cord injury. Fortunately, the overall incidence of neurologic injury in children suffering lap belt injuries is low, but it must be considered in any child injured by this mechanism.

6. **A** If a child has obvious peritonitis, then immediate laparotomy is the most appropriate treatment. More often, however, the child will have a normal or near normal abdominal examination and CT scan and will be admitted for observation and serial abdominal examination. Subsequently, the child will develop peritoneal signs and operation can be carried out at this time. Diagnostic peritoneal lavage (DPL) and diagnostic laparoscopy may have an adjunctive role to play in either the unconscious patient or one with equivocal findings.

7. **B** There is no evidence that small bowel injury diagnosed and treated on clinical grounds (rather than diagnosed by imaging study on admission) is associated with an increased rate of complications due to a delay in diagnosis. Thus, until a more accurate diagnostic test is discovered, these patients are probably best treated based on a reasonable index of suspicion of small bowel injury and findings on clinical examination.

BIBLIOGRAPHY

Eichelberger MR, Moront M. Abdominal trauma. In: O'Neill JA, Rowe MI, Gorsfeld JL, et al. eds. *Pediatric Surgery.* 5th ed. St. Louis: Mosby-Year Book; 1998.

Moss RL, Musemeche CA. Clinical judgment is superior to diagnostic tests in the management of pediatric small bowel injury. *J Pediatr Surg.* 1996; 31:1178–1182.

Newman KD, Bowman LM, Eichelberger MR, et al. The lap belt complex: intestinal and lumbar spine injury in children. *J Trauma.* 1990; 30:1133–1138.

A 4-YEAR-OLD GIRL WITH WHEEZING

HISTORY A 4-year-old girl developed onset of difficulty breathing and "wheezing" 24 hours ago. Her mother first noted the dyspnea when putting the child to bed last night. The child refused to lie down and demanded that she sleep on several pillows. She has otherwise been well except for a decreased activity level and poor appetite over the past few weeks. She has had no fever or cough. Her sister recently recovered from bronchiolitis.

EXAMINATION She is a frightened child in obvious respiratory distress with very loud "wheezing" upon expiration. Temperature 37.0°C, heart rate 133, blood pressure 100/58, and respiratory rate 38. Breath sounds are poor throughout and nearly absent on the right. It is difficult to hear wheezing on auscultation. She has significant supraclavicular and intercostal retractions. Her heart sounds are normal, and her abdomen is soft and nontender without masses or hepatosplenomegaly.

LABORATORY Hemoglobin 13.2, hematocrit 39, white blood cell count 14.2, platelet count 412,000. Urinalysis is normal. Oxygen saturation is 80% on room air and 92% on a high flow oxygen mask.

Please answer all questions before proceeding to discussion section.

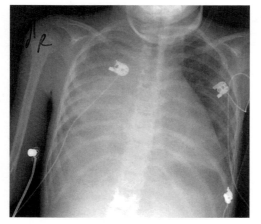

Figure 51–1. *Posterior-anterior view of the chest.*

✓ QUESTIONS

1. Initial evaluation should include all of the following *except:*
   A. Radiographic examination of the chest
   B. Administration of sedation to reduce anxiety
   C. Administration of oxygen via humidified face mask
   D. Administration of inhaled bronchodilators
   E. Admission to the intensive care unit

2. The posterior-anterior and lateral chest x-ray is shown in Figures 51–1 and 51–2, respectively. Which of the following is true?

A. The right lung has collapsed due to a mucous plug associated with the patient's asthma

B. The patient has a large, right pleural effusion

C. A large pulmonary emoblus can cause this radiographic appearance

D. The mediastinal structures are shifted to the left

3. Appropriate diagnostic maneuvers include:
   A. A computed tomography (CT) scan-guided needle biopsy of the mass
   B. A left thoracotomy and open biopsy of the mass
   C. A right thoracotomy and open biopsy of the mass
   D. A median sternotomy with cautious debulking and biopsy
   E. An ultrasound-guided right thoracentesis under local anesthesia

4. The most likely diagnosis is:
   A. Hodgkin disease
   B. Mediastinal teratoma
   C. Thymoma
   D. Neuroblastoma
   E. Lymphoblastic lymphoma

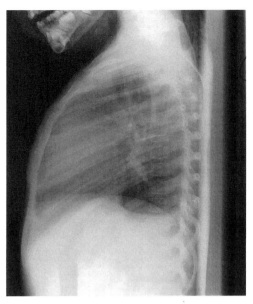

Figure 51–2. *Lateral chest radiograph.*

5. A diagnosis is made, and treatment is begun immediately with intravenous steroids, doxorubicin, vincristine, and methotrexate. The most likely early complication of therapy is:
   A. Renal failure
   B. Cardiomyopathy
   C. Neutropenic enterocolitis
   D. Airway obstruction
   E. Nerve damage

6. The patient's likelihood of cure is:
   A. Remote
   B. Ten percent
   C. Fifty percent
   D. Seventy-five percent
   E. Greater than 95%

ANSWERS AND DISCUSSION

1. **B** This little girl has evidence of acute respiratory failure. She should immediately receive oxygen by face mask and be monitored in an intensive care environment. Placement of a cardiac monitor and a pulse oximeter will provide continuous data regarding her status. Since she appears to have some type of airway obstruction, administration of bronchodilators is prudent as the diagnostic evaluation proceeds. The absence of wheezing on auscultation of the chest suggests obstruction of the large airways rather than bronchial obstruction. In any child with respiratory distress, posterior-anterior and lateral radiographs of the chest are the initial diagnostic studies of choice.

2. **D** These radiographs show a large right thoracic and anterior mediastinal mass that is markedly displacing the mediastinal structures to the left. If the opacity in the right hemithorax were due to lung collapse (**A**), the mediastinum would be shifted to the right due to vol-

ume loss. A pleural effusion (**B**) may cause this radiographic appearance with or without a mass, but a decubitus film is necessary to distinguish free fluid from a mass or loculated fluid.

Alternatively, a CT scan of the chest shows this distinction quite clearly. A pulmonary embolus causes hypoxia but does not cause radiographic changes.

Figure 51–3 shows a CT scan of a similar patient. A CT scan provides a lot information. It allows one to characterize the mass and determine whether it is solid or cystic. It reliably shows the degree of anatomic airway obstruction. It also will show whether or not there is an associated pleural effusion. This is very important diagnostically. If the patient can be stabilized, a CT scan is the appropriate study once a mass is identified on chest x-ray.

3. **E** Patients with large mediastinal masses and airway symptoms are at extremely high risk of developing complete airway obstruction. Symptoms do not occur until the airway is greater than 90% blocked, and the progression from "wheezing" to complete obstruction can be very rapid. These patients are better able to protect their own airway than by any invasive means. Administration of any sedation or anesthetic agents that may relax mediastinal structures can lead to acute airway obstruction. Therefore, any procedure requiring general anesthesia is extremely dangerous and must be avoided. In contrast to almost every other cause of acute respiratory failure, intubation is strictly contraindicated. This is because the mass obstructs the airway at the level of the carina or below. Therefore, the endotracheal tube will lie above the obstruction and be of little value. The necessary medications to allow intubation will take away the patient's conscious ability to protect his or her own airway.

The role of operation in this case is only to provide tissue for diagnosis. Resection or debulking is not clinically helpful and is not indicated. Needle biopsy is not likely to provide sufficient tissue for diagnosis. Futhermore, needle biopsy of a mass in this location can be dangerous. Injury to the lung can cause pneumothorax, or injury to one of the great vessels may cause massive hemorrhage.

4. **E** This presentation is almost diagnostic of lymphoblastic lymphoma. This rapidly growing neoplastic process produces an anterior mediastinal mass in about 70% of cases. Bone marrow involvement at diagnosis is common. Pleural effusions are common. Patients may present with superior vena cava syndrome; facial chest and upper extremity edema due to impaired venous return. Hodgkin disease will often present with a mediastinal mass, but the mass would rarely be this large or symptomatic. Patient's with Hodgkin disease typically have marked cervical adenopathy. Mediastinal teratoma is a rare and usually benign lesion. There is usually a significant cystic component, and the tumor is almost never symptomatic. Thymomas are rare in this age group and do not produce compressive symptoms. Neuroblastoma occurs in the site of sympathetic ganglia in the posterior mediastinum.

5. **A** Once the diagnosis of lymphoblastic lymphoma has been established, treatment is begun immediately. This tumor is exceedingly responsive to steroids. Upon initiation of treatment, the tumor undergoes rapid necrosis and literally "melts away." Figure 51–4 shows the appearance of a chest x-ray done 5 days after initiation of therapy. The most immediate danger to the patient is tumor lysis syndrome, causing elevated serum uric acid, lactate, and potassium levels. Unless the patient is carefully managed, hyperuricemic

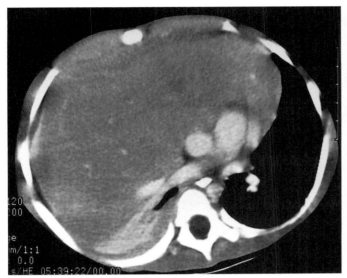

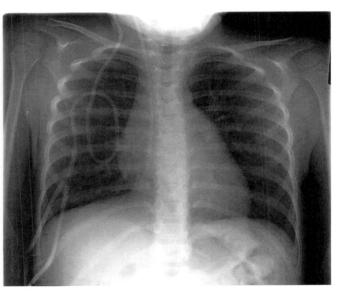

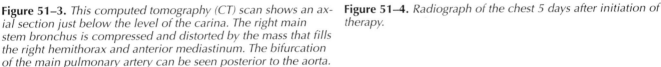

Figure 51–3. *This computed tomography (CT) scan shows an axial section just below the level of the carina. The right main stem bronchus is compressed and distorted by the mass that fills the right hemithorax and anterior mediastinum. The bifurcation of the main pulmonary artery can be seen posterior to the aorta.*

Figure 51–4. *Radiograph of the chest 5 days after initiation of therapy.*

nephropathy can cause acute renal failure. This is prevented by inducing an alkaline diuresis and giving allopurinol.

Cardiomyopathy is a complication caused by doxorubicin but occurs late. Patients receiving this drug should undergo baseline echocardiography at the beginning of treatment and serial echocardiography during treatment. Neutropenic enterocolitis may occur during therapy but is rare during induction. The risk of airway obstruction markedly decreases as soon as the mass begins to shrink. Neurotoxicity may be a late complication of vincristine.

6. **D** This tumor is very responsive to therapy. Despite its dramatic presentation, cure can be anticipated in about 75% of patients receiving therapy.

BIBLIOGRAPHY

Chaignaud BE, Bonsack TA, Kozakewich HP, et al. Pleural effusions in lymphoblastic lymphoma: a diagnostic alternative. *J Pediatr Surg.* 1998;33:1355–1357.

Ingram L, Rivera GK, Shapiro DN. Superior vena cava syndrome associated with childhood malignancy: analysis of 24 cases. *Med Pediatr Onc.* 1990;18:476–481.

King D, Patrick LE, Ginn-Pease ME, McCoy KS. Pulmonary function is compromised in children with mediastinal lymphoma. *J Pediatr Surg.* 1997;32:294–299.

Lewer BM, Torrance JM. Anaesthesia for a patient with a mediastinal mass presenting with acute stridor. *Anaesth Intens Care.* 1996;24:605–608.

Shamberger RC, Holzman RS, Griscom NT. CT quantitation of tracheal cross-sectional area as a guide to the surgical and anesthetic management of children with anterior mediastinal masses. *J Pediatr Surg.* 1991;26:138–142.

Whalen TV, LaQuaglia MP. The lymphomas: an update for surgeons. *Semin Ped Surg.* 1997;6:50–55.

52 CASE

AN INFANT WITH A DRAINING SKIN PIT IN THE NECK

HISTORY   An infant is noted at birth to have a small, right of midline skin pit in the lower neck. At 2 weeks of age, the mother notices spontaneous discharge of clear mucus from the skin pit, and the infant is referred for surgical opinion.

EXAMINATION   Examination reveals a healthy baby boy with clear mucus draining from a small ostium in the skin located anterior to the lower third of the right sternomastoid muscle. A cephalad running "cord" is palpable above the ostium and downward "milking" of the tract results in more mucus drainage.

   Please answer all questions before proceeding to discussion section.

✓ QUESTIONS

1. The lesion represents a:
   A. Thyroglossal duct fistula
   B. First branchial cleft fistula
   C. Second branchial cleft fistula
   D. Third branchial cleft fistula

2. Match the following anatomic pathways with their respective neck fistulae:
   A. Cephalad from skin, along the anterior border of the sternomastoid muscle, through the common carotid artery bifurcation, above the glossopharyngeal nerve (cranial nerve IX), and into the posterolateral pharynx at the level of the supratonsillar fossa
   B. Cephalad from skin, along the anterior border of the sternomastoid muscle, posterior to the internal carotid artery, above the hypoglossal nerve (cranial nerve XII), and into the piriform sinus

   C. Cephalad from skin, anterior to, and sometimes through, the midportion of the hyoid bone, and into the floor of the pharynx
   D. Cephalad and posterior from the skin ostium anterior to the pinna, over the facial nerve and its bifurcation, and into the external auditory canal
      i. Thyroglossal duct fistula
      ii. First branchial cleft fistula
      iii. Second branchial cleft fistula
      iv. Third branchial cleft fistula

3. Ninety percent of branchial cleft anomalies arise from the second branchial arch system:
   A. True
   B. False

4. The risks associated with untreated branchial cleft anomalies include:
   A. Infection
   B. Mass effect
   C. Development of carcinoma in adulthood
   D. All of the above

5. Which of the following statements regarding second branchial cleft anomalies is *false?*
   A. They occur more often on the right side than the left
   B. They may be bilateral in up to 10% of patients
   C. In children, sinuses and fistulae occur more commonly than cysts, while in adults the converse is true
   D. They have a relative male to female incidence of 2.5:1

6. Surgical excision of branchial cleft anomalies:
   A. May require parallel (stepladder) incisions, especially in adolescents
   B. Should not be done in the presence of acute infection
   C. May be facilitated by placement of a small probe in the fistulous tract
   D. Should not endanger the adjacent, vital neurovascular structures if the plane of dissection remains on the cyst or fistula wall
   E. All of the above

ANSWERS AND DISCUSSION

1. **C** Second, third, and fourth branchial cleft fistulae all have an external opening at the same approximate location that is at the anterior border of the sternomastoid muscle at the junction of the lower and middle thirds. Based on the rarity of the third and fourth branchial cleft derivatives (also known as piriform sinus fistulae), this almost certainly represents a second pouch fistula. First branchial cleft anomalies are rare lesions that may present with a cyst or draining fistula in a preauricular location. The internal opening is into the external auditory canal, and the tracts are notable for their proximity to the facial nerve and its branches. Thyroglossal duct derivatives are typically midline (although they can present off of midline) cystic neck masses adjacent to the hyoid bone.

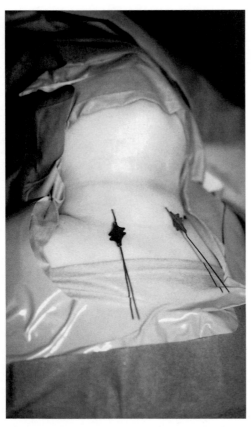

Figure 52–1. *Intraoperative photograph of a child with bilateral second branchial cleft fistulae. The external openings at the anterior border of the sternomastoid muscles have been cannulated and probes have been placed along the tracts to facilitate dissection.*

2. **A: iii, B: iv, C: i, D: ii**

3. **A** Greater than 90% of branchial cleft anomalies arise from the second branchial apparatus, while 8% arise from the first branchial apparatus. Third and fourth branchial arch malformations are exceedingly uncommon.

4. **D** Infection or a mass effect may be the initial presentation of a branchial cleft cyst. When infection occurs, it should be treated with antibiotics and, if necessary, needle aspiration. Incision and drainage should be avoided if possible, since scarring and anatomic distortion may make subsequent complete excision of the tract more difficult. The risk of carcinoma developing in the tract is likely related to chronic infection, and although a rare event in adulthood, certainly justifies childhood excision of these lesions.

5. **D** Branchial cleft malformations have a roughly equal gender incidence. The right side to left side incidence ratio is approximately 1.5:1. Frequency of bilaterality is reported to range from 2% to 10%. Since a fistula or sinus is externally apparent, it will more often be diagnosed in infancy, as opposed to a cyst, which may not become clinically evident until later in life.

6. **E** Surgical excision of a noninfected branchial cleft malformation is usually done at diagnosis. An exception is when the diagnosis is made in a newborn, in which case surgery is often deferred for 3 to 6 months. Definitive surgery should not be done in the presence of acute infection. Dissection of the ascending tract may be facilitated by placement of a small probe within, although injection of vital dyes, such as methylene blue, for tract identification may create problems if the tract is violated during the dissection (Figure 52–1). As long as the plane of dissection remains on the tract wall, the risk of inadvertent neurovascular injury is very low. In older children and adolescents, a second parallel "ladder" incision may be necessary to complete the cephalad portion of the dissection.

BIBLIOGRAPHY

Skandalakis JE, Gray SW, Todd NW. The pharynx and its derivatives. In: Skandalakis JE, Gray SW, eds. *Embryology for Surgeons.* 2nd ed. Baltimore: Williams & Wilkins; 1994.

Smith CD. Cysts and sinuses of the neck. In: O'Neill JA, Rowe MI, Grosfeld JL, et al. eds. *Pediatric Surgery.* 5th ed. St. Louis: Mosby-Yearbook; 1998.

A BOY WITH A MIDLINE CERVICAL MASS

HISTORY This 4-year-old boy is referred because of a lump in the neck of 2 weeks' duration. He has been well until 2 weeks previously, when he developed a "cold" and a sore throat. A mass appeared in the midline under his chin. There was erythema and tenderness, but the mass did not become fluctuant. After a course of amoxicillin from his pediatrician, the erythema resolved, but the mass did not diminish in size. In fact, it seemed to grow slightly larger.

EXAMINATION He is a well-developed, thin boy in no acute distress. Temperature is 37.5°C orally, pulse is 100/min, respirations 28/min, blood pressure is 86/54. There are no abnormalities of the eyes, ears, or nose. The mouth and tongue are normal; the pharynx is clear of erythema or exudates. A few tiny posterior cervical nodes are palpable bilaterally. The trachea is in the midline. A firm, slightly tender, 2.5-cm mass is noted in the midline (Figure 53–1; see also color plate), just below the hyoid bone. It is slightly movable. One examiner notes that the mass rises slightly when the patient protrudes his tongue. The lungs are clear to auscultation and percussion. No cardiac murmur is audible. The abdomen is soft without palpable masses. Rectum and genitalia are within normal limits.

LABORATORY Hemoglobin 13 gm%, hematocrit 43%, white blood cell count 9200/mm³, segments 58, lymphocytes 38, and monocytes 4. Urinalysis reveals yellow urine with a specific gravity of 1.015 and a pH of 6.0. Protein was negative, as was glucose and acetone. White blood cell count was 0 to 1/hpf, and the red blood cell count was 0/hpf. No casts were seen.

HOSPITAL COURSE Under general anesthesia, the mass, with its deep attachments, is excised (Figure 53–2; see also color plate). A small Penrose drain is left in the wound for 24 hours and removed the following morning. He makes an uneventful recovery.

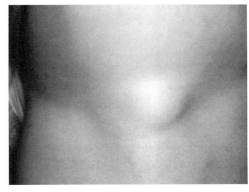

Figure 53–1. *Midline anterior cervical mass overlying the hyoid bone. (See also color plate.)*

255

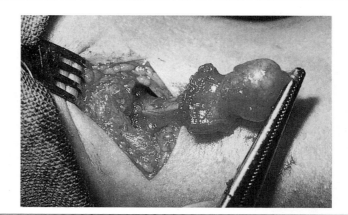

Figure 53–2. *Operative specimen showing thyroglossal duct cyst, middle one third of the hyoid bone, and suprahyoid tract. (See also color plate.)*

Please answer all questions before proceeding to discussion section.

✓ QUESTIONS

1. Which of the following has the highest risk of recurrence of a thyroglossal duct cyst?
   A. Associated lingual thyroid
   B. Double tracts, one of which is overlooked
   C. Retained hyoid segment
   D. Postoperative wound infection
   E. Use of nonabsorbable suture material

2. Total excision should *not* be performed for which one of the following cervical masses in children?
   A. Midline dermoid
   B. Midline ectopic thyroid
   C. Lateral aberrant thyroid
   D. Scrofula due to atypical mycobacteria
   E. Branchial cleft cyst

ANSWERS AND DISCUSSION

1. **C** A retained hyoid segment carries a 33% risk of recurrence of a thyroglossal duct cyst. The embryonic thryoglossal duct extends from the pyramidal lobe of the thyroid to the foramen cecum at the base of the tongue. Remnants anywhere along this pathway may develop into a cyst, sinus tract, or both. The standard operation, the Sistrunk procedure, includes removal of all remnants of the embryonic thyroglossal duct: the cyst, the infrahyoid tract, the central one third of the hyoid bone, and the suprahyoid tract, which ends in the muscles at the base of the tongue. The 33% recurrence rate for retained hyoid segment is based on a series cited by Gross; 9 out of 27 patients who had excision of the cyst without resection of the hyoid bone had recurrence (33%). Operation for a recurrence is always more difficult than the original operation. Lingual thyroid (**A**) is the most common variant of functioning ectopic thyroid. An association with thyroglossal duct cyst, however, is virtually impossible from an embryologic standpoint; an undescended (lingual) thyroid

would not give rise to a mass below it in the neck. A double tract (**B**) is possible but has not been reported in texts. Postoperative wound infection (**D**) occasionally occurs, but if excision was complete, the cyst should not recur. Perioperative antibotics are indicated for excision of a thyroglossal duct cyst because of majority of patients (like this one) have a history of infection in the cyst. The use of nonabsorbable suture material (**E**) is inadvisable because such sutures may form a nidus for granulomas and draining sinuses.

2. **B** Midline ectopic thyroid, when identified, should probably be preserved, as it is the child's only thyroid. In this situation, the midline mass should be bivalved before any lateral dissection is done, and the halves tucked into the strap muscles of the neck. Alternatively, the gland may be removed and autotransplanted into the rectus abdominis or quadriceps muscle. In any case, lifelong exogenous thyroid replacement will probably be necessary. Ideally, the diagnosis of midline ectopic thyroid should be suspected preoperatively in patients who have no palpable thyroid gland in the normal location. Ultrasound or I^{131} scan may be helpful in such cases, but these studies are *not* indicated routinely for all patients with thyroglossal duct cyst. Should the dilemma of midline ectopic thyroid arise at operation, Gross suggested that a second small incision be made inferiorly over the normal location of the thyroid to confirm its anatomic presence or absence. If the thyroid is there, then the midline mass can be removed no matter what the histology. Midline dermoids (**A**) are in the differential diagnosis of thyroglossal duct cyst. A midline dermoid cannot be ruled out until operation, when careful dissection discloses no tract leading upward toward the hyoid bone. Lateral aberrant thyroid (**C**) is a lymph node metastasis from a primary malignancy of the thyroid, usually papillary carcinoma. The histology may be deceptively well differentiated. Surgical excision is the preferred treatment for thyroid malignancies. Scrofula (ie, cervical lymphadenitis due to mycobacteria [**D**]) usually presents as a submandibular mass or masses and rarely is located in the midline. The involved lymph nodes may suppurate and develop cutaneous sinuses. Atypical mycobacteria do not respond to drug therapy; surgical extirpation is recommended for cure. Management of branchial cleft cyst (**E**), like that of thyroglossal duct cyst, requires excision of the entire anomaly (both cyst and deep connections leading toward the pharynx).

BIBLIOGRAPHY

Altman RP, Margileth AM. Cervical lymphadenopathy from atypical mycobacteria: diagnosis and surgical treatment. *J Pediatr Surg.* 1975;10:419–422.

Gross RE. *The Surgery of Infancy and Childhood.* Philadelphia: Saunders; 1953:936.

Smith CD. Cysts and sinuses of the neck. In: O'Neill JA Jr, Rowe MI, Grosfeld JL, et al. eds. *Pediatric Surgery.* 5th ed. St. Louis: Mosby-Year Book; 1998:757–771.

A TENDER NECK MASS IN A 4-YEAR-OLD GIRL

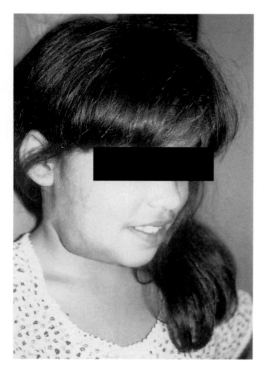

Figure 54–1. *A 4-year-old girl with a tender neck mass.*

HISTORY   A 4-year-old girl recently recovered from a sore throat, severe cough, and fever. Her father has noted a growing lump on the right side of her neck over the past 2 days. She has been somewhat listless but has had no difficulty breathing or swallowing. The family has many pets including two dogs, a cat, and seven goldfish.

EXAMINATION   The child is seen in Figure 54–1. She is fussy and apparently uncomfortable. Temperature 39.2°C, heart rate 145, blood pressure 110/70, respiratory rate 22. There is a 3-cm erythematous mass at the anterior border of the right sternomastoid muscle just under the mandible. This is fluctuant and exquisitely tender. There is moderate cervical adenopathy on both sides. The heart and lung examination is normal.

LABORATORY   None.
    Please answer all questions before proceeding to discussion section.

✔ QUESTIONS

1. The most likely diagnosis is:
    A. Suppurative infection of a cervical lymph node
    B. An infected branchial arch remnant
    C. Infection with atypical mycobacterium
    D. Esophageal rupture due to vigorous coughing
    E. Fibrosis in the sternomastoid muscle due to torticollis

2. Appropriate management may include:
    A. A magnetic resonance imaging (MRI) scan of the neck to further delineate anatomy
    B. Endoscopic examination of the trachea and upper esophagus

C. Needle aspiration of the mass
D. Incision and drainage under general anesthesia
E. C or D

3. Culture of the mass is most likely to reveal:
A. *Mycobacterium avium* intracellulare
B. *Streptococcus* or *Staphylococcus*
C. *Candida albicans*
D. The culture is usually sterile
E. Oral flora

4. Which of the following is true regarding cat-scratch disease?
A. The etiology is unknown
B. Excision of the suppurative node is required in up to 30% of cases
C. It accounts for 75,000 to 100,000 physician visits per year in the United States
D. It causes disease limited to the lymphatic system
E. Needle aspiration of the node is often curative

5. The child responds to your treatment, and you see her in the office 2 weeks later with apparent complete resolution of the problem. You should:
A. Initiate an evaluation of the child's immune function immediately
B. Wait 6 weeks then initiate an evaluation of immune function immediately
C. Repeat a purified protein derivative (PPD)
D. Obtain a chest radiograph
E. Do nothing further

6. When performing needle aspiration of an anterior cervical lymph node, one should be careful to avoid injury to which of the following nerves?
A. Spinal accessory nerve
B. Phrenic nerve
C. Recurrent laryngeal nerve
D. Vagus nerve
E. None of the above

ANSWERS AND DISCUSSION

1. **A** The history and physical findings are typical of cervical adenitis. This suppurative process most commonly occurs following an upper respiratory infection or an episode of tonsilitis. Branchial arch remnants (**B**) are subcutaneous fragments of cartilage that occur from developmental anomalies and present as subcutaneous nodules rather that infection. Branchial cleft cysts may present as suppurative masses, but there is usually a history of a preexisting cyst prior to suppuration. Infections with atypical mycobacteria (**C**) commonly occur in the anterior neck. In these infections, the involved node is firm, and the overlying skin may be often edematous. Acute suppuration with cellulitis and fever is very uncommon. Rupture of the cervical esophagus (**D**) is rare and would not present in this manner.

Torticollis (**E**) is a common problem in the newborn infant and presents as a painless neck mass without signs of infection.

2. **E** The diagnosis is usually apparent from clinical examination. If an imaging study is felt to be needed, an ultrasound will determine whether or not the center of the node is fluid or a computed tomography (CT) scan will nicely delineate the surrounding anatomy. An MRI scan (**A**) would not provide additional information. Endoscopic examination of the aerodigestive tract (**B**) is not indicated. Needle aspiration is an appropriate diagnostic maneuver and is often therapeutic as well. If the needle returns pus, the diagnosis is made. Cultures will guide antibiotic therapy. Often the needle aspiration must be repeated one or more times before the process completely resolves. If needle aspiration does not provide adequate drainage, incision and drainage should be effective. At this age, this is usually best done with the child under general anesthesia.

3. **B** Acute cervical adenitis is usually caused by *Streptococcus* or *Staphylococcus*. These organisms are thought to enter the node during an episode of pharyngitis or tonsillitis. Atypical mycobacterial infection (**A**) does not present in this manner (see answer 1). Further, these fastidious organisms are difficult to grow in culture. *Candida albicans* (**C**) does not cause lymphadenopathy in immunocompetent hosts.

4. **C** Cat-scratch disease is a very common cause of benign, self-limited lymphadenopathy. The lymph node is enlarged and may be tender but is not fluctuant and cellulitic. Most cases can be traced to contact with a cat, and the usual site of inoculation is the arm. Following inoculation, adenitis occurs in the lymph node group draining the site. This is most commonly the axilla but occurs in the cervical region in 25% of cases. Cat-scratch disease is caused by the organism *Bartonella henselae;* a pleomorphic gram-negative rod. Typically, the diagnosis is made clinically since removal of the involved node is rarely indicated. There is a test that will detect antibodies to the organism in the serum, but this is not positive until several weeks after infection. Lymphadenopthy usually resolves spontaneously within 6 to 8 weeks.

   Rarely, cat-scratch disease may produce systemic manifestations that can involve any organ. This can manifest as encephalopathy, peripheral nerve involvement, visceral organ involvement, or ocular abnormalities.

5. **E** Cervical adenitis typically occurs in normal healthy children. There is no reason to suspect an immune deficiency. Disorders of white blood cell function, such as chronic granulomatous disease, may present with recurrent subcutaneous abscesses, but adenitis is uncommon. A repeat PPD is not needed if an initial test was negative, and the clinical course and cultures confirm a bacterial infection. A chest radiograph would only be indicated in the case of adenitis caused by *Mycobacterium tuberculosis.*

6. E Needle aspiration of an anterior cervical node is a relatively safe procedure. One must remember the anatomy of the internal jugular vein and common carotid artery. These structures, however, are usually much deeper than the involved node. The spinal accessory nerve is in the posterior triangle of the neck and should be considered during procedures in this region. The phrenic nerve in the neck is on the anterior scalene muscle, much deeper than in the node chain. The recurrent laryngeal nerves originate in the chest and ascend in the tracheoesophageal grooves. The vagus nerve is in the carotid sheath deep to the jugular vein and carotid artery.

BILBIOGRAPHY

Kelly CS, Kelly RE. Lymphadenopathy in children. *Pediatr Clin North Am.* 1998;45:875–888.

Newman KD, Sato TT. Lymph node disorders. In: *Pediatric Surgery.* 5th ed. O'Neill JA, Rowe MI, Grosfeld JL, et al. eds. Mosby-Yearbook; St. Louis: 1998:737–741.

Rosenberg R. Systemic cat scratch disease: a brief case report and review of the literature. *Conn Med.* 1998;62:205–208.

Zangwill K. Therapeutic options for cat-scratch disease. *Pediatr Infect Dis J.* 1998;17:1059–1061.

Zbinden R. *Bartonella henselae*-based indirect fluorescence assays are useful for diagnosis of cat scratch disease. *J Clin Microbiol.* 1998;36:3741–3742.

A 3-YEAR-OLD GIRL WITH AN ENLARGING PAINLESS NECK MASS

HISTORY   You see a 3-year-old girl with a mass in the area of the angle of her mandible. Her parents thought she had "mumps," but the mass has persisted for 3 months and seems to be getting larger. The child is otherwise entirely healthy. She has not had a fever and is growing and developing normally. Her mother denies a history of recent upper respiratory infection or any chronic pulmonary complaints. The child has just completed a 10-day course of antibiotics prescribed by her pediatrician.

EXAMINATION   The child is healthy appearing. She is afebrile with normal vital signs. She has a firm mass wrapping around the angle of the mandible on the right. The mass is much firmer than typical lymph nodes and feels like hard rubber. The skin is a bit shiny over the mass and seems tethered to it. There is no erythema, and the mass is not fluctuant. It is nontender. There are no other masses in the neck. The lungs are clear to auscultation. The cardiac and abdominal examinations are normal.

A purified protein derivative (PPD) was placed by the child's pediatrician 48 hours ago. The test is not positive, but there is about 11 mm of faint induration. The *Candida* control skin test is positive.

Please answer all questions before proceeding to discussion section.

✓ QUESTIONS

1. The differential diagnosis of a mass in this location in a 3-year-old child includes:
   A. Bacterial adenitis
   B. Lymphoma
   C. Viral adenitis
   D. All of the above
   E. None of the above

2. The most likely diagnosis is:
   A. Bacterial adenitis
   B. Lymphoma
   C. Viral adenitis
   D. Atypical mycobacterial adenitis
   E. Tuberculous adenitis

3. Appropriate management options at this point include:
   A. Surgical excision
   B. Fine needle aspiration cytology
   C. Antibiotic therapy
   D. Surgical incision and drainage combined with antibiotics
   E. A or B

4. When you counsel the parents regarding possible complications of therapy, you discuss:
   A. Bleeding
   B. Recurrennce of the lesion
   C. Facial paralysis
   D. A and B
   E. All of the above

5. The expected recurrence rate following total surgical excision is:
   A. Almost zero
   B. Ten percent
   C. Thirty percent
   D. Sixty percent
   E. Surgical excision is not appropriate since antibiotic therapy is almost always effective

6. What do you tell the family regarding this child's future health?
   A. She is at moderate risk for persistent infections with unusual organisms
   B. She probably has a defect in white blood cell phagocytic function, and further testing is indicated
   C. She probably has a defect in lymphocyte function, but testing is not necessary unless she develops recurrent infection
   D. She is at particular risk for infection from *Pneumocystis carinii*
   E. Her immune function is probably normal

ANSWERS AND DISCUSSION

1. **D** There are several causes of neck masses in small children. The most common cause is acute cervical adenitis, which is caused by a bacterial infection of the involved lymph node. These infections are usually caused by *Staphylococcus* or *Streptococcus* species and usually present with fever, marked tenderness around the node, and erythema and fluctuance of the involved node. Nevertheless, sometimes these infections can present in a more indolent fashion. Lymphoma is quite unusual in a 3-year-old child, but it is a possibility whenever an enlarged, solitary lymph node or group of lymph nodes is seen. Viral adenitis is quite common. It is the most common cause of lymph node enlargement in small children. It is a diagnosis of exclusion, which can be made only after more serious causes have been

ruled out. Viral adenitis typically causes enlarged but soft and mobile nodes. It would be unlikely but possible for viral adenitis to produce a fixed mass such as is found in this patient. Other possible diagnoses in the differential diagnosis include atypical myobacterial adenitis, tuberculous adenitis, branchial cleft cyst, branchial arch remnant, or metastatic tumor.

2. **D** The history and physical findings strongly support the diagnosis of atypical mycobacterial adenitis. In contrast to tuberculous adenitis, atypical myobacterial adenitis is generally considered a local infectious process without systemic involvement. The most common causative organisms include *Mycobacterium avium*-entracellular, *M. scrofulaceum*, and *M. kansasii*. This infection usually occurs in healthy children with normal immune systems. The portal of entry is believed to be through the oropharynx. The infection most commonly occurs between ages 1 and 5 years. The enlarged nodes tend to be firm, rubbery, and fixed to the surrounding tissue. Skin changes, such as shiny skin over the lesion, are quite common. These infections almost always produce nontender enlargement of lymph nodes.

Infection with atypical mycobacteria typically produces a negative or weakly positive PPD test. This is due to cross-reactivity with antigens from *M. tuberculosis*. Specific atypical myobacterial antigens for skin testing have been developed, but they are not in wide clinical use.

3. **E** When diagnosis of atypical mycobacterial infection of a group of lymph nodes is likely, complete surgical excision is the management of choice. Atypical mycobacteria are highly resistant to antibiotic therapy, and even long-term treatment has not been reported to produce successful results. Data suggest that, if the diagnosis is in doubt, fine needle aspiration cytology may be helpful. Since surgical excision may result in some possible complications discussed in the next answer, it is helpful to confirm the diagnosis if it is in doubt.

Surgical incision and drainage is likely to be ineffective in treating the infection and usually results in a chronically draining sinus tract. One study compared 20 patients treated with surgical excision to 18 patients treated with incision and drainage. All patients in the surgical excision group were cured of the infection without recurrence. Sixteen of 18 patients treated with incision and drainage developed a persistent draining sinus. These data confirm that surgical excision is the treatment of choice.

4. **E** These infections typically occur high in the cervical lymph node chain near the angle of the mandible. It is not uncommon for these infections to envelop branches of the facial nerve. Since atypical mycobacterial infection is highly inflammatory and the involved lymph nodes tend to "stick" to the surrounding tissue, avoidance of injury to the facial nerve can be somewhat difficult. It is best to use an electrical neurostimulator during the dissection to avoid injury to the marginal mandibular branch of the facial nerve. If this nerve is injured, paralysis can be temporary or occasionally permanent. Recurrence of a lesion is possible, but fairly unlikely, following complete surgical excision (see answer 5). Bleeding can occur around inflammatory lesions in the neck.

5. **B** As already noted, surgical excision is the appropriate therapy. Most series report a recurrence rate of around 10%. If the lesion recurs, a reexcision is appropriate.

6. **E** Atypical mycobacterial infection occurs in healthy children with normal immune systems. The presence of one of these infections does not suggest any immune defect and does not imply a risk of further infections in the future. White cell function defects are not correlated with the presence of these infections, and testing of white cell function is not indicated.

BIBLIOGRAPHY

Evans MJ, Smith NM, Thornton CM, et al. Atypical mycobacterial lymphadenitis in childhood—a clinical, pathological study of 17 cases. *J Clin Pathol.* 1998;51:925–927.

Fergusson JA, Simpson E. Surgical treatment of atypical mycobacterial cerviofacial adenitis in children. *Aust N Z Surg.* 1999;69:426–429.

Margileth AM. Management of nontuberculous (atypical) mycobacterial infections in children and adolescents. *Pediatr Infect Dis.* 1985;4:119–121.

Taha AM, Davidson PT, Bailey WC. Surgical treatment of atypical mycobacterial lymphadenitis in children. *Pediatr Infect Dis.* 1985;4:664–667.

A 6-YEAR-OLD GIRL WHO FELL OFF HER BICYCLE

HISTORY A 6-year-old bicyclist swerved to avoid a car and was launched over her handlebars onto a grassy front yard. Initially winded, she felt better for a few hours until epigastric abdominal pain became worse and a bruise started to form just below the xiphisternum. That night she began to vomit food and later bilious material. Today (the next day) her father brings her to your office.

EXAMINATION Vital signs are stable with a borderline tachycardia of 100 bpm. Examination of the head, neck, chest, pelvis, and extremities is normal. The left upper quadrant of the abdomen is not tender, and Kerr's sign is negative. The epigastric region is mildly tender to superficial and deep palpation, but there are no peritoneal signs. The lower quadrants are benign.

LABORATORY Blood work demonstrates a hemoglobin of 10.4, and a white blood cell count that is elevated to 13,500. Electrolytes reveal a CO_2 level of 19 and are otherwise normal. Renal function and the serum glutamic pyruvic transaminase (SGPT) are normal. An amylase is slightly elevated at 210 IU. Two views of the abdomen demonstrate a dilated gastric bubble containing an air fluid level on the dependent view.

Please answer all questions before proceeding to discussion section.

✓ QUESTIONS

1. The most likely diagnosis is:
   A. Duodenal hematoma
   B. Pancreatic trauma
   C. Splenic laceration
   D. Liver laceration
   E. Occult jejunal perforation

2. Your next step would be to:
   A. Send off a blood gas to evaluate the alkalosis
   B. Cross-match two units
   C. Request lipase and trypsin levels
   D. Admit the patient, request placement of a PIC line, and nasogastric (NG) tube
   E. Request cervical spine, chest, and pelvic radiographic views

3. What would your next investigation be?
   A. Abdominal computed tomography (CT) scan with infusion and enteric contrast
   B. Upper gastrointestinal series
   C. Noncontrast abdominal CT scan
   D. Barium enema
   E. A or B

4. Assuming the patient's only problem is a duodenal hematoma, in approximately how long would you expect the lumen to reopen?
   A. Three days
   B. Two weeks
   C. One month
   D. Two months
   E. Six months

5. Which of the following is incorrect concerning duodenal hematoma?
   A. It usually involves the second or third stage
   B. Many children will have associated injuries
   C. This patient presented later than most
   D. A "coiled spring" appearance is classic on an upper gastrointestinal series
   E. If surgical therapy is required, incisions through serosa with hematoma evacuation should be sufficient

ANSWERS AND DISCUSSION

1. **A** The most likely explanation for the patient's symptoms is a duodenal hematoma. This injury occurs after blunt trauma to the epigastrium or midabdomen. A submucosal hematoma occurs in the third or fourth portion of the duodenum and obstructs the lumen. Patients typically present with bilious vomiting hours or days following injury. When they are isolated injuries, duodenal hematomas are relatively easy to care for. They may be associated, however, with much graver injuries, of which the worst listed is injury to the pancreatic duct. Duodenal perforation—not listed—is also of significant concern.

2. **D** This little girl needs resuscitation. She has clearly been vomiting and must be significantly volume depleted. It would also be a good idea to send blood for cross-match although directed donor blood should be discussed with available family members. Blood gas determination is painful, but often the CO_2 level from the electrolyte panel gives good information. While a chest x-ray would be a good idea at some point, the other films are unnecessary in a neurologically normal patient without symptoms.

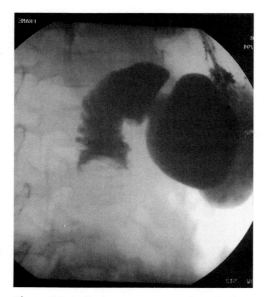

Figure 56–1. *Barium upper gastrointestinal series in a patient with a traumatic intramural hematoma of the duodenum. There is a completely obstructing mass at the junction of the second and third portions.*

3. **E** Duodenal hematoma is traditionally diagnosed by means of a barium upper gastrointestinal series (Figure 56–1). This study results in the "reverse intussusception sign." The hematoma impacts on the duodenal wall and causes a filling defect that seems to point proximally. Abdominal CT scan is an excellent alternative study and is becoming the study of choice. It clearly shows the hematoma and also allows one to evaluate for the presence of associated injury to the pancreas or other structures.

4. **B** Most series report spontaneous resolution within 2 to 3 weeks. Surgical intervention certainly should not be considered prior to this time. When operation is required for duodenal hematoma, most authors recommend making a serosal incision and evacuating the hematoma without entering the duodenal lumen. Figure 56–2 (see also color plate) shows the appearance of a duodenal hematoma at operation.

5. **C** In Touloukian's series of 12 children, presentation was delayed from 18 hours to 7 days in children with duodenal hematoma. The early findings are less impressive than with other handlebar injuries, which may include pancreatic transection, gastric perforation, splenic laceration, liver laceration, and bowel perforation.

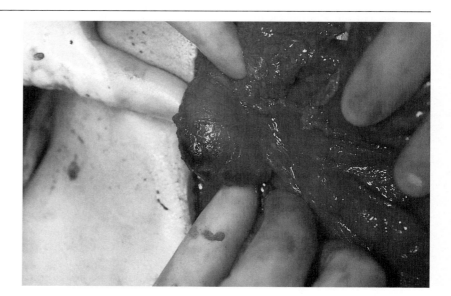

Figure 56–2. *Appearance of a traumatic duodenal hematoma at operation. The duodenum has been mobilized out of the retroperitoneum. The hematoma is at the bottom of the C-loop in the third portion. (See also color plate.)*

BIBLIOGRAPHY

Shilyansky J, Pearl RH, Kreller M, et al. Diagnosis and management of duodenal injuries in children. *J Pediatr Surg.* 1997;32:880–886.

Sidhu MK, Weinberger E, Healey P. Intramural duodenal hematoma after blunt abdominal trauma. *Am J Roentgenol.* 1998;170:38.

Touloukian RJ. Protocol for the nonoperative treatment of obstructing intramural duodenal hematoma during childhood. *Am J Surg.* 1983;145: 330–334.

Voss M, Bass DH. Traumatic duodenal haematoma in children. *Injury.* 1994;25:227–230.

A 14-MONTH-OLD GIRL WITH FEVER AND RESPIRATORY DISTRESS

HISTORY A 14-month-old girl with Down syndrome is referred for pediatric surgical evaluation. Four days ago she presented to the emergency room with fever, respiratory distress, and a right lower lobe infiltrate on x-ray. She was admitted to the pediatric service for pneumonia. She was treated with intravenous cefuroxime, nasal oxygen, and nebulizers. Admission blood culture was positive for *Streptococcus pneumoniae.* Chest x-ray (Figure 57–1) showed pleural fluid on the right, but thoracentesis yielded only 2 mL of a straw-colored fluid. A computed tomography (CT) scan (Figure 57–2) showed pleural thickening and fluid compressing the right lower lobe, but an attempt at CT-guided drainage of the fluid was unsuccessful. In spite of treatment, she continued to have daily fever spikes from 102°F to 103°F and grunting respirations.

EXAMINATION (FOURTH HOSPITAL DAY) The patient is a small, active, infant with the facies of Down syndrome. She is in moderate respiratory distress with grunting respirations at 41/min. Subcostal and suprasternal retractions are noted. Temperature is 100.8°F, blood pressure 90/64, pulse 126/min. Weight is 7.9 kg. A nasal oxygen catheter is in place. Dullness to percussion is noted over the right chest with decreased breath sounds. Coarse rhonchi are audible anteriorly on both sides of the chest. A grade II/VI systolic murmur is heard at the left sternal border. The abdomen is soft without masses or hernias. There is decreased tone in her extremities. Peripheral pulses are full.

LABORATORY (FOURTH HOSPITAL DAY) Hemoglobin 12.2 gm%, hematocrit 38%, white blood cell count 15.8/mm^3, with neutrophils 77, basophils 8, leukocytes 12, and monocytes 3. Pleural fluid (from thoracentesis) shows many white blood cells and occasional red blood cells. Gram stain reveals no bacteria. Pleural fluid culture has no growth. Chest x-ray is unchanged from Figure 57–1.

HOSPITAL COURSE An operation was performed on the fifth hospital day.

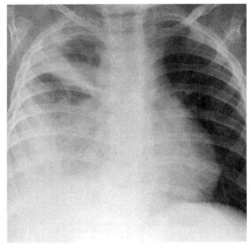

Figure 57–1. *Chest x-ray showing right lower lobe pneumonia and large right pleural effusion. Right upper lobe also has area of atelectasis/pneumonia.*

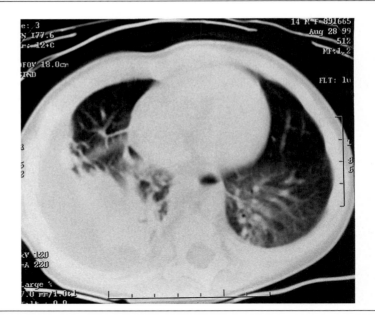

Figure 57–2. *Computed tomographic scan of chest showing large pleural effusion and compressed right lower lung.*

Please answer all questions before proceeding to discussion section.

✓ QUESTIONS

1. The diagnosis is:
   A. Parapneumonic effusion
   B. Chylothorax
   C. Tuberculosis
   D. Empyema
   E. Foreign body aspiration

2. Which of the following procedures is most appropriate for this patient?
   A. Bronchoscopy, aspiration, and insufflation of right lower lobe
   B. Insertion of trochar, tube thoracostomy
   C. Minithoractomy, limited pleural decortication
   D. Standard posterolateral thoracotomy, complete pleural decortication

3. Which of the following statements regarding empyema is most accurate?
   A. The most common pathogen in children is *Staphylococcus aureus*
   B. The incidence of empyema due to *Haemophilus influenzae* is rising
   C. The orgainzing phase is characterized by formation of pus and loculations
   D. The exudative phase generally lasts 5 to 7 days
   E. Empyema occurs most commonly among children with normal immune function

4. All of the following statements regarding empyema are true *except:*
   A. Minithoracotomy with limited pleural decortication is usually curative for empyema in the fibrinopurulent phase

B. Thoracoscopic decortication is usually curative for empyema in the fibrinopurulent phase

C. Anaerobic effusions loculate quickly and usually require aggressive surgical drainage

D. Antibiotics should be continued until pleural thickening resolves on x-ray

E. Most children who recover from empyema have no long-term deficit of pulmonary function

ANSWERS AND DISCUSSION

1. **D** Empyema is defined as pus (an exudate) in the pleural space. Most pediatric empyemas are postpneumonic; a few are post-traumatic. Parapneumonic effusion (**A**) is a more generic term that includes both transudates and exudates. Chylothorax (**B**), the most common pleural effusion in neonates, is less common in older infants. Chyle is sterile; a septic course would be unusual. Tuberculosis (**C**) in children may begin with pneumonia and pleural effusion. The initial blood culture positive for *S. pneumoniae,* however, points to this organism as the pathogen. Foreign body aspiration (**E**) may produce bronchopneumonia, which is not associated with large pleural effusions. About 90% of children who aspirate foreign bodies have a positive history.

2. **C** The optimal procedure is minithoracotomy, which consists of a limited incision directly over the empyema, drainage of the loculated pleural fluid, removal of fibrinous peel from the parietal and visceral pleural surfaces, and full expansion of the underlying lung. The procedure is done in the operating room under general anesthesia. In smaller children, a segment of rib is usually resected to permit optimal exposure through the small incision. (The rib grows back after subperiostal resection.) This procedure, termed "pleural debridement" or "limited decortication" by some authors, may also be performed thoracoscopically. It is effective for loculated empyema, but it may be less effective for advanced cases, which require a more extensive operation (ie, complete pleural decortication [**D**]). Foglia and Randolph found the CT scan helpful in the selection of patients for decortication. They recommended prompt decortication for children whose CT scan showed at least a 50% limitation of lung expansion by the products of empyema. Bronchoscopic suctioning with insufflation (**A**) is not likely to reexpand the right lower lobe because it does not address the primary problem (ie, a pleural mass that compresses the lobe). Trochars (**B**) are dangerous weapons that may perforate the lung and should be avoided in children (and probably in adults as well).

   Recently, thoracoscopic pleural debridement has been used in this setting. Proponents argue that it is less invasive than minithoracotomy. Uncontrolled observational data has shown that it may be an effective alternative.

3. **E** Most children with empyema were previously healthy and have normal immune function. (Lung abscess, in contrast, often occurs in chronically ill or immunocompromised children, especially after aspiration.) All of the other statements are false. Pneumonia and empyema due to *S. aureus* (**A**) reached a peak in children in the

1950s and 1960s but have since declined. The most common pathogen of pediatric empyema is *S. pneumoniae*. Culture of the pleural fluid, however, may be negative because of antibiotic treatment. Agglutination tests on the fluid may identify certain pathogens (eg, *S. pneumoniae*) in such cases. The occurrence of infections from *Haemophilus influenzae* (**B**), once a major pediatric pathogen, has dropped sharply following the introduction of a specific vaccine. Statements **C** and **D** are inaccurate descriptors of the pathology. The American Thoracic Society defined three phases of empyema: (1) exudative, characterized by an outpouring of watery, purulent fluid into the pleural space; (2) fibrinopurulent, characterized by development of thickened pus and fibrin loculations; and (3) organizing, characterized by development of a thick pleural peel, which is tightly adherent to the lung and chest wall because of ingrowth of fibroblasts. The exudative phase usually lasts up to 24 to 72 hours; the fibrinopurulent phase lasts 1 to 2 weeks; the organizing phase persists for weeks or months.

4. **D** Pleural thickening may persist for weeks or months following empyema. The patient recovers long before his or her chest x-ray returns to normal. Children with empyema are given intravenous antibiotics until the fever, leukocytosis, and respiratory impairment have resolved. Marked clinical improvement usually occurs in 48 to 72 hours after operative drainage. Most children are discharged from the hospital about a week after drainage and continued on oral antibiotics at home for another 10 to 14 days. All of the other statements are true. The pathologic phase of empyema determines the appropriate surgical treatment. The exudative phase is treated by thoracentesis or tube thoracostomy. The fibrinopurulent phase generally requires drainage by minithoracotomy (**A**) or by the thoracoscope (**B**). If surgical treatment is delayed until the organizing phase, an extensive operation is required. Removal of tightly adherent pleural peel may produce blood loss and pulmonary air leaks. Thus, the child with empyema benefits from early surgical referral before the process is advanced. Anaerobic effusions (**C**) tend to loculate more quickly then aerobic effusions, and almost always require open drainage. Recovery is complete in most children with no long-term deficit of pulmonary function (**E**).

BIBLIOGRAPHY

Bhattacharyya N, Umland ET, Kosloske AM. A bacteriologic basis for the evolution and severity of empyema. *J Pediatr Surg.* 1994;29:667–670.

Foglia RP, Randolph JG. Current indications for decortication in the treatment of empyema in children. *J Pediatr Surg.* 1987;22:28–37.

Kosloske AM, Ball WS Jr, Butler C, et al. Drainage of pediatric lung abscess by cough, catheter or complete resection. *J Pediatr Surg.* 1986;21:596–600.

Kosloske AM, Cartwright KC. The controversial role of decortication in the management of pediatric empyema. *J Thorac Cardiovasc Surg.* 1988; 96:166–170.

Kosloske AM, Cushing AH, Shuck JM. Early decortication for anaerobic empyema in children. *J Pediatr Surg.* 1980;15:422–429.

Reynolds M. Disorders of the thoracic cavity and pleura and infections of the lung, pleura, and mediastinum. In: O'Neill JA Jr, Rowe MI, Grosfeld JL, et al. eds. *Pediatric Surgery.* 5th ed. St. Louis: Mosby-Year Book; 1998:908–912.

A NEWBORN BOY WITH IMPERFORATE ANUS

HISTORY   A 3200 g male infant is born at term with Apgars of 9 and 9. He is sent to the well baby nursery where he feeds well. During his newborn screening examination, his nurse notes the absence of an anal opening.

EXAMINATION   General examination is normal with no evidence of dysmorphic features. The abdomen is moderately distended and soft. Examination of the perineum reveals a slightly flattened gluteal cleft with absence of an anal opening (Figure 58–1; see also color plate). There is no meconium seen on the perineum. Genitourinary examination is normal.

LABORATORY   Complete blood count (CBC) and electrolytes are normal. Urinalysis is cloudy, but there are no red or white blood cells. Leukocyte esterase is negative. Kidney, ureter, and bladder (KUB) and

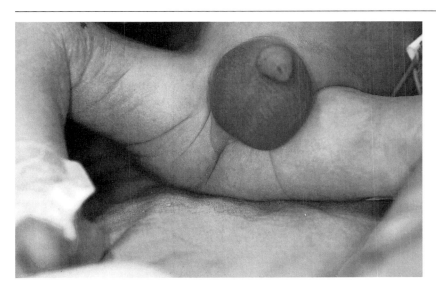

Figure 58–1. *Appearance of this newborn boy's perineum 4 hours after birth. (See also color plate.)*

upright abdominal films show increased bowel gas without fluid levels on the upright view.

Please answer all questions before proceeding to discussion section.

✓ QUESTIONS

1. How can you reliably determine whether imperforate anus in a newborn male is high or low?
   A. Administration of water soluble contrast by nasogastric tube with delayed images
   B. Ultrasound of the perineum
   C. Computed tomography (CT) scan of the pelvis
   D. Wait 24 hours, and observe the perineum for meconium
   E. Plain abdominal films with a radiopaque marker on the perineum

2. The next day, the baby's abdomen is distended and the perineum is unchanged. Appropriate management should include:
   A. Proximal sigmoid colostomy and mucous fistula
   B. Right transverse colostomy and mucous fistula
   C. Voiding cystourethrogram to evaluate for urinary fistula
   D. Transverse loop colostomy
   E. Sigmoid colostomy done as distally as possible

3. Associated anomalies include all *except:*
   A. Esophageal atresia with tracheoesophageal fistula
   B. Ventricular septal defect
   C. Malformation of the forearm
   D. Lipomeningocele
   E. Future risk of Wilms' tumor

4. Physical examination of the back is normal. Radiographs reveal a normal sacrum with five sacral vertebrae. Management includes:
   A. No further intervention
   B. Nerve conduction studies of the lower extremities
   C. Ultrasound of the spine
   D. A CT scan of the lumbosacral spine
   E. Serial neurologic examination at intervals of 6 months

5. The patient's chance for fecal continence in the future is best predicted by:
   A. The condition of the spinal cord
   B. The quality of neuromuscular development in the pelvis
   C. The height of the defect (high or low)
   D. The presence or absence of a urinary fistula
   E. The number of associated anomalies present

6. The most important anatomic study prior to repair is:
   A. Magnetic resonance imaging (MRI) of the pelvis
   B. Renal ultrasound
   C. Voiding cystourethrogram
   D. Nerve conduction studies in the pelvis
   E. Distal colostogram

ANSWERS AND DISCUSSION

1. **D** Determination of the height of the defect in imperforate anus is critical to management decisions. Low defects generally are amenable to "simple" perineal repair in the newborn period. High defects are generally associated with a urinary fistula. These defects are usually managed with a colostomy in the newborn period followed by definitive reconstruction at a later date. An abdominoperineal approach may be necessary. According to Pena, determination of the height of the defect may be made clinically 80% to 90% of the time (Figure 58–2). The best indicator of a low lesion is the presence of a perineal fistula (Figure 58–3; see also color plate). Frequently, these fistulae are not immediately apparent. Meconium may not appear on the perineum until the bowel has filled with gas and rectal peristalsis has pushed it through the fistula. The presence of a "bucket handle" perineum also suggests a low lesion. Flattening of the perineum as in this case suggests a high lesion. If there is doubt, an inverted abdominal x-ray may be taken after gas has reached the distal rectum. These studies are difficult to interpret even in experienced hands. It is the author's preference to do a colostomy in all male infants who do not have evidence of a perineal fistula. Other imaging studies are not helpful.

2. **A** This patient has a high lesion and should undergo a colostomy. This will relieve the obstruction, minimize the risk of urinary sepsis, and allow for contrast studies to delineate the anatomy. A loop colostomy is never indicated in imperforate anus. Loop colostomies are not completely diverting. Complications include urinary sepsis from continued contamination via the urinary fistula, marked dilation of the distal rectum due to inadequate diversion, prolapse of both limbs of the colostomy, and infection in the pelvis at the time of repair due to inadequate diversion. A transverse colostomy and mucous fistula avoid some of these problems but result in a long segment of defunctionalized colon, which can result in loose stools

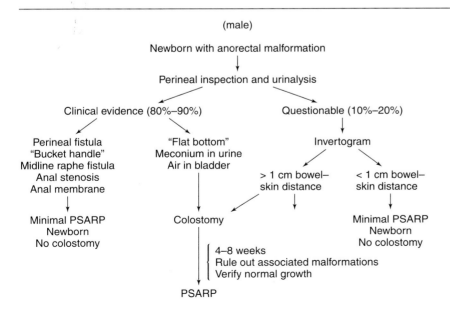

Figure 58–2. *Decision-making algorithm for the management of male patients. (From Pena A.* Atlas of Surgical Management of Anorectal Malformations. *New York: Springer-Verlag; 1990:9.)*

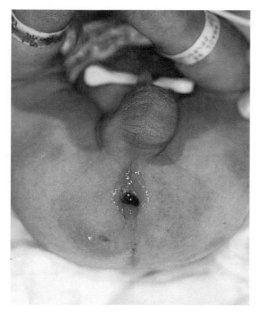

Figure 58–3. *Appearance of the perineum of a different patient at 24 hours of life. A small fistula is seen on the perineum anterior to the location of a normal anal opening. Frequently, these fistulae are not evident immediately after birth and only become apparent when colorectal peristalsis forces meconium through the tiny opening. The presence of a perineal opening correlates very strongly with a low lesion. (See also color plate.)*

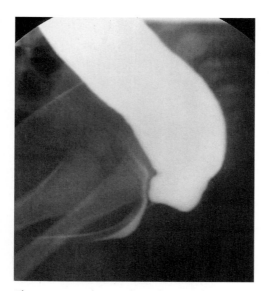

Figure 58–4. *This is a lateral view of a distal colostogram. A small fistula from the bottom of the rectum to the prostatic urethra can be seen. This defect may be successfully repaired via the posterior sagittal approach without a laparotomy.*

via the colostomy and diarrhea after colostomy closure because of disuse atrophy of the distal colon. A distal sigmoid colostomy may be too low. It may result in too short a length of distal bowel to pull-through and create a neoanus. A colostomy in the proximal sigmoid is "just right." In addition, the proximal bowel is fixed by the retroperitoneal attachments of the descending colon, thereby preventing prolapse.

3. **E** Imperforate anus is a component of the VACTERL syndrome. Anomalies include *V*ertebral and spinal cord abnormalities, *A*norectal malformations, congenital *C*ardiac disease, *T*racheoesophageal fistula and *E*sophageal atresia, *R*enal anomalies, and *L*imb defects, which usually include the radius. Affected infants may have one or any combination of these defects. Appropriate evaluation for associated anomalies may include ultrasound or MRI of the spine to exclude tethered cord or other occult spinal dysraphism, plain films of the spine to exclude vertebral anomalies, renal ultrasound to exclude malformations or hydronephrosis, echocardiogram to exclude congenital heart disease, and close clinical observation to exclude tracheoesophageal fistula and limb anomalies.

4. **C** Radiologic examination for occult spinal dysraphism is essential to the management of infants with anorectal malformations. It is possible to have significant disorders of the spinal cord with no symptoms or physical signs in infancy. When neurologic signs do appear later in life, the damage is usually irreversible. The incidence of occult spinal dysraphism with imperforate anus is at least 14%. High-resolution ultrasound is highly reliable up to around 3 months of age. At this point, ossification of the lumbosacral vertebrae begins to obscure resolution. An MRI is the best study for older children.

5. **B** The parents of these children must be counseled that *all* patients with imperforate anus have abnormal pelvic nerves and musculature. The range of abnormality is from mild to severe. After a proper repair, the likelihood of continence depends primarily on the quality of nerves and muscles in the pelvis. In general, higher defects are associated with poor development of these structures while low lesions tend to correlate with better neuromuscular development in the pelvis. This correlation is not absolute, and the height of the defect alone will not necessarily predict continence. An untreated spinal cord abnormality can impair continence, but many incontinent patients have a normal spinal cord. The presence of a urinary fistula or the number of associated anomalies do not affect continence.

6. **E** Prior to anoplasty the surgeon must answer two questions. First, can the defect be repaired via a posterior perineal approach or is a laparotomy necessary? Next, is there a urinary fistula and at what level is it? A properly done distal colostogram will answer these questions. Contrast is instilled into the distal stoma under enough pressure to fully distend the distal rectum and visualize the fistulae when present (Figure 58–4).

BIBLIOGRAPHY

Ditesheim JA, Templeton JM. Short-term v long-term quality of life in children following repair of high imperforate anus. *J Pediatr Surg.* 1987; 22:581–587.

Langemeijer RATM, Molenar JC. Continence after posterior sagittal anorectoplasty. *J Pediatr Surg.* 1991;26:587–590.

Nakayama DK, Templeton JM Jr, Zeigler MM, et al. Complications of posterior sagittal anorectoplasty. *J Pediatr Surg.* 1986;21:488–492.

Pena A. Posterior sagittal anorectroplasty: results in the management of 332 cases of anorectal malformations. *Pediatr Surg Inter.* 1988;3:94–104.

Pena A. *Atlas of Surgical Management of Anorectal Malformations.* New York: Springer-Verlag; 1990.

Pena A. Anorectal malformations. *Semin Pediatr Surg.* 1995;4:35–47.

Tsakayannis DE, Shamberger RC. Association of imperforate anus with occult spinal dysraphism. *J Pediatr Surg.* 1995;30:1010–1012.

A NEWBORN WITH AN ABNORMAL CHEST X-RAY

HISTORY You are asked to see a 10-hour-old female infant who was born at term. Her Apgar scores were 6 at 1 minute and 8 at 5 minutes. Because of some irritability, she was admitted to the neonatal intensive care unit to rule out sepsis. A chest x-ray was taken, and you are asked to evaluate the abnormality. The baby has been in no apparent respiratory distress. She was delivered vaginally via a low forceps delivery.

EXAMINATION Vital signs are temperature 37.0°C, heart rate 160, blood pressure 85/60, respiratory rate 36. The baby is resting comfortably with no evidence of respiratory distress. Specifically, there is no nasal flaring or retractions. Breath sounds are clear and equal on both sides with good air movement. The heart tones are normal, and the point of maximal impulse is in a normal location. The abdomen is nondistended and soft with no masses or hepatosplenomegaly. The extremities are normal.

LABORATORY Posterior-anterior and lateral chest x-ray is shown in Figure 59–1.

Please answer all questions before proceeding to discussion section.

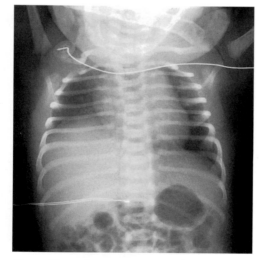

Figure 59–1. *Posterior-anterior chest radiograph with evidence of elevation of the right hemidiaphragm with underlying compressive atelectasis versus consolidation.*

✓ QUESTIONS

1. Which of the following conditions are associated with this disorder?
   A. Erb-Duchenne palsy
   B. Klumpke palsy
   C. Iatrogenic injury to the phrenic nerve
   D. Congenital defect in nerve development
   E. All of the above

2. The most appropriate management of this patient is:
   A. Immediate thoracotomy

278

    B. Exploratory thoracoscopy
    C. Elective repair via an abdominal approach
    D. Elective repair via a thoracic approach
    E. No intervention, repeat chest x-ray in 2 months

3. If the baby had an associated Erb-Duchenne palsy you would:
    A. Be more likely to recommend early repair
    B. Choose an abdominal approach for repair to avoid exacerbating the extremity problem
    C. Place the child on oxygen
    D. Tell the family that the prognosis for recovery is very good
    E. Recommend a combined repair with the orthopedic surgeon to avoid the need for two anesthetics

4. Which is an indication for repair in the asymptomatic patient?
    A. Presence of associated congenital anomalies
    B. Marked elevation with loss of 50% of thoracic volume
    C. Family history of asthma
    D. Lack of radiographic evidence of improvement over 3 months
    E. The family anticipates frequent airline travel

5. What are the advantages of repair through the chest compared to the abdomen?
    A. The phrenic nerve branches may be seen and preserved
    B. The hospital stay is shorter
    C. The recurrence rate is lower
    D. Commonly associated extralobar pulmonary sequestrations may be readily removed
    E. The incidence of liver injury is lower

6. Important technical aspects of the repair include:
    A. Use of absorbable sutures to avoid suture granuloma formation
    B. Resection of the involved portion of the diaphragm
    C. Fixation of the liver to the diaphragm to avoid torsion of the inferior vena cava
    D. Performance of a fundoplication to minimize the incidence of postoperative gastroesophageal reflux
    E. Moderate overcorrection of the deformity to avoid recurrence when the diaphragm stretches

ANSWERS AND DISCUSSION

1. **E** The chest x-ray shows evidence of elevation of the right hemidiaphragm with underlying compressive atelectasis versus consolidation. This is highly suggestive of eventration of the hemidiaphragm. The hemidiaphragm can be further examined with fluoroscopy or ultrasound. These studies would be likely to show either absence of depression of the affected portion of the hemidiaphragm on inspiration, or they may show paradoxical movement as the floppy section of diaphragm is drawn upward into the chest with negative intrathoracic pressure.

    Eventration of the diaphragm may be either from a congenital defect in the development of the muscle or of neurogenic origin. Congenital eventration of the diaphragm may occur in a focal area

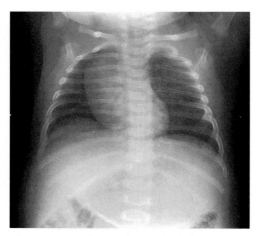

Figure 59–2. *Chest radiograph of the same patient as in Figure 59–1 at 3 months of age.*

or it can affect the entire diaphragm, leaving only a pleuroperitoneal membrane in its place. In these cases, distinction between eventration and a diaphragmatic hernia with a sac is semantic. Congenital eventration has been reported more commonly on the left side. A few bilateral cases have been reported.

Eventration is more commonly neurogenic in origin. Its most common cause is a traction injury to the phrenic nerve during delivery. This baby's history of a forceps delivery is consistent with this. Commonly associated traction nerve injuries include Erb-Duchenne palsy, which is caused by traction of the shoulder from the neck. In this disorder, the proximal limb muscles are affected, and the limb tends to be held in an extended, adducted, and internally rotated position. Klumpke palsy is caused by upward traction on the limb or compression in the region of the thoracic outlet. The distal limb muscles (ie, intrinsic muscles of the hand) are affected. Eventration is also a recognized complication of intrathoracic procedures, particularly cardiac procedures where phrenic nerve injury may occur.

2. **E** This baby has a moderate eventration, which is currently asymptomatic. The history of a forceps delivery increases the likelihood that the eventration is due to a traction injury to the phrenic nerve. In these cases, prognosis for complete recovery is excellent. In a newborn with an asymptomatic eventration, no intervention is indicated. The baby should be followed with serial radiographic examinations to determine whether the abnormality will resolve, remain stable, or worsen. If the baby develops any respiratory symptoms in the interim, then prompt investigation is, of course, indicated. Operation for eventration of the diaphragm is never an emergency, and immediate thoracotomy is certainly not indicated. If the decision has been made to repair an eventration, the lesion may be approached either through the thoracic or abdominal approach (see following answers).

Figure 59–2 shows the appearance of this patient's chest x-ray at age 3 months. There has been improvement in the appearance of the right hemidiaphragm and an increase in thoracic volume. Figure 59–3 shows the chest x-ray at 2 years, which is essentially normal.

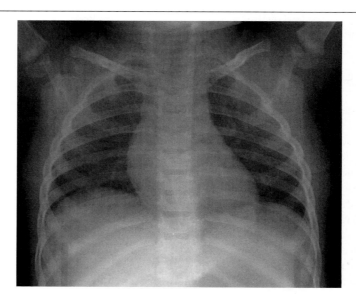

Figure 59–3. *Posterior-anterior chest x-ray at age 2 years. The appearance of the chest is essentially normal.*

3. **D** As mentioned already, when eventration is caused by a traction injury to the phrenic nerve, the patient not uncommonly will have an associated brachial plexus palsy from the same mechanism. Prognosis for recovery from these injuries is quite good. The presence or absence of associated brachial plexus palsy would not dictate the method of repair when it is done. Oxygen is only indicated in the presence of inadequate arterial oxygen tension. The prognosis for recovery of a brachial plexus palsy is very good, and no orthopedic surgical intervention is indicated, therefore, a combined procedure is out of the question.

4. **B** Most authorities agree that eventration of the diaphragm, *when symptomatic,* should be repaired. Some controversy exists regarding the indications for intervention in asymptomatic lesions. Children have the ability to grow alveoli in their lungs up to about age 8 years. If significant loss of thoracic volume persists through childhood, pulmonary hypoplasia will be permanent. Most experts agree that if there is marked elevation of the hemidiaphragm that does not improve over time, then diaphragmatic plication is indicated. Eventration of the diaphragm is not associated with other congenital anomalies. A family history of asthma would not influence the decision for repair. Lack of radiographic improvement over 3 months probably suggests that further improvement is unlikely. If the eventration is fairly minor, however, most experts would not intervene. Frequent airline travel should not pose any particular risk to this patient and is not a factor in deciding whether or not to recommend an operation.

    Figure 59–4 shows an example of an eventration in a 19-month-old child who has failed to improve with observation.

5. **A** Eventration of the hemidiaphragm may be repaired either via the chest or the abdomen. Most authorities prefer the thoracic approach because the phrenic nerve branches may be directly visualized and avoided during suture placement. Nevertheless, repair has been

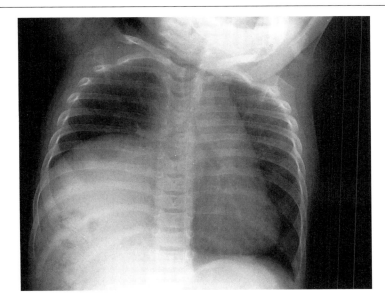

Figure 59–4. *A 19-month-old child with tachypnea.*

completed successfully via the abdominal approach. There is no reported difference in hospital stay or recurrence rate. Extralobar pulmonary sequestration is not associated with eventration of the diaphragm. The incidence of liver injury is essentially nil with either approach.

6. **E** Correction of eventration of the hemidiaphragm is by means of plication. The diaphragm should be folded upon itself and held in place with sutures. The diaphragm should be overcorrected a bit and stretched fairly flat as it typically stretches a bit postoperatively and returns to a normal contour. If this overstretching is not done, the eventration tends to recur. It is very important to use nonabsorbable sutures. When absorbable sutures are used, recurrence typically happens as the suture dissolves. It is not necessary to resect the involved portion of the diaphragm. It should simply be folded upon itself. It is also not necessary to fix the liver to the diaphragm as normal hepatodiaphragmatic attachments will prevent the liver from twisting.

Eventration of the hemidiaphragm does not involve the esophageal crura or hiatus. Gastroesophageal reflux is not an expected postoperative complication and fundoplication is not indicated.

BIBLIOGRAPHY

de Vries TS, Loens BL, Vos A. Surgical treatment of diaphragmatic eventration caused by phrenic nerve injury in the newborn. *J Pediatr Surg.* 1998;33:602–605.

Kizilcan F, Tanyel FC, Hicsonmez A, Buyukpamukcu N. The long-term results of diaphragmatic plication. *J Pediatr Surg.* 1993;28:42–44.

Smith CD, Sade RM, Crawford FA, Othersen HB. Diaphragmatic paralysis and eventration in infants. *J Thorac Cardiovasc Surg.* 1986;91:490–497.

Symbas PN, Hatcher CR Jr, Waldo W. Diaphragmatic eventration in infancy and childhood. *Ann Thorac Surg.* 1977;24:113–119.

A TEENAGE BOY INVOLVED IN A GARAGE EXPLOSION

HISTORY   A 15-year-old boy is brought to the emergency department following a gas explosion in his parents' garage. Paramedics report significant fire and smoke damage within the enclosed space. The boy is wearing burned clothing, has an obvious flame burn to his face with soot and singed facial hair, and is complaining of abdominal pain.

EXAMINATION   Heart rate 120, blood pressure 110/70, respirations 32, oxygen saturation 90% on 10 liters per minute of oxygen by face mask. He is alert and conversant but has a notably hoarse voice. His lungs are clear. He has a mildly distended and tender abdomen. His burned clothing is removed revealing second and third degree burns to his anterior trunk and perineum with a circumferential third degree burn to his left upper extremity.

Please answer all questions before proceeding to discussion section.

✓ QUESTIONS

1. Which of the following represents the ideal initial management sequence of this patient?
   A. Humidified 100% oxygen by rebreather mask; right arm antecubital venous access and rapid infusion of 1000 mL of Ringer's lactate; abdominal computed tomography (CT) scan; and left upper extremity escharotomy
   B. Endotracheal intubation and mechanical ventilation with 100% oxygen; right arm antecubital venous access and infusion of 1000 mL of Ringer's lactate; abdominal CT scan; and left upper extremity escharotomy
   C. Endotracheal intubation and mechanical ventilation with 30% oxygen (to keep oxygen saturations above 93%); right arm antecubital venous access and rapid infusion of 1000 mL Ringer's lactate; left upper extremity escharotomy; and abdominal CT scan

    D. Right arm antecubital venous access and infusion of 1000 mL of Ringer's lactate; endotracheal intubation and mechanical ventilation with 100% oxygen; left upper extremity escharotomy; and abdominal CT scan

2. Which of the following statements regarding inhalation injuries is true?
    A. Carbon monoxide poisoning is the primary determinant of mortality in patients with inhalation injury
    B. The absence of signs of inhalation injury at presentation is a reliable predictor of the absence of airway injury (high specificity)
    C. Bronchoscopy plays an important role in patients at risk for airway injury based on history but in whom there are no clinical signs of injury at presentation
    D. Prophylactic antibiotics should be started in any patient with endoscopic evidence of mucosal injury below the glottis

3. Assuming the boy is of adult body proportions and weighs 60 kg, a rough estimate of his total fluid requirements over the next 24 hours is:
    A. 7700 mL with half given over the first 8 hours and the remainder over the next 16 hours
    B. 10,000 mL equally divided over the 24-hour period
    C. 5500 mL with half given over the first 8 hours and the remainder over the next 16 hours
    D. Intravenous line to run at 120 mL per hour with 500 mL boluses for low urinary output

4. Which of the following statements regarding infection control and burns is *false?*
    A. Silver sulfadiazene application to burns reduces the incidence of burn wound sepsis
    B. Quantitative burn wound biopsies should be used to guide the use of systemic antibiotics in the absence of bacteremia
    C. There is no correlation between the percentage of body surface area burned and the incidence of burn wound sepsis
    D. Early administration of enteral rather than parenteral nutrition is associated with a lower incidence of sepsis and a decreased mortality rate

5. Which of the following statements pertaining to third degree burns (Figure 60–1; see also color plate) is *false?*
    A. Always require excision and skin grafting
    B. Are usually very painful
    C. Contain no viable epithelial elements
    D. May result from second degree or partial thickness burns that become infected

6. Recombinant growth hormone administration in massively burned pediatric patients is associated with decreased protein catabolism, accelerated graft donor site healing, and shortened hospital stay:
    A. True
    B. False

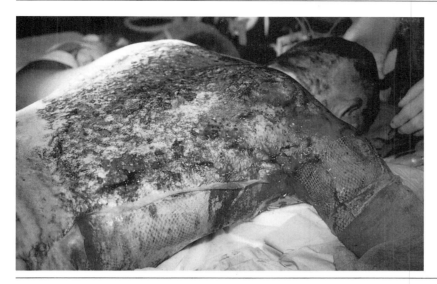

Figure 60–1. *Patient with extensive full thickness burn to back. (See also color plate.)*

ANSWERS AND DISCUSSION

1. **B** Burn patients are just like any other trauma patient and are subject to the same ABCs of resuscitation. The history of a gas explosion within an enclosed space and the clinical signs provided (singed hair, soot, and voice change), put this patient at very high risk for a serious heat and smoke inhalation injury with imminent airway obstruction and carbon monoxide poisoning. His airway should be managed by prompt endotracheal intubation with 100% oxygen administration (initially) to facilitate prompt elimination of carbon monoxide. There is no role for airway strategies that do not involve endotracheal intubation in this patient. Fluid resuscitation should be provided through a nonburned extremity and should be calculated according to the Parkland formula, which takes into account body weight and percentage of body surface burned (see answer 3). The blast mechanism puts this child at risk for cervical spine, head, torso, and extremity injuries, and after intubation, initiation of resuscitation and cervical spine, chest, and pelvis x-rays, other clinically indicated studies (in this case, an abdominal CT scan) should be performed. The circumferential nature of his upper extremity burn mandates that an escharotomy be done prior to his departure from the trauma room, particularly if transfer to a burn center is required.

2. **C** Inhalation injury is the primary factor responsible for death in burn patients. Burns in children that are complicated by an inhalation injury have an associated mortality rate of approximately 40%. Although exhaust inhalation in an enclosed space can lead to fatal carbon monoxide poisoning, it is the lung and small airway injury mediated by heat and toxic gas or combustion products that leads to the principle pulmonary morbidity and mortality associated with significant inhalation injuries. The absence of clinical signs of an inhalation injury should not preclude consideration of intubation in patients with a high risk mechanism. Fiberoptic bronchoscopy may be helpful in identifying patients with subclinical airway injuries in whom swelling will lead to delayed presentation with airway obstruction. These patients should all undergo elective endotracheal

intubation. Inhalation injuries produce hypoxia, decreased compliance, and increased pulmonary vascular resistance. Shed mucosa, polymorphs, and fibrinous exudate produce airway "casts," which cause atelectasis. Positive end-expiratory pressure (PEEP), aggressive pulmonary toilet with humidified oxygen, mucolytics (*N*-acetyl cysteine), and nebulized heparin are essential in avoiding secondary pneumonia. Antibiotics are indicated only in the presence of clinical or bacteriologic evidence of pneumonia and have no role to play in prophylaxis.

3. **A** Fluid requirements in burn patients are often massive, and must be calculated by formulas that take into account size and percentage of body surface burned (BSB). For adults and older children, the Parkland formula is appropriate: the total volume of resuscitative and maintenance fluids for the first 24 hours postburn equals 4 mL/kg × body weight (kg) × % BSB. One half of the calculated fluids are given in the first 8 hours and the remainder over the ensuing 16 hours. Standard burn assessment charts are used to estimate % BSB, which for adults, or adult-sized children, uses the "Rule of Nines," where the head and neck account for 9%, the torso 36%, upper extremities 9% each, lower extremities 18% each, and perineum 1%. For smaller children, the Parkland formula is less useful because of the increased surface to mass ratio. For infants and smaller children, fluid calculations should be based on surface area rather than weight, and % BSB estimates should be determined from age-specific burn diagrams that take into account the differences in body proportions between adults and children.

4. **C** The incidence of burn wound sepsis is directly correlated with the percentage of body surface burned, therefore, the prevention or early detection of burn wound sepsis is critical to the outcome of the patient with extensive second and third degree burns. Topical agents, such as silver sulfadiazene, are used in burn wound dressings to reduce the bacterial concentration and, therefore, decrease the indicence of burn wound sepsis. Early recongition of invasive burn infection is facilitated by quantitative wound biopsies, for which a small wedge of eschar is excised. One piece is submitted for histology, and a second piece is incubated for 24 hours, and then a quantitative bacterial count is performed. In addition to documented bacteremia, pneumonia, or urinary tract infections, systemic antibiotics are indicated when signs of sepsis are present and a burn wound biopsy demonstrates histologic evidence of viable tissue invasion or greater than 10^5 organisms per gram of eschar by quantitative culture, or both. The high catabolic rate associated with burns mandates that adequate nutrition be provided early to avoid protein wasting. It has been shown that enteral feedings are associated with a significantly lower incidence of septic complications than parenteral feedings, presumably by reduction of bacterial translocation across the gut. It is recommended, therefore, that enteral feedings by gavage tube be instituted as soon as possible (usually within a few hours of the burn), in an amount that is likely to approximate the patient's increased metabolic need.

5. **B** Third degree of full thickness burns are painless because of thermal destruction of cutaneous nerves. Burns that are initially partial

thickness may be converted to full thickness by infection. All third degree burns require excision and skin grafting.

6. A

BIBLIOGRAPHY

Hansborough JF, Hansborough W. Pediatric burns. *Pediatr Rev.* 1999; 20:117–123.

Herndon DN, Rutan R, Rutan T. Management of the pediatric patient with burns. *J Burn Care Rehab.* 1993;14:3–8.

Judkins K, Pike H. Prevention and rehabilitation: the community faces of burn care. *Burns.* 1998;24(7):594–598.

Sheridan RL. The seriously burned child: resuscitation through reintegration—2. *Curr Probl Pediatr.* 1998;28(5):139–167.

Wolf SE, Debroy M, Herndon DM. The cornerstones and directions of pediatric burn care. *Pediatr Surg Int.* 1997;12:312–320.

A 13-YEAR-OLD BOY WITH SEVERE GROIN PAIN

HISTORY You receive a call at 10 PM to see a 13-year-old boy in the emergency department with a 4-hour history of severe scrotal pain and two episodes of vomiting. He reports having experienced similar pain of short duraton 2 weeks earlier. When you see the boy, he is in severe pain despite a dose of morphine. He has swelling redness and warmth in the left hemiscrotum (Figure 61–1), and attempts to palpate the testis are associated with exquisite discomfort. You diagnose testicular torsion and call the radiologist to obtain a confirmatory study. The radiologist informs you that his car is in the shop for repairs, and he will have to come in by bicycle, which will take at least 60 minutes.

Please answer all questions before proceeding to discussion section.

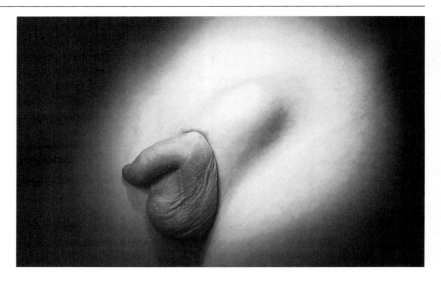

Figure 61–1. *Appearance of the groin of a 13-year-old boy with left groin pain.*

✓ QUESTIONS

1. You decide to:
   A. Wait for the radiologist to come in and perform a Doppler ultrasound to assess left testicular blood flow
   B. Call the nuclear medicine technician since it looks like you may be able to get a nuclear scan more quickly
   C. Attempt external detorsion
   D. Proceed directly to the operating room for scrotal exploration

2. The differential diagnosis in this child would include all of the following *except:*
   A. Scrotal trauma with fat necrosis
   B. Epididymoorchitis
   C. Strangulated inguinal hernia
   D. Acute hydrocele

3. At exploration, you find a viable testis except for a small area of necrosis at the superior pole. The correct diagnosis is:
   A. Testicular trauma with focal hemorrhage
   B. Hydatid of Morgagni (appendix testis) torsion
   C. Henoch-Schönlein purpura
   D. None of the above

4. A decision to leave a testis of doubtful viability in situ following detorsion:
   A. May threaten future spermatogenesis of the contralateral testis in an adolescent
   B. May be influenced by intraoperative Doppler studies
   C. May be appropriate in a prepubertal child
   D. All of the above
   E. None of the above

5. Extravaginal torsion occurs more commonly than intravaginal torson:
   A. True
   B. False

ANSWERS AND DISCUSSION

1. **D** The left testis is retracted up toward the inguinal canal. The history and physical findings strongly suggest acute testicular torsion. A clinical diagnosis of testicular torsion is adequate in a setting such as this. The patient has been symptomatic for 4 hours, and an additional treatment delay may compromise testicular salvage. Experience with external detorsion under sedation is variable, but it does not obviate the need for surgical exploration and orchidopexy. If a diagnostic test is desired, then both Doppler ultrasound and radioisotope scanning can accurately determine whether or not there is blood flow to the testis.

2. **D** The presence of tenderness, redness, and warmth imply that if this is not testicular torsion, then it must be something associated with inflammation. Although an acute hydrocele may be painful, it

should not cause scrotal redness or warmth, as would the other conditions listed.

3. **B** The appendix testis, or hydatid of Morgagni, believed to be an embryologic remnant of the cranial end of the müllerian duct is present in 90% of males. Prior to puberty, torsion of a testicular appendage is more common than torsion of the testicle itself. Differentiating the two may be difficult because the history is similar, although typically the pain associated with a torsed testicular appendage is less severe. Ocasionally, the torsed appendage will be visible through the skin as a dark bluish spot at the upper pole of the testis, known as the "blue dot sign."

4. **D** After operative detorsion, it may be difficult to determine whether or not the testis is viable, especially if there has been secondary hemorrhage. The testicle should be observed for a few minutes for return of perfusion, and diagnostic adjuncts, such as intraoperative Doppler, may be helpful in assessing its survivability. There is evidence that an ischemic injury to the blood–testis barrier in adolescence can result in the formation of sperm agglutinating antibodies, which might impair future fertility. The risk of ischemic autoimmunization against one's own spermatogonia is low in boys less than 10 years because there is no blood–testis barrier, and spermatogenesis has not yet begun. This observation justifies leaving in situ, doubtfully viable testes in boys under the age of 10 and orchiectomy in boys older than 10. Contralateral orchidopexy should always be performed to prevent torsion of the similarly predisposed testis (Figure 61–2; see also color plate).

5. **B** The most common form of testicular torsion is intravaginal. An unusually high investment of the tunica vaginalis on the spermatic cord (the so-called bell clapper deformity) creates a long and unsupported intravaginal spermatic cord, which is predisposed to twisting. This form of torsion occurs at puberty and is thought to be initiated by the cremaster mediated elevation and rotation that often occurs during sleep. A rare variant of intravaginal torsion occurs between the testis and epididymis when the two are separated by an elongated mesorchium. Extravaginal torsion occurs exclusively during the perinatal period and is probably responsible for cases of absent testis when a blind ending vas is encountered during groin exploration for cryptorchidism.

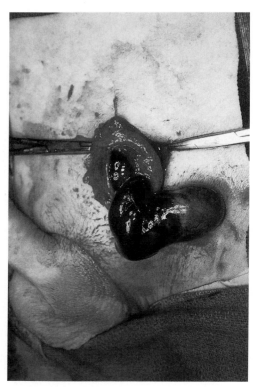

Figure 61–2. *This is a photograph (from a different patient) showing a clearly necrotic testicle due to torsion. This patient was explored via an inguinal incision because of diagnostic concern regarding testicular tumor. (See also color plate.)*

BIBLIOGRAPY

Hutson JM. Undescended testis, torsion and varicocele. In: O'Neill JA, Rowe MI, Grosfeld JL, et al. eds. *Pediatric Surgery.* 5th ed. St. Louis: Mosby-Yearbook; 1998.

Kass EJ, Lundak B. The acute scrotum. *Pediatr Clin North Am.* 1997; 44:1251–1266.

A 2-MONTH-OLD BABY WITH A WET UMBILICUS

HISTORY   A 2-month-old baby girl is sent to your office by her pediatrician because of a lesion in the umbilical fold that secretes a clear, viscid liquid, which is yellowish when it dries on the child's clothes. She had a three vessel cord, which fell off after treatment with triple dye solution.

EXAMINATION   Deep in the folds of the umbilicus an 8-mm round pinkish lesion with a sessile stalk can be moved painlessly with sterile cotton applicators (Figure 62–1; see also color plate).
Please answer all questions before proceeding to discussion section.

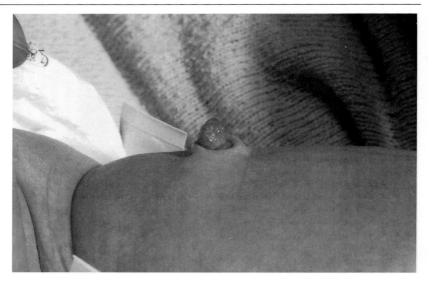

Figure 62–1. *A 2-month-old girl with an umbilical mass. (See also color plate.)*

✓ QUESTIONS

1. Prior to sending the patient to your office, you suggest the referring pediatrician:
   A. Try using steriod cream
   B. Try using silver nitrate (AgNO$_3$)
   C. Perform an abdominal ultrasound
   D. Perform a Meckel's scan
   E. Perform a voiding cystourethrogram

2. You offer the mother medical therapy or surgical excision, and she opts for the surgical approach. To prepare the child you:
   A. Anesthetize the skin with marcaine and a fine needle
   B. Take the child to the amulatory care unit and ask anesthesia for a caudal block
   C. Prepare the skin with a betadine solution
   D. Send the child to ultrasound to rule out remnants of the urachal and vitelline duct systems
   E. Make plans to perform repair in the operating room the following week, as there is no sign of omphalitis

3. When the time comes to treat the lesion, you do not:
   A. Ligate the base with a 2.0 silk
   B. Send the mass to pathology
   C. Perform a supraumbilical incision to approach the lesion at the level of the linea alba
   D. Tell the mother the granuloma will turn purple within 2 hours and fall off in 24 to 48 hours
   E. Recommend bathing of the site

4. Concerning the etiology of umbilical granulomas:
   A. Some believe they result from irritation and chronic inflammation at the old site of cord insertion
   B. Some believe they are similar to umbilical polyps, which are considered remnants of the vitelline (omphalomesenteric) duct system
   C. They present little threat to the infant, and often, repeat AgNO$_3$ treatment is successful
   D. When cauterizing with AgNO$_3$, one must warn parents that it permanently stains clothes black
   E. When cauterizing with AgNO$_3$, placing Vaseline on adjacent skin minimizes the chances of burning it inadvertently
   F. All of the above

ANSWERS AND DISCUSSION

1. **B** This baby has an umbilical granuloma. This consists of granulation tissue that appears following separation of the cord. Most commonly, these lesions have no specific cause and respond to local application of silver nitrate. If the lesion is uncomplicated, as this one is, there is no need for sophisticated investigations. When cauterization with silver nitrate is not effective, surgical excision is necessary (see answer 3). Rarely, an umbilical granuloma is a sign of a patent

urachus. The family should be questioned about the presence of watery umbilical discharge (urine).

2. **C** The umbilicus is scar tissue that is painful to anesthetize—more painful than ligation of the stalk. Rectal acetaminophen given before the procedure, followed by oral acetaminophen once or twice afterwards, is usually sufficient. Antibiotics would be overkill unless there is reason to suspect immunosuppression.

3. **C** The mass is uncomplicated, and there is no risk of malignancy. Nothing else the pathologist tells you will change therapy. The lesion usually consists of granulation tissue with abundant fibroblasts and capillaries. The site should be kept relatively dry between baths by keeping it above the diaper line. The ligated granuloma will necrose and fall off within a few days.

4. **F**

BIBLIOGRAPHY

Chamberlain JM, Gorman RL, Young GM. Silver nitrate burns following treatment for umbilical granuloma. *Pediatr Emerg Care.* 1992;8:29–30.
Lee CN, Cheng WF, Lai HL, et al. Perinatal management and outcome of fetuses with single umbilical artery diagnosed prenatally. *J Maternal Fetal Med.* 1998;8:156–159.

CARDIAC FAILURE IN A 1-WEEK-OLD PREMATURE INFANT ON A VENTILATOR

HISTORY   This 990 g male infant was born to a gravida 2, para 1, 19-year-old mother, who smoked cigarettes during early pregnancy and missed several of her prenatal appointments. Premature labor began at 31 weeks and progressed rapidly. Delivery was vaginal. Apgars were 5 at 1 minute and 7 at 5 minutes.

EXAMINATION   The infant is a 990 g male infant in moderate respiratory distress. Gestational age by examination is 30 weeks. The pulse is 164, mean arterial pressure 48, respiratory rate 65/min. There are no anomalies noted of the head, eyes, ears, palate, or extremities. Moderate intercostal retractions are present. Breath sounds are decreased bilaterally, but no rales are audible. No cardiac murmur is heard. The abdomen is normal. Testes are palpable in the inguinal canals bilaterally. Peripheral pulses are full and synchronous.

LABORATORY   Hemoglobin 14.7 gm%, hematocrit 56%, white blood cell count 14,000/mm³, polymorphonuclear leukocytes 62, bands 2, lymphocytes 32, monocytes 4. Platelets are 120,000/mm³. Urinalysis is unremarkable. The arterial blood pH is 7.30, P_{CO_2} is 43, P_{O_2} is 40, and F_{IO_2} is 40% (in oxyhood). The chemistry results (mg/dL) or (mmol/L) are glucose 70; sodium 137; potassium 4.0; creatinine 0.2; blood, urea, nitrogen 20; chloride 95; and carbon dioxide 23. The chest x-ray is shown in Figure 63–1.

HOSPITAL COURSE   An umbilical arterial catheter is inserted for monitoring. Respiratory distress becomes progressively more severe over the next 3 to 4 hours, with grunting, nasal flaring, and intercostal retractions. The infant is intubated and placed on a ventilator in 80% oxygen. Surfactant is administered via the endotracheal tube. His oxygen requirement gradually decreases from 80% to 50% over the next 72 hours. On the fourth hospital day, a faint holosystolic murmur is audible in the left infraclavicular area. The baby's intravenous fluid volume is restricted; he

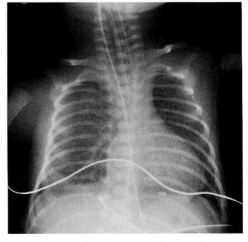

Figure 63–1. *Chest x-ray at 2 hours of age showing early reticulogranular infiltrates in the lungs characteristic of neonatal respiratory distress syndrome (RDS).*

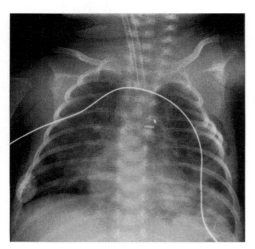

Figure 63–2. *Chest x-ray on the fifth day of life showing worsening pulmonary inflitrates and cardiomegaly.*

receives a transfusion of packed red cells for anemia and phototherapy for jaundice. On the fifth day, the murmur is harsh (grade 3/6) and audible over the entire left precordium. Bounding peripheral pulses are noted. Echocardiogram shows a patent ductus arteriosus (PDA), with a left-to-right shunt that is hemodynamically significant. Repeat chest x-ray is shown in Figure 63–2. Indomethacin is administered. After the third (final) dose of indomethacin, he develops oliguria; serum creatinine rises to 1.3; platelet count falls to 68,000. The cardiac murmur disappears for 24 hours, but then returns.

Surgical consultation is obtained for ligation of the PDA. At operation, the diameter of the ductus is observed to be equal to that of the descending aorta. Postoperatively, his oxygen requirement gradually decreases to room air, his carbon dioxide retention improves, and he is weaned from the ventilator. He develops pneumonia 10 days postoperatively but is finally extubated in the third hospital week. He is transferred to the "growers" unit and is discharged at 6 weeks of age.

Please answer all questions before proceeding to discussion section.

✓ QUESTIONS

1. Closure of the ductus arteriosus may result from:
   A. Oxygen
   B. Indomethacin
   C. Aspirin
   D. A and B
   E. A, B, and C

2. The most constant physical finding in infants with patent ductus arteriosus is:
   A. Continuous murmur
   B. Bounding peripheral pulses
   C. Cardiomegaly
   D. Hepatomegaly
   E. Differential cyanosis

3. Contraindications to indomethacin therapy in the premature infant include all of the following *except:*
   A. Intracranial hemorrhage
   B. Renal failure (creatinine concentration > 1.2 mg/dL)
   C. Severe thrombocytopenia
   D. Necrotizing enterocolitis
   E. Progressive increase in ventilator settings

4. Which *one* of the following procedures is indicated for assessment of a PDA in a premature infant?
   A. Serial electrocardiograms
   B. Echocardiogram with Doppler flow
   C. Cardiac catheterization
   D. Aortogram via the umbilical arterial catheter
   E. Dye dilution studies for quantitation of shunt

5. Bronchopulmonary dysplasia (end-stage pulmonary disease in infants) is associated with:
   A. High levels of inspired oxygen

    B. High ventilator pressures
    C. Pulmonary immaturity
    D. Pulmonary overcirculation from left-to-right shunts
    E. All of the above

6. Anatomic variants or abnormalities of the great vessels create a risk for certain technical mishaps during which a vessel other than the PDA is ligated. Which of the following is most likely?
    A. Ligation of anterior branch of double aortic arch
    B. Ligation of main pulmonary artery
    C. Ligation of left pulmonary artery
    D. Ligation of left subclavian artery
    E. Ligation of aberrant right subclavian artery

7. Which of the following techniques is/are appropriate for surgical closure of a PDA in a 1000 g infant?
    A. Double ligatures
    B. Double application of clips
    C. Double clamping, division of PDA, oversewing the ends
    D. A and B
    E. A, B, and C

ANSWERS AND DISCUSSION

1. **E** All of the agents listed may initiate ductal closure. In the normal neonate, ductal closure is related to increasing oxygen tension as fetal circulation shifts to the adult form. Prostaglandin E_1 produces dilation of the ductus arteriosus in newborn lambs and humans and has been used in neonates with cyanotic congenital heart disease in whom patency of the ductus arteriosus was necessary to maintain oxygen saturation. Conversely, prostaglandin inhibitors, such as indomethacin and aspirin, produce ductal closure.

2. **B** Bounding peripheral pulses are a constant finding in patients with PDA and significant left-to-right shunting. A continuous murmur (**A**) is exceptional; loud crescendo murmurs are far more common. Cardiomegaly (**C**) and hepatomegaly (**D**) may occur in infants with overt congestive failure, but congestive failure is not always present with PDA. Differential cyanosis (**E**) of the lower part of the body could occur in the infant who was shunting right-to-left through the ductus, but this would be a late, infrequent finding.

3. **E** Progressive increase in ventilator settings is not a contraindication to indomethacin. It is, rather, more likely to be clinical evidence of pulmonary overcirculation from the PDA shunt, indicating the *need* for indomethacin. Intracranial hemorrhage (**A**), renal failure (**B**), and severe thrombocytopenia (**C**) are standard contraindications to indomethacin as cited by Zakha and Patel (1997). The possible relationship of indomethacin, a potent vasoconstrictor, to (**D**) necrotizing enterocolitis (NEC), a syndrome of ischemic bowel, makes many experts reluctant to use the drug in the face of acute NEC; however, the interrelationships between NEC, PDA, and indomethacin remain controversial. A retrospective analysis by Grosfeld and associates (1996) documented that infants with NEC who received in-

domethacin had worse outcomes than infants with NEC who did not receive the drug. Skeptics could argue, however, that since all of the infants who received indomethacin also had PDA, they were a sicker group and would be expected to have worse outcomes.

4. **B** Echocardiogram with Doppler directional flow, a noninvasive study, is now the gold standard for evalution of PDA in premature infants. Increasing size of the left atrium compared to the aortic root is indicative of an increasing shunt across the ductus. Doppler color flow determines volume and direction of the shunt. Cardiac catheterization (**C**), a more invasive study, is rarely needed for documentation of PDA in this fragile patient population. Serial electrocardiograms (**A**) are of little value. Retrograde aortogram (**D**) and dye dilution studies (**E**) were used in the past, but they are surpassed by modern echocardiography.

5. **E** All the factors and agents cited may contribute to development of bronchopulmonary dysplasia (BPD). In Northway and coworkers' classic article (1967) describing BPD, inspired oxygen concentration was thought to be the critical causative factor. More recently, however, evidence has accumulated showing that positive pressure, pulmonary immaturity, and duration of ventilatory support are important etiologic factors as well. Prolonged pulmonary overcirculation from a PDA may contribute to development of BPD.

6. **C** Ligation of the left pulmonary artery (LPA), misidentified as the ductus, is a rare technical complication that is probably underreported. How could such a complication happen? Typically, the ductal anatomy is beautifully visualized through the transparent neonatal pleura. Two deceptive scenarios exist, however. The first is when a huge PDA runs anterior and parallel to the arch, covering the arch, which may be mistaken for the arch. The second scenario involves a huge main pulmonary artery that covers both the arch and the PDA. In both cases, the vessel coursing downward is the LPA not the ductus. The greatest risk seems to occur in two groups: in infants with other congenital cardiac lesions (eg, pulmonic stenosis) in which the pulmonary artery may be markedly dilated, or in infants with a history of pneumonia in whom the pleura is opacified. Adhesions may further impede the dissection. To avoid this complication, the surgeon's two caveats are (1) always dissect thoroughly enough to identify the recurrent laryngeal nerve. If the nerve does not course underneath the vessel, do *not* ligate it; and (2) palpate the thrill before ligation and its disappearance after. Do not close until the thrill is gone! Any ligature discovered on the LPA should be removed. Reestablishment of flow has been reported with removal of LPA ligatures 1 week after they were placed. None of the other answers has proven to be a technical risk in this operation.

7. **D** The techniques of choice for closure of the PDA in the premature infant are (**A**) double ligation with heavy nonabsorbable ligatures (eg, 2.0 or 0.0 silk), or (**B**) double application of clips. A gentle dissection is *de rigeur*. The two ligatures or clips are placed a few millimeters apart. A single ligature or clip is inadequate because of a small risk of subsequent recanalization of the ductus. Thorascoscopic closure of the PDA has been reported, but most

neonatal surgeons prefer the standard operation, via a limited thoracotomy, that allows direct control of bleeding and takes only about 30 minutes. **C**, a standard technique of vascular surgery, is used in older children with PDA but is inappropriate for the short, friable ductus of the premature infant, which tears too easily to permit application of clamps.

BIBLIOGRAPHY

Bancalari E: Neonatal chronic lung disease. In: Fanaroff AA, Martin RI, eds. *Neonatal-Perinatal Medicine: Diseases of the Fetus and Infant.* St. Louis: Mosby; 1997:1074–1089.

Fleming WH, Sarafian MN, Kugler JD, Nelson RM Jr. Ligation of patent ductus arteriosus in premature infants: importance of accurate anatomic definition. *Pediatrics.* 1986;71:373–375.

Grosfeld JL, Chaet M, Molinari F, et al. Increased risk of necrotizing enterocolitis in premature infants with patent ductus arteriosus treated with indomethacin. *Ann Surg.* 1996;224:350–357.

Northway WH Jr, Rosan RC, Porter DY. Pulmonary disease following respiratory therapy of hyaline membrane disease: bronchopulmonary dysplasia. *New Engl J Med.* 1967;276:357.

Pegoli WJ Jr. Pericardium and great vessels. In: Oldham KT, Colombani PM, Foglia RP, eds. *Surgery of Infants and Children: Scientific Principles and Practice.* Philadelphia: Lippincott-Raven; 1997:1001–1004.

Pontius RG, Danielson GK, Noonan JA, Judson JP. Illusions leading to surgical closure of the distal left pulmonary artery instead of the ductus arteriosus. *J Thorac Cardiovasc Surg.* 1981;82:107–113.

Zahka KG, Patel CR. Patent ductus arteriosus. In: Fanaroff AA, Martin RJ, eds. *Neonatal-Perinatal Medicine: Diseases of the Fetus and Infant.* St. Louis: Mosby; 1997:1155–1157.

64 CASE

A 5-YEAR-OLD BOY WITH CEREBRAL PALSY AND VOMITING

HISTORY   A 5-year-old boy with cerebral palsy and developmental delay is hospitalized with right lower lobe pneumonia. He has been hospitalized five times with pulmonary problems over the past 2 years. His parents report that he vomits frequently at home. He is fed via a combination of spoon feeding and gastrostomy tube. He has a seizure disorder that is moderately well controlled on phenobarbitol.

EXAMINATION   Vital signs are temperature 38.6°C, heart rate 110, blood pressure 110/60, respiratory rate 31. His weight is below the fifth percentile for age. Breath sounds are very coarse bilaterally and diminished in the left lower lung field. There is a considerable amount of upper airway congestion. The heart tones are normal without a murmur. His abdomen is flat and nondistended without masses. A percutaneously placed gastrostomy tube is a few centimeters below the left costal margin. He has marked spasticity of all four extremities and significant scoliosis. He is nonverbal but does respond to discomfort with a facial grimace.

LABORATORY   Chest x-ray shows mild to moderate scarring in both lungs with right lower lobe consolidation and a small right pleural effusion. Hematocrit is 35, white blood cell count is 15.8 with an increased fraction of bands.

Please answer all questions before proceeding to discussion section.

✓ QUESTIONS

1. Possible causes for the patient's pneumonia include:
   A. Community acquired pneumococcus
   B. Oropharyngeal aspiration
   C. Gastroesophageal reflux with aspiration

D. Secondary infection of atelectatic lung due to poor secretion clearance

E. All of the above

2. You are asked to see the patient because of possible gastroesophageal (GE) reflux. A barium upper gastrointestinal series has been done and is shown in Figure 64–1. Which of the following is/are true?

A. The image confirms the presence of GE reflux

B. Barium swallow is roughly 85% sensitive for detecting GE reflux

C. The study is not complete unless the ligament of Treitz is visualized

D. This study is a useful means to assess the swallowing mechanism and rule out oropharyngeal aspiration

E. All of the above

3. The most sensitive study to evaluate for the presence of GE reflux is:

A. Barium esophogram

B. Gastroesophageal scintigraphy

C. Twenty-four hour esophageal pH monitoring

D. Upper gastrointestinal endoscopy

E. Bronchoscopy

4. By means of a combination of the tests in question 3, you determine that the patient has significant GE reflux. What is the natural history of the disease in this patient?

A. It is likely to improve with age

B. He has a 25% chance of developing Barrett's epithelium in the distal esophagus if reflux is uncontrolled for 4 years

C. If he is placed on a proton pump inhibitor, he is likely to do well without further intervention

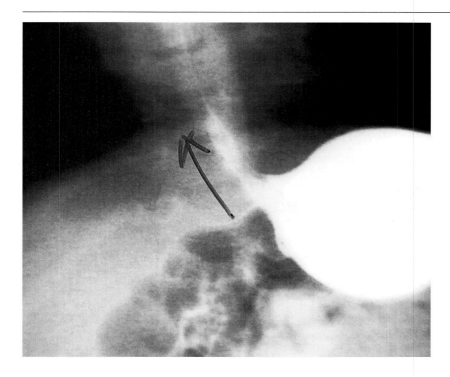

Figure 64–1. *Appearance of an upper gastrointestinal series from a 5-year-old boy with cerebral palsy and vomiting.*

   D. His reflux is not likely to improve
   E. He is at higher risk for gastric cancer than the general population

5. In a patient on maximal medical management, which of the following is *not* considered a strong indication for operation for GE reflux?
   A. Barrett's epithelium
   B. Esophagitis seen at endoscopy and confirmed by esophageal biopsy
   C. Failure the thrive on continuous tube feedings in the absence of esophagitis
   D. Apnea and cyanotic spells coincident with low esophageal pH on a 24-hour study
   E. Recurrent aspiration pneumonia in a patient exclusively fed via gastrostomy tube

6. A video swallowing study shows no evidence of oropharyngeal aspiration and a 24-hour pH study is strongly suggestive of severe GE reflux. When discussing possible operation with the family you tell them:
   A. You are confident that he will be able to continue to be fed by mouth after the operation and perhaps will tolerate oral feeding better when his reflux is controlled
   B. You plan to do a partial fundoplication as studies have shown that this is more effective for neurologically impaired patients
   C. He will require yearly endoscopic examination to ensure that reflux has not returned
   D. Doing the fundoplication laparoscopically has been shown to improve short- and long-term results
   E. There is a 30% chance that the operation will no longer be effective within 5 years

7. What is the natural history of severe GE reflux in a term newborn without neurologic abnormality?
   A. The majority will require fundoplication within 1 year
   B. Thirty percent of infants will develop subglottic stenosis within the first year of life
   C. The reflux will resolve spontaneously in almost all cases
   D. The child will likely develop episodes of pneumonia, but chronic pulmonary disease is not likely
   E. About one fifth of these children will be found to have Hirschsprung disease

8. What is the role of pyloroplasty in conjunction with fundoplication?
   A. It is absolutely indicated if gastric emptying is delayed by greater than 50%
   B. It should never be done
   C. It should be done when there is an esophageal stricture
   D. It might be useful in cases of failed fundoplication and confirmed delayed gastric emptying
   E. It should be done if dumping syndrome is present

ANSWERS AND DISCUSSION

1. **E** Patients with developmental delay can contract pneumonia for many reasons. While GE reflux with aspiration is a common cause of

pneumonia in this population, it is by no means the only cause. Pneumonia is more likely to be caused by gram-negative organisms in a developmentally delayed child than in the general population. The majority of pneumonias in developmentally delayed children, however, are caused by common organisms, such as pneumococcus. Aspiration penumonia in developmentally delayed children may be cause by GE reflux, but it also may be caused by aspiration of oral secretions due to a poorly functioning swallowing mechanism. If a patient such as this one is suspected to have aspiration pneumonia, it is important to evaluate swallowing function with video fluoroscopy in order to investigate the possibility that the pneumonia is secondary to aspirated food or oral secretions. If this is the cause, then elimination of reflux by either medical or surgical means will not prevent further episodes of pneumonia. Children with significant oropharyngeal aspiraton must refrain from oral feeding and be fed via gastrostomy tube.

Patients who are bedridden and immobile have poor clearance of pulmonary secretions. Even in the absence of aspiration, such patients are at risk for recurrent episodes of pneumonia. Regardless of the cause of this patient's pneumonia, it is necessary to wait for clinical stability prior to proceeding with the investigations listed.

2. **C** Figure 64–1 reveals an esophogram with contrast filling the distal esophagus and stomach. The shape of the gastroesophageal junction is somewhat abnormal and in the configuration of an upside-down funnel. This anatomy correlates highly with severe GE reflux. This is a single static image from a real-time study. In order to determine whether or not reflux is present on an upper gastrointestinal series, one must either be present and witness the entire study or speak to the radiologist who performed it. On this single image, one cannot be sure whether the contrast in the esophagus is swallowed contrast on the way down to the stomach or whether it is contrast that is refluxed up from the stomach. Even if you know it is refluxed contrast, you are still not in a position to diagnose GE reflux. A certain amount of reflux is present in normal individuals and can be seen on normal gastrointestinal series. It is important to know the number of episodes of reflux and the time period studied to determine whether or not pathologic reflux is present. A barium swallow is a fairly insensitive test for GE reflux. Its sensitivity is estimated to be anywhere from 30% to 75%, depending on the series. On the other hand, an upper gastrointestinal (GI) series is quite specific. When GE reflux is seen, this is considered diagnostic.

Any time a barium study is done for suspected GE reflux, it is very important to visualize the entire stomach, duodenum, and ligament of Treitz. In some cases, malrotation or gastric outlet obstruction can be causing the patient's vomiting. A standard barium upper GI series is not an effective means of assessing oropharyngeal function. Swallowing must be assessed by a high-speed video examination of the neck while the patient swallows barium of various consistencies. If oropharyngeal swallowing dysfunction is suspected, then this test should be done in addition to the upper GI series.

3. **C** A 24-hour esophageal pH monitoring is considered to be the most sensitive and accurate indicator of GE reflux. First introduced in 1974, this technique measures the duration and frequency of episodes in which the esophageal pH falls below 4. A 24-hour

esophageal pH monitoring is considered the gold standard in the diagnosis of GE reflux. It is reported to be 87% to 93% sensitive and 93% to 97% specific.

The parameters that correlate most highly with clinically important GE reflux are the total percentage of time during the 24 hours where the esophageal pH is less than 4 and the number of reflux episodes that exceed 5 minutes in duration.

A critical aspect of esophageal pH monitoring is confirmation that there actually is acid in the stomach. At the beginning of the study, the probe should be advanced into the stomach to confirm that gastric pH is indeed below 4. If gastric pH is abnormally high secondary to H_2 blockers or proton pump inhibitors, reflux will not be detected by the pH probe. It is, of course, necessary to discontinue the use of these acid-blocking drugs prior to the study. There is mixed evidence whether or not continuous tube feedings will buffer the gastric pH and decrease the sensitivity of the pH study. Jolley and others (1981) have suggested feeding with apple juice during the study in order to obviate this possibility.

As mentioned previously, a barium esophogram is a very insensitive measure of GE reflux. Gastroesophageal scintigraphy is used primarily to evaluate gastric emptying. Nevertheless, it is a reasonably good test for reflux. The scanner is placed over the esophagus, and the isotope is counted within the esophagus. Sensitivity of this study is probably between 50% and 60%. Upper gastrointestinal endoscopy is an important study to evaluate the status of the distal esophagus. Esophagitis can easily be seen visually and can be confirmed by esophageal biopsy. Esophagitis provides confirmation of the presence of GE reflux, but it is not a reliable indicator of its severity. Esophagitis alone seen on endoscopy is not necessarily an indication for surgical therapy. Bronchoscopic examination is sometimes done in infants suspected of having severe GE reflux. A finding of erythema in the glottic and subglottic areas strongly correlates with GE reflux. A normal bronchoscopy, however, by no means rules out the presence of reflux.

4. **D** It is important to understand the natural history of GE reflux in order to select patients properly for surgical therapy. Both the patient's age and neurologic status markedly influence the natural history of GE reflux. The younger the patient, the more likely the reflux will improve over time. The natural history of GE reflux in most infants is one of continued improvement. In a 5-year-old child such as this, further improvement is less likely. Neurologic status is an equally important determinant of natural history. The natural history of GE reflux in neurologically normal children is one of continued improvement in most cases. In children with severe neurologic delay such as this child, GE reflux tends to worsen over time.

Barrett's epithelium occurs when the normal squamous mucosa of the esophagus changes to a columnar-type of mucosa in response to severe and continued acid irritation. Barrett's epithelium is thought to be a precursor for esophageal cancer. It occurs occasionally in children with severe GE reflux, but its incidence is nowhere near the 25% suggested in **B**. Proton pump inhibitors, such as omeprezole, are a highly effective means of reducing the acidity of the stomach. It is important to remember that these drugs reduce or eliminate acid, but they do little to affect GE reflux. In a patient such as this whose primary problem is pulmonary aspiration, elimination of gastric acid is not the answer. Medications, such as cissapride and metaclopramide, increase the rapidity of gastric emptying and may increase lower esophageal sphincter tone. These drugs are effective in controlling reflux in many children. Children with GE reflux have not been shown to be at an increased risk for gastric cancer (**E**).

5. **B** Maximal medical management may include a variety of different measures. Most gastroenterologists recommend that patients with GE reflux be placed on cissapride or metaclopramide for reasons already stated. Patients are also treated with gastric acid inhibitors in an effort to reduce damage to the distal esophagus. Infants with GE reflux should be placed in the prone and 45-degree upright position for 30 to 45 minutes after feeding to use gravity as a means to prevent reflux. Older children should avoid excessively large meals and refrain from lying down immediately after eating.

   Any child considered to have persistent symptomatic reflux despite maximal medical therapy may be considered for operation. Since reflux improves over time in many patients, however, only patients with severe symptoms or those with specific indications are advised to proceed with surgical therapy.

   Barrett's metaplasia in the distal esopagus is indicative of severe and persistent GE reflux and is considered an indication for operation. Failure to thrive despite maximal medical management can lead to severe nutritional compromise. If growth cannot be maintained because of intractable vomiting due to GE reflux, then surgical therapy should be undertaken, even in the absence of other complications of reflux, such as esophagitis or pulmonary disease. Gastroesophageal reflux can cause a laryngospasm and apnea in infants. These spells can lead to cyanosis and are considered life threatening. If apnea spells can be correlated with reflux, the patient should undergo fundoplication. Recurrent aspiration pneumonia due to GE reflux that cannot be controlled medically is also considered an indication for operation.

6. **E** The cornerstone of surgical therapy for GE reflux includes fundoplication of the fundus of the stomach around the distal esophagus. This may include a 360-degree wrap, such as a Nissen fundoplication, or a partial wrap, such as a Thal or Boix-Ochoa operation. Proponents of Nissen fundoplication, the most commonly done procedure, argue that it is the most effective means of preventing GE reflux. Detractors of Nissen fundoplication argue that it has an unacceptably high rate of dysphagia and poor esophageal emptying. This is a particular problem in children with esophageal dysmotility or poor esophageal clearance. Proponents of partial fundoplication argue that it is more physiologic and will allow the child to burp or vomit. They argue that gas-bloat syndrome and dysphagia are much less common after these operations. Critics argue that partial wrap operations are less effective in controlling GE reflux.

   Many children with developmental delay, such as this patient, have abnormal esophageal motility. Fundoplication can affect function of the distal esophagus and esophageal emptying. It is quite possible that a child who tolerated a small amount of oral feedings prior to fundoplication will no longer tolerate them after operation. Families should be made well aware of this possibility, as oral feeding is often one of the greatest pleasures in life for these children. The results of all types of fundoplications are significantly worse in neurologically delayed children than in neurologically normal children. Yearly endoscopic examination is not necessary. In fact, no periodic investigation is necessary unless the child develops clinical evidence of recurrent GE reflux after fundoplication. Laparoscopic fundoplication has been introduced in recent years. While this procedure shows promise and may have a decreased length of stay for neurologically normal patients, its results in this population remain to be seen.

Fundoplication is, at best, an imperfect solution to GE reflux. Even in the best of hands, the rate of recurrent reflux is significant. The best long-term series have shown a 30% reoperation rate over a 5-year period.

7. **C** Gastroesophageal reflux is very common in term infants. Even when it is very severe, it almost always resolves in time. For this reason, these patients should be treated very conservatively. A combination of proper positioning after feedings and medications usually will improve symptoms until the reflux resolves spontaneously. Only a small percentage of these children will ultimately require fundoplication. It is very unlikely that these children will develop pneumonia, and it is virtually unheard of for them to develop subglottic stenosis. Hirschsprung disease causes a distal intestinal obstruction associated with abdominal distention and bilious vomiting. It should not be confused with GE reflux.

8. **D** Most authorities believe that poor gastric emptying is at least a partial cause of GE reflux in some children. Pyloroplasty can increase gastric emptying at the expense of inducing dumping syndrome and other complications in a subset of patients. Gastric emptying is best assessed by a nuclear medicine gastric emptying study. Interpretation of the study's results, however, varies widely. Some authors recommend that pyloroplasty should be done in all children when nuclear medicine gastric emptying is abnormal, and others recommend that pyloroplasty should never be done except in cases of failed fundoplication. There are data to support both of these positions. There is some evidence to suggest that patients undergoing reoperative fundoplication who have markedly prolonged gastric emptying on nuclear study may benefit from pyloroplasty.

BIBLIOGRAPHY

Ashcraft KW, Holder TM, Amoury RA. Treatment of gastroesophageal reflux in children by Thal fundoplication. *J Thorac Cardiovasc Surg.* 1981; 82:706.

Boix-Ochoa J, Casasa JM. Surgical treatment of gastroesophageal reflux in children. In: Nyhus LM, ed. *Surgery Annual.* Norwalk, CT: Appleton & Lange; 1989.

Campbell JR, Gilchrist BF, Harrison MW. Pyloroplasty in association with Nissen fundoplication in children with neurologic disorders. *J Pediatr Surg.* 1989;24:375.

Caniano DA, Ginn-Pease ME, King DR. The failed antireflux procedure: analysis of risk factors and morbidity. *J Pediatr Surg.* 1990;25:1022.

Dahms BB, Rothstein FC. Barrett's esophagus in children: a consequence of chronic gastroesophageal reflux. *Gastroenterol.* 1984;86:318.

Fonkalsrud EW. Nissen fundoplication for gastroesophageal reflux disease in infants and children. *Sem Pediatr Surg.* 1998;7:110–114.

Fonkalsrud EW, Ellis DG, Shaw A, et al. A combined hospital experience with fundoplication and gastric emptying procedure for gastroesophageal reflux in children. *J Am Coll Surg.* 1995;180:449–455.

Georgeson KE. Laparoscopic fundoplication. *Curr Opin Pediatr.* 1998; 10(3):318–322.

Jolley SG, Herbst JJ, Johnson DG. Esophageal pH monitoring during sleep identifies children with respiratory symptoms. *Gastroenterol.* 1981;80:1501.

Orenstein SR. Gastroesophageal reflux. *Pediatr Rev.* 1999;20(1):24–28.

A LARGE INFANT WITH GRUNTING RESPIRATIONS

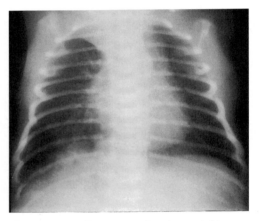

Figure 65–1. *Chest x-ray showing a right lower lobe density. The right upper lobe density represented an azygous lobe.*
From Nicolette LA, Kosleske AM, Bartow SA, et al. *J Pediatr Surg.* 1993;28:802–805.

HISTORY   A 39-week, large for gestational age boy presents shortly after birth with tachypnea and grunting.

EXAMINATION   He is an active male infant in moderate respiratory distress. His respiratory rate is 70/min with intercostal retractions. Temperature is 98.8°F rectally; pulse is 120/min, blood pressure is 74/50. Weight is 3.8 kg. There are no abnormalities of the head, palate, or extremities. Breath sounds are decreased over the right lower lung fields. A grade I/VI systolic murmur is most prominent over the right posterior thorax. The remainder of the physical examination is within normal limits.

LABORATORY   Hemoglobin 14.4 gm%, hematocrit 49%, white blood cell count 11,000/mm^3. Urinalysis is normal. The chest x-ray is shown in Figure 65–1. The oxygen saturation is 88% on room air. Arterial blood gas is pH 7.45, PCO_2 45, PO_2 49, and FIO_2 23%.

HOSPITAL COURSE   Nasal oxygen is administered. Oxygen saturation rises to 92, on 25% oxygen, and respiratory distress decreases. Echocardiogram shows an enlarged left atrium with high ventricular output. Cardiac catheterization is subsequently performed. The aortogram is shown in Figure 65–2. The venous phase of the injection shows normal venous return through a pulmonary vein to the left atrium. No cardiac anomaly is identified. Over the next few days, his dyspnea resolves, although he remains tachypneic. An operation is performed at 3 weeks of age.

Please answer all questions before proceeding to discussion section.

✔ QUESTIONS

1. The primary diagnosis is:
   A. Extralobar pulmonary sequestration
   B. Intralobar pulmonary sequestration
   C. Lobar emphysema
   D. Right upper lobe atelectasis
   E. Right lower lobe pneumonia

2. All of the following statements regarding sequestration are true *except:*
   A. Preoperative angiography is essential for identification of the arterial blood supply
   B. Because of their foregut derivation, sequestrations occasionally communicate with the esophagus or stomach
   C. Intralobar sequestration usually presents with recurrent pulmonary infection
   D. Extralobar sequestration is often associated with congenital diaphragmatic hernia
   E. Both types of sequestration are more common on the left side

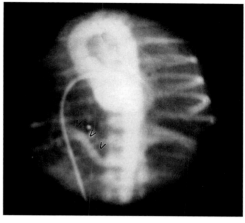

Figure 65–2. *Aortogram showing a large artery (arrow) arising from the descending aorta supplying the anomalous portion of right lower lobe.*
From Nicolette LA, Kosleske AM, Bartow SA, et al. *J Pediatr Surg.* 1993;28:802–805.

ANSWERS AND DISCUSSION

1. **B** The primary diagnosis is intralobar pulmonary sequestration. Pulmonary sequestration is defined as a mass of lung tissue that does not communicate with the tracheobronchial tree through a normal bronchus. The two types of sequestration are intralobar and extralobar. An intralobar sequestration is located within the parenchyma of the lung, whereas an extralobar sequestration (**A**) is separate from the normal lung and enclosed within its own pleural investment. An extralobar sequestration has the gross appearance of a pancake of airless lung tissue located below the lower lobe. The characteristics of the two types of sequestration are summarized in Table 65–1. Lobar emphysema (**C**) has both its arterial supply and venous drainage via the pulmonary vessels, although these vessels are often compressed and tiny from hyperinflation of the lobe. Neither right upper lobe atelectasis (**D**) nor right lower lobe pneu-

Table 65–1. CHARACTERISTICS OF PULMONARY SEQUESTRATION

	Extralobar	Intralobar
Anatomy	Separate from lung	Within lung parenchyma
Location	Below lower lobe	Within basal segments
Predominant side	Left	Left
Age	60% < 1 yr of age	50% > 20 yr
Presentation	Mass at operation or on x-ray	Infection
Male:female ratio	4:1	1:1
Artery	Systemic	Systemic
Vein	Systemic (azygous)	Central (pulmonary veins)
Associated anomalies	Frequent (CDH)	Rare

CDH, congenital diaphragmatic hernia.

monia (**E**) is associated with an aberrant blood supply from the aorta (as shown in Figure 65–2). Neither atelectasis nor pneumonia was found in this case. The right upper lobe density that looked like atelectasis proved to be an azygous lobe, and the sequestration, unlike most of the intralobar variety, was not infected.

2. **A** Angiography is no longer considered essential to the work-up of sequestration. Although the arterial blood supply for both types of sequestration originates from below the diaphragm in up to 20% of patients, other less invasive studies (eg, Doppler flow ultrasound) have supplanted angiography in the work-up. The aberrant vessels traverse the inferior pulmonary ligament; meticulous dissection of this structure is required in the surgery of sequestration. All of the other statements are true. Communication with the gastrointestinal tract (**B**) is found in approximately 10% of sequestrations. Intralobar sequestrations, although lacking their own bronchus, may communicate with adjacent normal lung tissue and typically present with infection (**C**). In general, the older the patient with intralobar sequestration, the more severe the inflammatory change. Nicolette and associates documented the clinical and pathologic spectrum of intralobar sequestration in four patients ranging in age from 3 weeks (mild symptoms and no inflammation) to 6 years (recurrent pneumonia and severe inflammation with bronchiectatic changes). The two children of intermediate ages (3 months, 7.5 months) had intermediate severities of clinical symptoms and inflammatory changes in the pathologic specimen. About 10% to 15% of infants with congenital diaphragmatic hernia (**D**) have an extralobar sequestration discovered during repair of the hernia. Excision is the recommended management for both types of sequestration. Ninety percent of extralobar sequestrations and 60% of intralobar sequestrations occur on the left (**E**). Other features of the two types of sequestration are compared in Table 65–1.

FOLLOW-UP   The operation performed at 3 weeks of age was a right thoracotomy. The medial and anterior basal portions of the right lower lobe were airless and congested with a clear demarcation from the normal appearing portion of the right lower lobe (Figure 65–3; see also color plate). A large artery in the inferior pulmonary ligament (Figure 65–4; see also color plate) was doubly ligated and divided. Stapled wedge

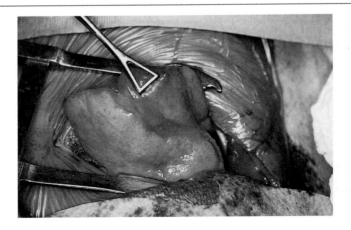

Figure 65–3. *Operative photograph, right lower lobe, showing intralobar sequestration well demarcated from normal lung. (See also color plate.)*

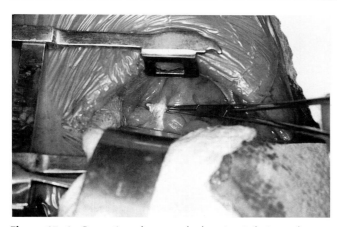

Figure 65–4. *Operative photograph showing inferior pulmonary ligament containing large artery that supplies sequestration. (See also color plate.)*

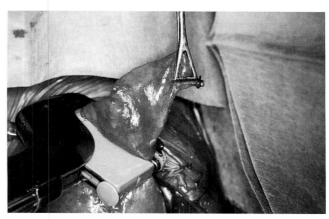

Figure 65–5. *Operative photograph, intralobar sequestration showing stapled wedge resection. (See also color plate.)*

resection was carried out (Figure 65–5; see also color plate). The infant was also noted to have a right upper azygous lobe that was left intact. He made an uncomplicated recovery and was discharged on the sixth postoperative day.

BIBLIOGRAPHY

de Lorimier AA. Respiratory problems related to the airway and lung. In: O'Neill JA Jr, Rowe MI, Grosfeld JL, et al. eds. *Pediatric Surgery.* 5th ed. St. Louis: Mosby-Year Book; 1998:873–897.

Gilbert EF, Opitz JM. Malformations and genetic disorders of the respiratory tract. In: Stocker JT, ed. *Pediatric Pulmonary Disease.* New York: Hemisphere Publishing Corporation; 1989:29–100.

Nicolette LA, Kosloske AM, Bartow SA, et al. Intralobar pulmonary sequestration: a clinical and pathological spectrum. *J Pediatr Surg.* 1993; 28:802–805.

Oldham KT. Lung. In: Oldham KT, Colombani PM, Foglia RP, eds. *Surgery of Infants and Children: Scientific Principles and Practice.* Philadelphia: Lippincott-Raven; 1997:935–970.

CASE

AN 11-MONTH-OLD GIRL WITH A PROTRUDING UMBILICUS

HISTORY   A mother brings her 11-month-old daughter to your office because she is concerned about a protruding umbilicus, which seems to cause pain. Her pediatrician has said it will get better by itself but the mother feels it is too large and ugly, and she worries that her daughter will have an "outie" unless something is done.

EXAMINATION   The patient's abdomen is shown in Figure 66–1. You detect a 2- to 3-cm mound of bowel beneath the umbilical skin, which is temporarily reducible. The abdomen is otherwise normal without masses or tenderness.
  Please answer all questions before proceeding to discussion section.

✓ QUESTIONS

  1. In Figure 66–2 the umbilical mamelon corresponds to which letter?

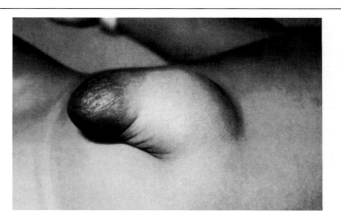

Figure 66–1. *A painless umbilical protrusion in an 11-month-old girl.*

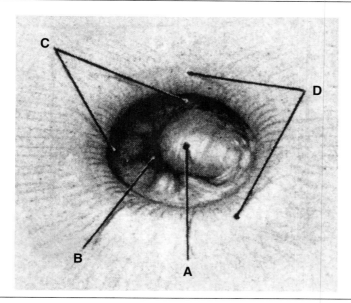

Figure 66–2. *Umbilical structures. See question 1.*

2. A cross-section of a term infant's umbilical cord will never contain:
   A. Wharton's jelly
   B. Amnion
   C. Right umbilical vein
   D. Urachus
   E. Yolk sac

3. Which of the following statements concerning umbilical hernias in children is true?
   A. They occur in 10% of Caucasian newborns and more frequently in African-American children
   B. Spontaneous closure occurs in 85% of children by the age of 5 years and seldom thereafter
   C. They occur with equal frequency in boys and girls
   D. Incarcerated hernias are rare and always contain small bowel
   E. It is a funicular type of hernia and, therefore, prone to incarceration

4. Criteria for operative closure of umbilical hernias may include all but:
   A. Defect greater than 1.5 cm
   B. Age ≥ 5 years
   C. Vitelline or urachal duct remnants present
   D. Incarceration
   E. A "long" sac with a small neck

5. Fine points of the surgical repair of an average umbilical hernia include:
   A. Vest-over-pants fiscial closure
   B. Avoidance of wound infection, the most common complication
   C. Imbrication of the sac
   D. Fluff gauze and tacking suture in the umbilicus
   E. Laparoscopic repair

6. A two vessel umbilical cord:
   A. Should be investigated with an abdominal ultrasound in the newborn
   B. Is due to an absent vein in 1% of live births
   C. May be associated with trisomy, thalidomide use, or maternal diabetes
   D. Is associated with congenital anomalies in 24% of children
   E. Usually presages preterm birth and is associated with an increased rate of fetal demise

7. The umbilical cord should separate:
   A. By 2 weeks following vaginal delivery
   B. Earlier following cesarean delivery
   C. By 10 days; later separation may indicate neutrophil dysfunction
   D. And if it does not, it predisposes the infant to omphalitis
   E. By 2 weeks but if it has not, it may be ligated without further investigation

8. Which of the pairings is unrelated?
   A. Omphalolith—poor hygiene
   B. Sister Mary Joseph—Halsted
   C. Vitelline duct—omphalomesenteric duct
   D. Allantois—urachus
   E. Two Horned Red Monster—omphalomesenteric duct

9. Which of the pairings is unrelated?
   A. Meckel's diverticulum—bladder diverticulum
   B. Omphalomesenteric cyst—urachal cyst
   C. Omphalomesenteric fistula—patent urachus
   D. Umbilical polyp—allantois
   E. Infected urachal cyst—Meckel's diverticulitis

10. In the newborn, possible umbilical secretions and their investigation include all but:
    A. Blood—umbilical artery sinus, local exploration
    B. Urine—patent urachus, Foley catheter
    C. Mucous—patent vitelline duct, sinogram
    D. Pus—omphalitis, umbilical vein excision
    E. Stool—patent omphalomesenteric duct, surgical exploration

ANSWERS AND DISCUSSION

1. **A** Other labels include the cicatrix (**B**), furrow (**C**), and cushion (**D**).

2. **C** The normal umbilical cord contains the left umbilical vein and Wharton's jelly; urachal remnants are sometimes found. Yolk sac remnants are rare. The outer layer of cord epithelium is made up of amnion. The right umbilical vein is thought to obliterate early. When this event occurs late in gestation it may explain the abdominal wall defect of gastroschisis.

3. **C** The finding of an umbilical hernia is weight and gestation dependent: ≥ 80% children under 1.2 kg will have hernias at least transiently; at least 4% of Caucasian and 13% of African-American chil-

dren under 6 weeks of age will have umbilical hernias. Spontaneous closure probably occurs in over 95% of Caucasian patients by age 5 (although accurate longitudinal figures are lacking) and often thereafter, but many surgeons repair them at that age to prevent a source of embarrasment at school. Although umbilical hernias are funicular and predisposed to incarceration in adults, this is a rare event in childhood (~1:1500). When it does occur, the hernia may contain small bowel or omentum.

4. **E** The only hernia that absolutely needs repair in childhood is the incarcerated or strangulated one. This is rare. All other indications are relative. Length of the sac, however, is irrelevant; the diameter of its neck is the rate-limiting factor. Thus, large "proboscis" hernias with narrow necks tend to close spontaneously (even when a "mound" of bowel is present), and those with wide necks do not. Most "outie" belly buttons in adult life are caused by scarring or subcutaneous fat, not a hernia. The only umbilical hernias that predispose to an outie appearance are those with incarcerated omentum.

5. **D** Simple closure with absorbable or nonabsorbable sutures suffices for the initial repair of a typical pediatric umbilical hernia. Some recommend overlapping the fascia with a double line of stitches (vest-over-pants or Mayo technique) when the hernia is particularly large or recurrent. Wound hematoma is the most frequent complication, and it may lead to infection or the appearance of an outie belly button. While sac imbrication may work, most surgeons stress the importance of removing the sac down to healthy linea alba to obtain secure closure and a strong repair. A fluffed gauze compress prevents hematoma and, along with a tacking suture from fascia to skin, encourages an inward appearance of the healed repair. If laparoscopy is being performed for other reasons, it may also be used for repair of an umbilical hernia; otherwise, it is overkill.

6. **C** A single umbilical artery is responsible for the 1% incidence of two vessel cords and should prompt no investigations in the absence of clinical findings. There is, however, an over 50% incidence of associated congenital anomalies including most systems, and these anomalies lead to an increased rate of fetal demise (tenfold) and preterm delivery (tenfold), although most pregnancies still go to term. If detected antenatally, a mother should be offered genetic counseling. Amniocentesis should probably be performed when associated anomalies are detected.

7. **A** Cesarean delivery retards the usual separation of the umbilical cord (by approximately 3 days), which occurs by 2 weeks. Neutrophil dysfunction is infrequent but may be heralded by delayed cord separation. Omphalitis is associated with home deliveries, septic deliveries, low birth weight, and umbilical catheterization but not delayed cord separation. Delayed cord separation may be treated with cord ligation ofter 3 weeks only if there is thin cord with no unusual contents. If the cord is thick, ductal remnants are possible (vitelline, allantois), and it is prudent to perform cord ultrasound to eliminate these possibilities.

8. **B** An omphalolith is dirt found in the umbilicus. Sister Mary Joseph was Mayo's nurse; she noted the association of a prominent umbili-

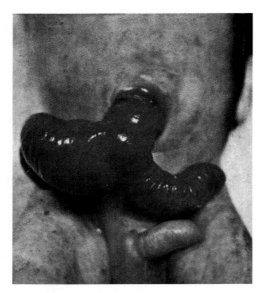

Figure 66–3. *Appearance of a prolapsed omphalomesenteric duct fistula.*

cus with metastatic abdominal cancer. The structures in **C** are synonyms. The allantois divides into the rectum and the urachus, which becomes the bladder. A patent omphalomesenteric duct that prolapses through the umbilicus forms a "T" shape of pink mucosa given the moniker listed (Figure 66–3).

9. **D** Considering the vitelline and urachal systems in parallel does much to simplify the concepts and nomenclature as well as explain findings at or below the umbilicus. (Figures 66–4 and 66–5). Some aspects of each system are unique though. For example, many think that umbilical polyps, which have a pink exterior and secrete mucous, are probably remnants of the vitelline system. They are a nuisance but pose no long-term risks except infection. In contrast, an undetected urachal remnant contains transitional epithelium, which may develop malignancy in later life. The allantois gives rise to both urachal and vitelline systems. It is a precursor of an umbilical polyp.

10. **C** As a general approach to this problem, early operation is preferred to multiple investigations. A section of artery that remains

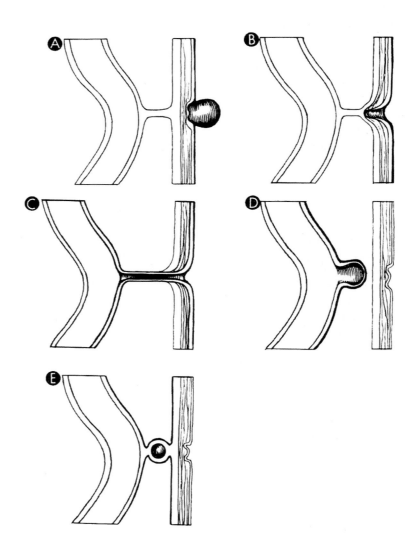

Figure 66–4. *Vitelline duct remnants.* **A,** *granuloma;* **B,** *sinus;* **C,** *fistula (patent omphalomesenteric duct);* **D,** *diverticulum (Meckel's);* and E, cyst.*

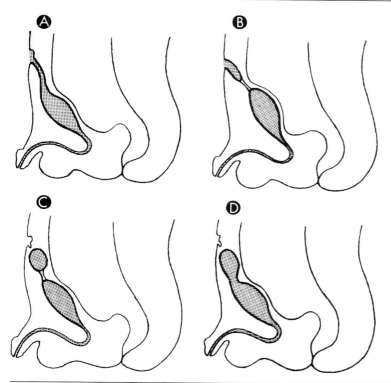

Figure 66–5. *Urachal duct remnants. **A**, fistula (patent urachus); **B**, sinus; **C**, cyst; and **D**, diverticulum (bladder).*

patent may rebleed and should prompt a search for infection. Clear fluid emanating from the umbilicus may be tested for creatinine (this is seldom done), which is diagnostic for a patent urachus (PA). Before undertaking repair of a PA one must assure continuity of the lower genitourinary tract as evidenced by micturition or passage of a Foley catheter. A patent vitelline duct may rarely permit the passage of stool; more often mucous discharge is observed. Few—at most an ultrasound—or no investigations are indicated. A macerated umbilical stump is sometimes confused with pus; however, the latter is diagnostic of omphalitis and should receive immediate antibiotic therapy and aggressive debridement.

This should include the umbilical vein that otherwise provides a diirect route to the venous system. Sometimes infection of an underlying urachal cyst will be found.

BIBLIOGRAPHY

Cullen TS. *Embryology, Anatomy, and Diseases of the Umbilicus Together with Diseases of the Urachus.* Philadelphia: WB Saunders; 1916.

Gill FT. Umbilical hernia, inguinal hernias, and hydroceles in children: diagnostic clues for optimal patient management. *J Pediatr Health Care.* 1998;12:231–235.

Scherer LR 3rd, Grosfeld JL. Inguinal hernia and umbilical anomalies. *Pediatr Clin North Am.* 1993;40:1121.

Skinner MA, Grosfeld JL. Inguinal and umbilical hernia repair in infants and children. *Surg Clin North Am.* 1993;73:439–449.

A 2-YEAR-OLD GIRL WITH JAUNDICE

HISTORY You are asked to see a 2-year-old girl with jaundice. She was born at term and has been entirely healthy until 2 weeks ago when she became fussy and began to eat poorly. She has vomited once or twice a day since that time, and her mother noticed that her eyes were yellow. She has had a few episodes of low grade fever, but her temperature has never been higher than 38.0°C.

EXAMINATION Vital signs are temperature 37.0°C, heart rate 108, blood pressure 110/60, respiratory rate 21. Breath sounds are clear and equal on both sides. The heart tones are normal without a murmur. Her abdomen is full but not markedly distended. It is soft, with mild diffuse tenderness. The liver edge is 1.5 cm below the costal margin. Rectal examination reveals grayish stool that is guaiac negative.

LABORATORY The hematocrit is 31, white blood cell count 14.5 with a normal differential, platelet count 187,000. Total bilirubin is 6.2 with a direct fraction of 4.4. Aspartate transaminase (AST) is 190, alanine transaminase (ALT) is 232, alkaline phosphatase is 456. Prothrombin time is 11.5 with INR of 1.1.
   Please answer all questions before proceeding to discussion section.

✓ QUESTIONS

1. Which of the following is most consistent with the findings?
   A. Acute hepatitis A infection
   B. Acute hepatitis B infection
   C. Chronic hepatitis B carrier state with hepatic fibrosis
   D. Obstructive jaundice
   E. Extrahepatic biliary atresia

2. The most appropriate diagnostic test at this point is:
   A. Abdominal computed tomography (CT) scan with intravenous and oral contrast
   B. Abdominal ultrasound
   C. Upper gastrointestinal endoscopy
   D. Serum for hepatitis panel
   E. A and C

3. You obtain the study shown in Figure 67–1. You advise the child's family that:
   A. Urgent operation is indicated because of biliary tract obstruction
   B. The child should undergo a nuclear medicine study of biliary excretion
   C. Antibiotics are indicated to treat cholangitis. If the child does not improve, operation may be necessary
   D. An abdominal CT scan will be necessary for diagnosis
   E. None of the above

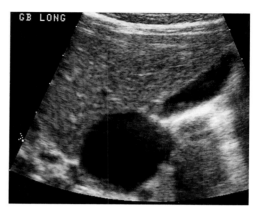

Figure 67–1. *Ultrasound examination of the baby's abdomen.*

4. Many variants of choledochal cyst have been described using several different classification systems. Which of the following is *not* considered a variant of choledochal cyst?
   A. Diverticulum of the common bile duct
   B. Intraduodenal cystic dilation at the ampulla of Vater (choledochocele)
   C. Cystic dilation of the common bile duct
   D. Dilation of both intra- and extrahepatic bile ducts
   E. Dilation of the gallbladder with normal-sized common bile duct

5. Theories regarding the etiology of choledochal cyst include:
   A. Presence of a long common channel between the common bile and pancreatic ducts causing pancreaticobiliary reflux
   B. Congenital factors that cause a marked female predominance of the disease
   C. In utero obstruction of the common bile duct
   D. A and C
   E. All of the above

6. A hepato-iminodiacetic acid (HIDA) scan confirms that this patient has a type I choledochal cyst. Acceptable management options include:
   A. Complete excision of the cyst with Roux-en-Y hepaticojejunostomy
   B. Cyst duodenostomy
   C. Drainage of the cyst with a Roux-en-Y limb of jejunum
   D. Transhepatic biliary drainage followed by cyst excision after the dilation has resolved
   E. All of the above

7. With regard to malignant degeneration of a choledochal cyst, which is true?
   A. It has been reported to occur following drainage of the cyst with a Roux-en-Y limb of jejunum
   B. It typically occurs 2 to 4 years after the onset of jaundice
   C. After cyst excision, malignancy occurs in about 5% of cases

D. The incidence is 5% to 8% after cyst excision, but it is usually resectable when it occurs

E. Squamous carcinoma is the most common histologic variant

8. You do the appropriate operation, and the patient has a very smooth postoperative course. Three years later the patient develops fever, abdominal pain, and jaundice. The most likely diagnosis is:
   A. Cholangiocarcinoma
   B. Acute cholecystitis
   C. Pancreatitis and secondary obstruction of the anastamosis
   D. Caroli disease
   E. Biliary stricture

ANSWERS AND DISCUSSION

1. **D** The most important initial observation in a patient with jaundice is to determine whether the jaundice is due to a blockage of the bile duct (usually a surgical problem) or to a problem with bilirubin conjugation and excretion (usually a medical problem). The preponderance of direct bilirubin on serum testing argues strongly that this patient has biliary obstruction. The finding of acholic stools further supports the provisional diagnosis of obstructive jaundice.

   Infectious hepatitis can occur at any age. Acute viral hepatitis causes jaundice, abdominal pain, and vomiting. The liver, however, is usually enlarged and tender, and the transaminase levels are markedly elevated due to necrosis of hepatocytes. The AST and ALT levels are usually in the thousands rather than the hundreds. Chronic hepatitis B infection with fibrosis can lead to slowly progressive jaundice, but the indirect fraction is typically predominant. Extrahepatic biliary atresia causes obstructive jaundice in the first 3 months of life. It is not in the differential diagnosis of a previously well 2 year old.

2. **B** Abdominal ultrasound is an extremely useful test in the evaluation of the patient thought to have obstructive jaundice. It is a readily available and noninvasive means of determining the size of the extra- and intrahepatic bile ducts, the status of the gallbladder, and the condition of the liver parenchyma. An abdominal CT scan is a less effective means of imaging the bile duct and is not an effective way to image the gallbladder. It also requires radiation exposure. Upper gastrointestinal endoscopy is of little use in the evaluation of jaundice. A hepatitis panel is unlikely to be helpful for reasons already mentioned.

3. **B** This longitudinal image through the liver shows the gallbladder next to a large cystic structure in the porta hepatis. The liver parenchyma appears normal, and there is no dilation of the intrahepatic ductal system. These findings are most consistent with the diagnosis of type I choledochal cyst (cystic dilation of the common bile duct). Other cystic masses that could occur in this region include duodenal or gastric duplication, omental or mesenteric cysts, or choledochocele. Intestinal duplications usually have an echogenic wall on ultrasound and are not typically associated with biliary obstruction. Omental or mesenteric cysts are similarly unrelated to

jaundice and typically do not occur near the porta hepatis. Choledochoceles are rare and may cause jaundice, but they are rarely as large as this lesion.

To confirm your diagnostic suspicions, you would like to demonstrate that the dilated cystic structure is indeed part of the biliary tree. The best way to do this is by means of a nuclear medicine biliary excretion study—a HIDA or DISIDA scan. In this study, a radio-labeled isotope is given that is taken up by the liver and excreted in the bile. The isotope should be seen filling the entire cystic structure prior to its appearance in the intestine.

Operation for choledochal cyst is never an emergency except in rare cases of cyst rupture. Antibiotics are appropriate to treat cholangitis when present. Abdominal CT scan is not useful for reasons already mentioned.

4. **E** Alonzo-Lej and colleagues (1959) and Todani and associates (1984) are responsible for the widely used classification system of choledochal cysts (Figure 67–2). These varieties are type I, cystic or fusiform dilation of the extrahepatic bile duct with normal intrahepatic ducts; type II, diverticulum of the extrahepatic duct; type III, choledochocele (cystic dilation within the duodenal wall at the ampulla of Vater); type IV, multiple cysts of both the intra- and extraheaptic biliary tree; and type V, intrahepatic biliary cystic disease (also called Caroli disease when associated with hepatic fibrosis).

Type I is the most common abnormality. There is no known entity that causes congenital dilation of the gallbladder.

5. **E** Theories abound regarding the etiology of choledochal cysts. All of them provide useful clues to the pathogenesis, but none of them explains all of the facets of the disease. Cholangiography of these patients confirms that, in the majority, the pancreatic duct enters the

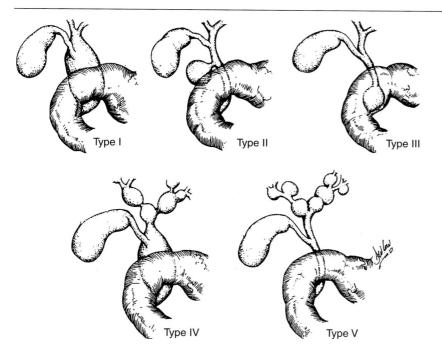

Figure 67–2. *The classification system for choledochal cysts (see text). (Redrawn from O'Neill JA. Choledochal cyst.* Curr Probl Surg. *1992;29:372.)*

common bile duct well proximal to the sphincter of Oddi. Therefore, pancreatic juice may reflux into the common bile duct during development and weaken the wall, predisposing to dilation. Some patients with choledochal cyst, however, do not have this pancreaticobiliary anatomy. Furthermore, up to 10% of patients without choledochal cyst who undergo endoscopic retrograde cholangiopancreatography (ERCP) are found to have this anatomic variant.

Other investigators believe that intrauterine bile duct obstruction is a cause of choledochal cyst. Experimental obstruction in neonatal lambs produces a lesion similar to choledochal cysts. Choledochal cysts are now frequently diagnosed by prenatal ultrasound examination, however. Most of these patients are asymptomatic, and many never develop jaundice after birth. The disease is much more common in girls, and some type of sex-linked genetic factor has been suggested.

6. **A** Proper treatment of a type I choledochal cyst incudes complete excision of the cyst wall with biliary enteric reconstruction. Any procedure that simply drains the cyst will predispose the patient to two problems: recurrent cholangitis and bile duct cancer. Long-term follow-up of patients undergoing cyst drainage suggests that 20% to 40% of patients will develop episodes of cholangitis. This compares to a 2% to 3% incidence after excision of the cyst. Malignancy has been reported following drainage in multiple cases (see answer 7). Transhepatic biliary drainage has been used to treat cholangitis refractory to antibiotics. This is rarely necessary. In most cases, this one included, it is not necessary.

Prior to operative resection of the cyst, the surgeon should place a small tube in the gallbladder and do a cholangiogram. This study defines the cyst anatomy in relation to the liver and the pancreatic duct. It also allows the surgeon to determine the status of the right and left hepatic ducts and the intrahepatic ducts. If the disease extends above the bifurcation of the common hepatic duct, the surgeon may elect to excise this area and anastomose the right and left ducts to the jejunum separately. If there is significant intrahepatic disease (type IV), the patient's prognosis is markedly altered. Figure 67–3 shows the operative cholangiogram in this case.

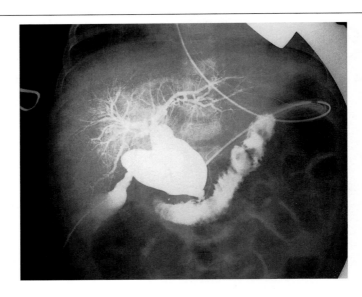

Figure 67–3. *Operative cholangiogram for this patient. A tube has been surgically placed in the gallbladder. A nasogastric tube is in the stomach. There is a large cystic dilation of the extrahepatic bile duct up to the level of the bifurcation. At this point, the ducts become normal in caliber. The structure and arborization pattern of the intrahepatic ducts appear normal. There is flow of contrast into the duodenum. The pancreatic duct enters the common bile duct proximal to the sphincter of Oddi forming a "long common channel."*

After cyst resection, the biliary tree may be drained by several means. Roux-en-Y hepaticojejunostomy is the most widely practiced. Some authors advocate hepaticoduodenostomy while others use a valved jejunal conduit from the liver to the duodenum. None of these methods have been proven superior to the others.

7. **A** Numerous authors have reported the occurrence of malignant degeneration of choledochal cysts treated by drainage alone. Malignancy typically occurs 15 to 20 years following drainage of the cyst. Most of these cancers are not resectable and prove fatal. There are no reports of bile duct cancer after excision of a choledochal cyst. The histologic type is adenocarcinoma.

8. **E** Long-term complications after successful cyst excision and Roux-en-Y hepaticojejunostomy occur in less than 5% of patients. When jaundice occurs late, it is usually the result of a stricture in the right or left hepatic duct or at the anastomosis. The initial test of choice is an abdominal ultrasound. If all or part of the biliary tree is dilated, it may be investigated via percutaneous transhepatic cholangiography.

   Carcinoma has not been reported following cyst excision. Acute cholecystitis is not possible since the gallbladder was removed along with the choledochal cyst. Pancreatitis is uncommon, and the pancreas is anatomically remote from the anastomosis. Caroli disease is very unlikely since the cholangiogram at the time of resection showed a normal intrahepatic biliary tree.

BIBLIOGRAPHY

Alonzo-Lej F, Revor WB, Pessagno DJ. Congenital choledochal cyst, with a report of 2, and an analysis of 94 cases. *Surg Gynecol Obstet Internat Abst Surg.* 1959;108:1.

Fieber SS, Nance FC. Choledochal cyst and neoplasm: a comprehensive review of 106 cases and presentation of two original cases. *Am Surg.* 1997;63:982–987.

Miyano T, Yamataka A. Choledochal cysts. *Curr Opin Pediatr.* 1997;9:283–288.

Mori K, Akimoto R, Kanno M, et al. Anomalous union of the pancreaticobiliary ductal system without dilation of the common bile duct or tumor: case reports and literature review. *Hepatogastroenterology.* 1999;46:142–147.

O'Neill JA Jr. Choledochal cyst. *Curr Probl Surg.* 1992;29:361–410.

Todani T, et al. Anomalous arrangement of the pancreaticobiliary ductal system in patients with choledochal cyst. *Am J Surg.* 1984;147:672.

A 2-WEEK-OLD BABY WITH A RIGHT PLEURAL EFFUSION

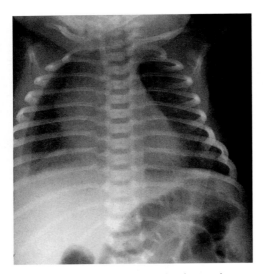

Figure 68–1. *Chest radiograph of a newborn infant with tachypnea.*

HISTORY   An infant is born following a difficult and prolonged labor requiring high forceps delivery. He is admitted to the nursery for observation and sepsis work-up. His blood cultures are negative, and apart from a cephalohematoma, he appears well. On his planned day of discharge, he is noted to be tachypneic, and a chest radiograph is obtained (Figure 68–1).

Please answer all questions before proceeding to discussion section.

✓ QUESTIONS

1. The most likely cause of this pleural effusion is:
   A. Traumatic hemothorax
   B. Unrecognized esophageal perforation
   C. Traumatic chylothorax
   D. Pulmonary lymphangiomatosis

2. Appropriate initial treatment would consist of:
   A. Chest tube placement, intravenous antibiotics
   B. Chest tube placement, contrast esophagogram
   C. Chest tube placement, cessation of enteral nutrition with full parenteral nutritional support
   D. None of the above

3. Confirmation of the diagnosis can be obtained by:
   A. Thoracoscopy
   B. Thoracotomy
   C. Pulmonary lymphangiography
   D. Cellular and biochemical analysis of the fluid

4. Complications of nonoperative treatment of this condition include:
   A. Malnutrition
   B. Lymphopenia
   C. Hyponatremia
   D. All of the above

5. Which of the following statements is *false?*
   A. Patients undergoing chylous drainage should be treated with immune stimulants to reduce susceptibility to infection from lymphocyte depletion
   B. Failure of conservative therapy may be due to central venous thrombosis
   C. Somatostatin (octreotide) may be useful in the treatment of chylothorax, which is refractory to initial conservative therapy
   D. Surgery is indicated in patients in whom a chylous leak persists after 2 to 4 weeks of conservative therapy

6. Which of the following statements regarding surgical therapy for chylothorax is true?
   A. Bilateral thoracotomies are usually required
   B. A pleuroperitoneal shunt may be required
   C. Surgery is necessary in most cases of postoperative chylothorax
   D. None of the above

ANSWERS AND DISCUSSION

1. C Chylothorax occurs when chyle escapes from the thoracic duct into one or both pleural spaces. The causes of chylothorax include congenital lymphatic malformations, trauma (both surgical and nonsurgical), and neoplastic conditions, most commonly lymphoma. A number of children will have no discernable cause for their chylothorax. Surgical procedures in the chest result in disruption of the thoracic duct or its branches represent the most common cause of chylothorax. It is estimated that postoperative chylothorax complicates approximately 1% to 2% of cardiothoracic procedures performed in children. Birth trauma, the presumed cause in this child, results when stretching, shearing, or sudden intrathoracic pressure changes causes thoracic duct rupture. Chylothorax may also result when thrombosis of the left subclavian vein causes lymphaticovenous obstruction.

2. C The appropriate initial treatment of chylothorax involves pleural drainage and reduction of chylous flow. This is best achieved by thoracostomy tube placement and restriction of dietary fat to either lipids in total parenteral nutrition or orally administered medium chain triglycerides (MCT), both of which result in minimal lymph flow in the thoracic duct.

3. D The diagnosis of chylothorax is confirmed by pleural fluid analysis. Typically, the fluid is creamy white and odorless with benign cytology and sterile cultures. The cellular composition is predominantly white blood cells, almost all of which are lymphocytes. The triglyceride content is high, usually in the range 400 to 4000 mg/dL, while the lipoprotein profile demonstrates a predominance of chylomicrons. There is a condition in which pleural fluid has an appearance similar to that seen in chylothorax that results from long-standing pleural inflammation and fibrosis. This condition, called "pseudochylothorax," produces fluid with a high cholesterol content but no triglycerides or chylomicrons.

4. **D** The complications associated with leakage of chyle out of mediastinal lymphatics are related acutely to pulmonary compression from accumulated fluid, which causes respiratory compromise. Nutritional deficiencies as well as fluid and electrolyte disorders (typically hyponatremia) result from the loss of the protein, fat, vitamin, and electrolyte components of chyle. Immune compromise may occur in response to prolonged lymphocyte (and hence T-cell) depletion.

5. **A** Although prolonged chylous drainage results in lymphocyte depression and transient immune compromise, there is no role for immune stimulating therapy. Rather, these patients should be considered conservative treatment failures and should undergo operation for definitive therapy. Another group of patients in whom early surgical intervention should be considered are those with subclavian vein or superior vena caval thrombosis, in whom the high resistance to lymphatic flow into the venous circulation makes it unlikely that a distal lymphatic leak will close spontaneously. Although recommendations for duration of conservative therapy vary, it would seem that a 2 to 4 week trial should be sufficient, as long as adequate nutrition by modified enteral or parenteral routes is provided. There is reported anecdotal success with the use of somatostatin in the conservative treatment of chylothorax refractory to chest drainage and total parenteral nutrition.

6. **B** Although the majority of cases of spontaneous, traumatic, or postoperative chylothorax will respond to conservative measures, operation is required for the occasional nonresponder. Until recently, surgical procedures mandated a thoracotomy, however, there now is considerable experience with video-assisted thoracoscopic surgery (VATS) for identification and obliteration of leak sites. Identification of the leak site is often difficult, but it may be facilitated by the adminstration of milk or a fatty meal prior to surgery. Direct suture techniques, thoracic duct ligation, and multiple suture ligatures placed in the mediastinal pleura, as well as application of fibrin glue, chemical or talc pleurodesis, and apical pleurectomy have all been described. Pleuroperitoneal shunts offer a good surgical alternative for patients in whom pulmonary comorbidity makes thoracotomy a formidable undertaking.

BIBLIOGRAPHY

Engum SA, Rescorla FJ, West KW, et al. The use of pleuroperitoneal shunts in the management of persistent chylothroax in infants. *J Pediatr Surg.* 1999;34:286–290.

Merrigan BA, Winter DC, O'Sullivan GC. Chylothorax. *Br J Surg.* 1997;84:15–20.

Miller JI. Diagnosis and management of chylothorax. *Chest Surg Clin North Am.* 1996;6:139–148.

A 15-YEAR-OLD FEMALE
WITH ABDOMINAL PAIN

HISTORY: A 15-year-old female has been admitted to the gastroenterology service for workup of abdominal pain and distension, bloody stools, and fever. She had been completely well until 3 days earlier, when upon her return from a camping trip with friends, she developed anorexia, malaise, and crampy abdominal pain, then profuse loose and now bloody stools. No one else from the camping trip has developed similar symptoms. Her past medical history includes a recent episode of sinusitis for which she was prescribed a week's course of augmentin. There is no family history of inflammatory bowel disease. She is lethargic and dehydrated on admission, but after 2000 mL of resuscitative crystalloid, feels considerably better. A surgical consultation is requested.

EXAMINATION Temperature is 39.4°C, pulse is 120, and blood pressure is 120/70. She is pale and warm. Her abdomen is distended, quiet, and diffusely tender. You observe one of her stools, which is loose and contains mucus and streaks of blood. Laboratory investigations include a hematocrit of 32, WBC 18,000, platelets of 350,000, and an erythrocyte sedimentation rate (ESR) of 60 mm/hour. Abdominal plain films are ordered, but without your knowledge the radiologist does a contrast enema instead (Figure 69–1).

Please answer all questions before proceeding to discussion section.

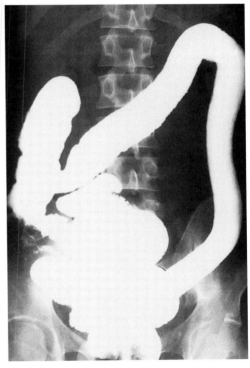

Figure 69–1. The contrast enema reveals a tubular colon, without haustrations, and with fine ulcerations throughout its entire length. These changes are caused by edema, ulceration, and altered motility due to inflammation. The barium has a granular, flocculent quality due to edema, mucus, blood, and exudate. The fuzziness of the luminal margin is due to mucus and ulcerations, and when pronounced, gives the surface a serrated border.

✓ QUESTIONS

1. The differential diagnosis in this girl includes all of the following except:
   A. Acute infectious colitis
   B. Crohn's colitis
   C. Neutropenic enterocolitis
   D. Fulminant ulcerative colitis

After stool and blood cultures are obtained, the child is started on intravenous ampicillin, gentamicin, and flagyl. Two days later her stool cultures are all negative. She undergoes a cautious flexible sigmoidoscopy with limited insufflation, which demonstrates diffuse mucosal friability and ulceration with extensive loss of epithelium, extending to the limit of the examination (Figure 69–2; see also color plate). No biopsies are taken for fear of perforating the colon. Although her abdominal pain has decreased somewhat, she remains distended and febrile with bloody mucoid stools.

2. At this juncture, the most appropriate course of treatment is:
   A. Nothing by mouth, central or peripheral hyperalimentation, and high dose intravenous steroids
   B. Intravenous vancomycin for probable pseudomembranous colitis (antibiotic associated)
   C. Mesalamine enemas
   D. None of the above

3. After 3 days of intensive medical therapy, her condition has not improved significantly. Her stool cultures have grown yeast, and she continues to spike fevers while still receiving triple antibiotics. Abdominal x-rays show pancolonic mural thickening and thumbprinting without colonic dilation, but no intramural or free air. Her abdomen remains soft, her hematocrit is stable at 27, and she has not yet received a blood transfusion. At this point, you elect to:
   A. Repeat colonoscopy, this time with biopsies
   B. Obtain and abdominal CT scan to look for microperforation with abscess formation
   C. Continue present medical therapy
   D. Proceed to laparotomy for total colectomy

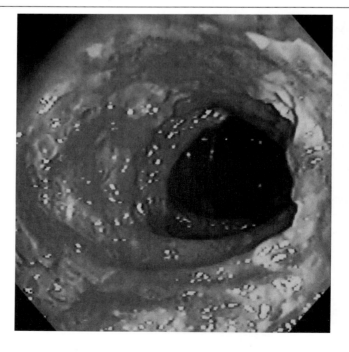

Figure 69–2. *Endoscopic appearance of the colon. The mucosa is severely inflamed with exudative, bloody mucus, and ulcerations. The folds appear thickened and nondistensible from swelling and spasm. No pseudomembranes are present. These changes are nonspecific, and could be seen in acute infectious colitis or inflammatory bowel disease. (See also color plate.)*

4. After 7 days of intensive medical therapy, there is a definite clinical improvement with defervescence, resolution of abdominal distension, and fewer bloody stools. Repeat colonoscopy demonstrates pancolitis, with mild inflammation in the last 2 or 3 cm of distal ileum. Biopsies are obtained from throughout the colon, and representative histopathology is shown in Figure 69–3 (see also color plate). Before you have a chance to review the slides yourself, the pathologist calls you to tell you he sees an abundant inflammatory process in the lamina propria, with frequent crypt abscesses. No granulomas are apparent. The most likely diagnosis is:
   A. Crohn's disease
   B. Ulcerative colitis
   C. Pseudomembranous colitis
   D. Amebic dysentery

5. After continued improvement the girl is discharged on 40 mg of prednisone and 4 g of salazopyrine daily. Over the next few months, several attempts to wean her dose of steroid have resulted in a symptomatic flare with bloody diarrhea. An upper GI series with follow-through does not demonstrate any abnormality of the small bowel. A repeat colonoscopy confirms acute pancolitis, with no evidence of granulomas. At this point you recommend that the patient undergo:
   A. Total proctocolectomy with end ileostomy
   B. Total abdominal colectomy
   C. Total abdominal with ileoproctostomy
   D. Total abdominal colectomy, endorectal mucosectomy, and ileal J-pouch pull through

6. Six months following complete surgical reconstruction with a J-pouch, the girl develops symptoms of crampy pelvic pain, fever, and loose watery stools. The most likely diagnosis is:
   A. Pelvic inflammatory disease
   B. "Pouchitis"
   C. Crohn's disease
   D. None of the above

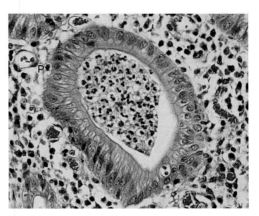

Figure 69–3. *High-powered cross-section through a colonic gland demonstrating pus in the lumen, with occasional polymorphs (P) near the basement membrane, consistent with a crypt abscess. (See also color plate.)*

ANSWERS AND DISCUSSION

1. **C** This girl appears to have acute colitis, the differential diagnosis of which includes infectious colitis (*Salmonella, Shigella, Campylobacter, Yersinia*), antibiotic associated colitis (*Clostridium difficile*), ischemic colitis, and inflammatory bowel disease. With a normal or elevated WBC, by definition she could not have neutropenic enterocolitis.

2. **A** The initial therapy for all patients with acute colitis is supportive and includes broad spectrum antibiotics, until an infectious etiology has been excluded. Early, cautious diagnostic endoscopy with limited insufflation should be performed, and in cases where inflammatory bowel disease is suspected, the patient should be treated aggressively with high-dose intravenous steroids and bowel rest. Patients with fulminant pancolitis on high steroid doses are at risk for acute colonic complications including perforation, hemorrhage, and toxic dilation, and must be followed very closely, both clinically and radiologically. High doses of opiates or anticholinergics, electrolyte disturbances such

as hypokalemia, and contrast or therapeutic steroid enemas should be avoided to minimize the risks of precipitating toxic megacolon.

3. **C** This patient continues to have symptomatic acute colitis of uncertain etiology, however the continued negative stool culture results increase the likelihood that this represents inflammatory bowel disease (IBD), most likely ulcerative colitis. In the absence of complicating factors, this patient should be maintained on aggressive medical therapy in the hopes of inducing a clinical remission, which typically occurs in three quarters of patients presenting with acute ulcerative pancolitis. Those patients that do not respond to systemic corticosteroids generally proceed to colectomy. Recently, reports of induced remission with cyclosporin A (CsA) after a failed trial of steroids have led to consideration of this therapy for patients with severe acute colitis refractory to steroids. In most reports, the remission is short lived, with less than half of all patients retaining their colons 6 months after treatment with CsA.

4. **B** Ulcerative colitis (UC) is characterized by chronic mucosal inflammation involving the rectum and a variable contiguous length of proximal colon, depending on disease extent. Patients with pancolitis usually have adjacent inflammation in the distal few centimeters of ileum; so called backwash ileitis. An inflammatory cellular infiltrate, composed primarily of neutrophils and lymphocytes, with varying amounts of plasma cells (depending on disease chronicity), and macrophages resides within the lamina propria. Crypt abscesses are collections of pus within the mucous gland crypts, and epithelial regeneration after crypt abscess formation often results in branched glandular architecture. Granulomas are the hallmark finding in "granulomatous" (Crohn's) colitis, and are never seen in UC. In some patients, the differentiation of Crohn's disease from UC cannot be made with certainty. This had led to the term "indeterminate colitis," which is used to describe colectomy specimens in which the predominant features are those of UC, except for the presence of a significant number of transmural lymphoid aggregates. Rather than being a separate disease, indeterminate colitis represents a histologic overlap, in which the behavior of the disease seems to more closely resemble UC than Crohn's disease, although it may be associated with a higher complication rate following restorative proctocolectomy than in patients with unequivocal UC.

Pseudomembranous colitis is an infectious disease usually associated with antibiotics and acquired *Clostridium difficile* infection. The spectrum of manifest symptoms range from the asymptomatic carrier to the patient with fulminant colitis or toxic megacolon. The classic endoscopic finding is that of yellow-white plaques of pseudomembranes which are adherent to inflamed mucosa in approximately 25% of patients. Treatment for peudomembranous enterocolitis is either metronidazole or vancomycin, preferable by the enteral route.

5. **B** The tendency for symptomatic relapse with attempted steroid reduction is quite characteristic of ulcerative pancolitis. Colectomy provides definitive therapy for patients with ulcerative colitis, and until 20 years ago this meant total proctocolectomy and end ileostomy. Nowadays, most patients are offered restorative proctocolectomy, in which the entire colon and the mucosal lining of the

rectum are removed, and a reservoir constructed from ileum (J- or S-pouch) is pulled through to the dentate line. This operation can be done in one, two, or three stages. Although there is experience with one-stage colectomy and ileal pouch reconstruction without temporary proximal fecal diversion, most surgeons would opt for a staged reconstruction, beginning with total abdominal colectomy, in patients with severe inflammatory disease on high dose steroids, or in anyone in whom the diagnosis of UC versus Crohn's disease is uncertain.

6. **B** Approximately 25% of patients undergoing restorative proctocolectomy develop symptomatic inflammation of their ileal reservoir. The typical symptoms are crampy abdominal pain, fever, rectal bleeding, and diarrhea, either in the form of acute intermittent attacks or a chronic "pouchitis" syndrome. The etiology of this pouchitis is probably multifactorial, involving genetic, immune, microbial, and toxic mediators. The histologic features are those of acute and chronic inflammation, and villous atrophy. Occasionally a patient thought to have ulcerative or indeterminate colitis will prove to have Crohn's pouchitis, however this diagnosis requires the identification of granulomata on biopsy. Approximately 80% of patients with pouchitis will respond to metronidazole. Occasionally pouchitis is so severe and difficult to control, that temporary ileostomy diversion and ultimately, pouch excision is required.

BIBLIOGRAPHY

Bickston SJ, Cominelli F. Inflammatory bowel disease: Short- and long-term treatments. *Dis Mon.* 1998;44:144–172.

Durno C, Sherman P, Harris K, et al. Outcome after ileoanal anastomosis in pediatric patients with ulcerative colitis. *J Pediatr Gastroenterol Nutr.* 1998;27:501–507.

Nicholls RJ, Banarjee AK. Pouchitis: Risk factors, etiology, and treatment. *World J Surg.* 1998;22:347–351.

Roy MA. Inflammatory bowel disease. *Surg Clin North Am.* 1997;77:1419–1431.

A LARGE ABDOMINAL MASS IN A 20-MONTH-OLD GIRL

HISTORY   A 20-month-old girl was referred by her pediatrician after the discovery of a large abdominal mass. She had been well until 3 weeks ago. Since then, she has experienced decreased appetite with intermittent vomiting, vague abdominal pain, and lethargy.

EXAMINATION   The girl is an irritable 20 month old. Sclerae are clear with no lymphadenopathy. Her abdomen is distended, and there is a firm, immobile, nontender upper abdominal mass extending from the right costal margin, across the midline in the epigastrium, inferiorly to the right iliac crest. There are prominent superficial veins across the upper abdominal wall.

LABORATORY   Hematocrit 27, platelets 300,000. Liver function tests are normal with the exception of mild elevation of serum transaminases (serum glutamic oxaloacetic transaminase 78, serum glutamic pyruvic transaminase 90). An abdominal computed tomography (CT) scan is shown in Figure 70–1. After open tumor biopsy, the patient received

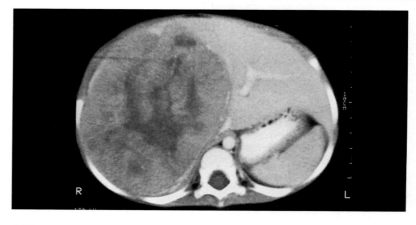

Figure 70–1. *Large tumor arising from the right liver lobe, which displaces and distorts the inferior vena cava. Although resectable, an extended right lobectomy (trisegmentectomy) would be required for complete tumor removal.*

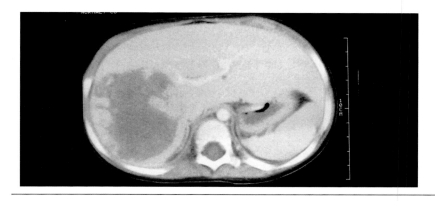

Figure 70–2. *The same patient as shown in Figure 70–1, after four cycles of cisplatin, vincristine, and 5-fluorouracil. The tumor has been reduced significantly in size and is now amenable to complete resection by right hepatic lobectomy.*

multiagent chemotherapy, and her post-treatment CT scan is shown in Figure 70–2. She then underwent right hepatic lobectomy (Figure 70–3).
 Please answer all questions before proceeding to discussion section.

✓ QUESTIONS

1. The most common primary hepatic tumor of childhood is:
   A. Hepatocellular carcinoma (HCC)
   B. Hepatoblastoma (HB)
   C. Hemangioma
   D. Mesenchymal hamartoma

2. Which of the following are *not* risk factors for the development of HB?
   A. Beckwith-Weidemann syndrome
   B. Hemihypertrophy
   C. Hepatitis B infection
   D. A genetic mutation involving the short arm of chromosome 11

3. Which of the following statements regarding the presentation of hepatoblastoma is *true?*
   A. Boys are more commonly affected than girls

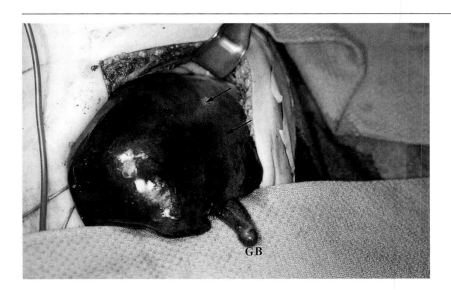

GB

Figure 70–3. *Operative photograph of the same patient during right hepatic lobectomy after portal dissection and division of the right hepatic artery and right portal vein. Note the area of vascular demarcation (arrows) in line with the mobilized gallbladder (GB).*

  B. Age at presentation is usually greater than 3 years
  C. Tumor location is distributed equally between right and left lobes
  D. Jaundice is a frequent presenting symptom

4. Which of the following are appropriate preoperative studies in this patient?
  A. Abdominal CT scan
  B. Chest x-ray
  C. Serum alpha-fetoprotein level
  D. All of the above

5. Which of the following statements regarding treatment of hepatoblastoma is *false?*
  A. Multiagent chemotherapy is administered adjuvantly to patients with stages I and II disease and as initial therapy after tumor biopsy to patients with (unresectable) stage III and (metastatic) stage IV disease
  B. Cisplatin-based multiagent chemotherapy is the standard for hepatoblastoma
  C. Liver transplantation may be indicated for tumors that remain unresectable after chemotherapy
  D. Radiation therapy plays an important primary role in the treatment of unresectable hepatoblastomas

6. Completely resectable hepatoblastomas with "pure fetal" histology have a better prognosis than do other histologic subtypes:
  A. True
  B. False

ANSWERS AND DISCUSSION

1. **B** Although primary liver tumors in children are uncommon, approximately 75% of them are malignant. Of pediatric liver cancers in North America and Europe, roughly 65% are hepatoblastomas (HB) and 25% are hepatocellular carcinomas (HCC). Other primary liver malignancies are extremely unusual and include such rare entities as rhabdomyosarcoma, angiosarcoma, and malignant germ cell tumors. The most frequently encountered benign liver neoplasms are vascular tumors, of which hemangioendothelioma is the most common. These patients may present before 6 months of age with life-threatening hepatomegaly or the Kasabach-Merritt syndrome (thrombocytopenia from platelet sequestration or consumption within the vascular tumor). Mesenchymal hamartomas are believed to derive from a "mesenchymal rest" composed primarily of connective tissue stroma (mesenchyme), bile ducts, and blood vessels that differentiates independently from the rest of the liver. These tumors, which can be predominantly cystic or vascular, usually present with hepatomegaly before age 2.

2. **C** There is an apparent association between hepatoblastoma and Beckwith-Weidemann syndrome, hemihypertrophy, and other embryonal neoplasms, such as Wilms' tumor and rhabdomyosarcoma. The association points to a common genetic mutation, and the prime candidate is the short arm of chromosome 11 (the 11p re-

gion). A specific gene locus (11p15.5) has been mapped, and loss of allelic heterozygosity at this locus is frequently demonstrated in children with hepatoblastoma. Unlike the association between hepatitis B infection and HCC, no such association exists for hepatoblastoma.

3. **A** Hepatoblastoma affects boys more frequently than girls with a ratio of 3:2. The age at diagnosis is almost always less than 3 years, and 50% present before 18 months. Hepatoblastomas typically present as an abdominal mass arising from the right liver lobe, which is involved three times more often than the left lobe, and only rarely is jaundice a presenting symptom.

4. **D** Preoperative studies are done to determine the organ of origin of the tumor to assess its resectability, and to predict tumor stage. A child presenting with an apparent liver tumor requires abdominal imaging (either a CT or magnetic resonance imaging [MRI] scan) and a chest x-ray to exclude lung metastases. Serum tumor markers are useful in differentiating the various pediatric liver tumors. Alpha-fetoprotein (AFP) produced by embryonal endoderm is elevated in 90% of children with hepatoblastomas. Yolk sac tumors and pregnancy may give similar AFP elevations. Serial AFP measurement is important in the assessment of response to treatment (either as a determinant of the completeness of surgical resection or response to chemotherapy) and as an early indicator of tumor recurrence. The half-life of AFP is 4 to 8 days, and in the absence of residual tumor, it will take four to five half-lives (3 to 6 weeks) for the serum level of AFP to reach its nadir after tumor resection. Contrast enhanced CT scans usually provide sufficient information to determine the organ of origin of an abdominal tumor and may give enough anatomic information to predict its resectability. Magnetic resonance imaging (MRI) and magnetic resonance angiography (MRA) have found increasing acceptance as reliable imaging modalities for the assessment of liver tumors and their vascularity and have greatly diminished the need for preoperative angiography. Abdominal ultrasound may be useful in defining the organ of origin or an abdominal mass and when determining whether it is cystic or solid. It may also be useful for tumor localization for percutaneous biopsy if that is necessary and appropriate.

5. **D** Complete resection of tumor remains the mainstay of treatment for hepatoblastoma. Refinements in adjuvant chemotherapy (in particular, the consistent use of cisplatin-based combination therapy) have increased in 5-year survival of stage I (confined to the liver and completely resected) and stage II (stage I with microscopic residual disease) disease to greater than 90%. Some centers advocated routine use of preoperative ("neoadjuvant") chemotherapy to shrink large, resectable tumors prior to surgery in an attempt to reduce the extent of hepatic resection required. Stage III hepatoblastoma are unresectable at presentation, based on the extent of hepatic disease or lymph node involvement, while stage IV disease implies distant metastases, most commonly to lung and brain. Stage III and IV tumors should be biopsied and treated with multiagent chemotherapy, which should enable complete tumor resection in more than 80% at the time of second-look laparotomy. Therapy for stage III and IV patients who are still not resectable at second look, may include liver

transplantation, if their metastatic disease can be controlled. Although hepatoblastoma is often radiosensitive, radiation therapy is reserved for stage III and IV patients who remain unresectable after standard chemotherapeutic regimens.

6. **A** The histology of hepatoblastoma is classified as fetal, embryonal, undifferentiated, and mixed histology. Tumors with pure fetal histology tend to be less primitive and, in at least stage I disease, have a better prognosis than do hepatoblastomas with nonfetal histology.

BIBLIOGRAPHY

Bleacher JC, Newman KD. Hepatoblastoma. In: Andrassy RJ ed. *Pediatric Surgical Oncology.* Philadelphia: WB Saunders; 1998:213–220.

Ehrlich PF, Greenberg ML, Filler RM. Improved long-term survival with preoperative chemotherapy for hepatoblastoma. *J Pediatr Surg.* 1997;32: 99–1002.

King DR. Liver tumors. In: O'Neill JA, Rowe MI, Grosfeld JL, et al. eds. *Pediatric Surgery.* St. Louis: Mosby-Year Book; 1998:421–430.

RESPIRATORY FAILURE IN A 4-MONTH-OLD INFANT

HISTORY A 4-month-old infant is transferred to the pediatric intensive care unit at the children's hospital with fever, cough, and respiratory distress of 3 days' duration. He was previously a healthy, term infant prior to developing an upper respiratory infection with wheezing. He was admitted to a local hospital and treated with intravenous ampicillin, nasal oxygen, and nebulizers with no improvement. On admission to the intensive care unit, he is in mild to moderate respiratory distress with retractions and wheezing. Respiratory rate is 50/min, and an oxygen saturation is 89%. He is treated with nebulized bronchodilators, cefuroxime, steroids, and a humidified oxygen hood. Chest x-ray (Figure 71–1) shows evidence of bronchiolitis with hyperinflation of both lungs.

He improves initially, but he develops spiking fevers to 104°F. Over the next 48 hours, his respiratory status worsens. Surgical consultation is obtained. An endotracheal tube is inserted and a chest x-ray is done (Figure 71–2), and mechanical ventilation is begun.

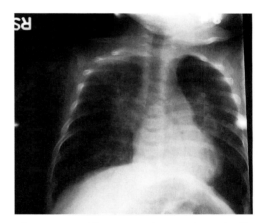

Figure 71–1. *Chest x-ray showing bronchiolitis with hyperinflation of both lungs. The trachea is midline.*

EXAMINATION (THIRD HOSPITAL DAY) The patient is a well-developed male infant with an endotracheal tube in place and multiple monitors. His pulse is 190/min, temperature 102°F, blood pressure 86/66. Ventilator rate is 26/min. Weight is 6.5 kg. There is no cyanosis. Eyes, ears, and throat are unremarkable. The trachea is midline. There are no cervical masses. The right hemithorax is hyperresonant to percussion. Breath sounds are decreased on the right. Heart sounds are maximal at the left sternal border with no cardiac murmur audible. The abdomen is mildly distended but soft and without masses or hernias. The extremities are well perfused.

LABORATORY Hemoglobin 10.3 gm%, hematocrit 34%, white blood cell count 18,400. The differential is segments 60, basophils 8, leukocytes 24, and monocytes 8. Electrolytes are normal. Culture of nasopharynx is positive for respiratory syncytial virus (RSV). Aterial blood gases are F_{IO_2}

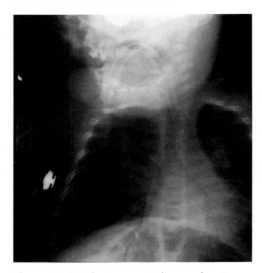

Figure 71–2. *Chest x-ray 48 hours after Figure 71–1 showing marked emphysema on the right. Trachea and mediastinum are shifted to the left. Endotracheal tube is too high in trachea.*

70%, pH 7.30, Pco_2 50, and Po_2 110. Chest x-ray is shown in Figure 71–2.

HOSPITAL COURSE   The endotracheal tube is repositioned and the ventilator settings are adjusted. He receives a bolus of intravenous fluid and a Tylenol suppository. His pulse decreases to 162/min, his temperature falls to 98.6°F, and his respiratory status stabilizes. Later on the third day, an operation is performed.

Please answer all questions before proceeding to discussion section.

✓ QUESTIONS

1. Which of the following is the most likely diagnosis?
   A. Congenital lobar emphysema
   B. Acquired lobar emphysema
   C. Tension pneumothorax
   D. Congenital cystic adenomatoid malformation
   E. Aspirated foreign body

2. Which of the following procedures is recommended prior to thoracotomy?
   A. Right tube thoracostomy
   B. Bronchoscopy
   C. A computed tomography (CT) scan of the chest with intravenous contrast
   D. A magnetic resonance imaging (MRI) scan of the chest
   E. Ventilation perfusion scan

3. Which of the following statements is *most* accurate regarding neonatal lobectomy for *congenital* lobar emphysema?
   A. Pathologic examination usually demonstrates dysplasia of the bronchial cartilage
   B. Lower lobectomy is more commonly performed than upper lobectomy
   C. Stapling is the technique of choice for bronchial closure
   D. There is a life-long decrease in ipsilateral lung volume of 20% to 35%
   E. There is no long-term functional impairment

ANSWERS AND DISCUSSION

1. **B** Acquired lobar emphysema is the most likely diagnosis in this 4-month-old infant. He was asymptomatic until he developed bronchiolitis with RSV, a virus that may cause severe and prolonged injury to the airways. The smallest of the lobar bronchi, the middle lobe bronchus proved to be the most vulnerable with ectasia, distal air-trapping, mediastinal shift, and respiratory failure. Congenital lobar emphysema (**A**) is attributed to dysplasia of the cartilage of the affected bronchus. It does not result from infection, as occurred in this infant. About half of cases of congenital lobar emphysema present with respiratory distress in the first few days of life; the remainder occur by 6 months of age. There is overlap between congenital and acquired lobar emphysema, so a definitive diagnosis is not always possi-

ble. Tension pneumothorax (**C**) may be difficult to differentiate from lobar emphysema, as both may produce mediastinal shift and catastrophic respiratory difficulty. The chest x-ray may show distinguishing features. Tension pneumothorax is characterized by collapse of the entire affected lung into the hilum, whereas lobar emphysema, which usually involves an upper lobe, produces collapse of an adjacent lobe, usually a lower lobe, at the base of the thorax. Congenital cystic adenomatoid malformation (CCAM) (**D**) with a single dominant cyst may also be mistaken for lobar emphysema. Because their surgical management is similar, however, preoperative differentiation of these two lesions is not as crucial as preoperative differentiation of tension pneumothorax from lobar emphysema, which requires different surgical management. Aspirated foreign body (**E**) can produce air-trapping from partial bronchial obstruction; however, this diagnosis is not likely in a 4-month-old infant who lacks the manual dexterity to put an object, such as a peanut, in his mouth. Further, an aspirated foreign body usually lodges in a mainstem bronchus or the bronchus intermedius and rarely obstructs the middle lobe bronchus only.

2. **B** If the child is stable, bronchoscopy is recommended to rule out a bronchial lesion that might be reversible (eg, bronchial stenosis, mucous plug, foreign body). Some pediatric surgeons might argue that, in this case, the emphysematous changes in the middle lobe are already advanced and irreversible. In any case, none of the other procedures is necessary in an infant with respiratory failure from lobar emphysema. Right tube thoracostomy (**A**) should not be done, as the chest x-ray shows lung markings indicating that the diagnosis is not tension pneumothorax. A CT scan (**C**), MRI scan (**D**), or ventilation perfusion scan (**E**) may be useful for confirmation of the diagnosis (emphysema of the middle lobe and compression/collapse of the right upper and lower lobes) in an elective situation, but the scans are not needed in an emergency as they will not change the definitive treatment.

3. **E** Because of compensatory lung growth in the neonate, there is no long-term functional impairment following neonatal lobectomy for congenital lobar emphysema. Pulmonary function studies in adults who have undergone neonatal lobectomy for congenital lobar emphysema have shown no deficit. All of the other statements are false. Congenital lobar emphysema is attributed to dysplasia of bronchial cartilage, producing a ball-valve type of bronchial obstruction. Pathologic examination, however, shows no abnormality (**A**) in about 50% of cases. Lobar emphysema rarely involves the lower lobes (**B**). The affected sites are distributed as follows: left upper lobe, 40% to 50%; (right) middle lobe, 30% to 40%; right upper lobe, 20%; lower lobes, 1%; and multiple sites, the remainder. Although stapled closure of the bronchus (**C**) is recommended in adults, a hand-sewn bronchial closure is technically superior in infants and small children. The stapling instruments and the staples themselves are generally too larger for accurate and secure closure of the neonatal bronchus. There is no deficit in lung volume (**D**) in adults who have undergone neonatal lobectomy for congenital lobar emphysema. Actual lung volumes were measured at 90% to 100% of predicted values with perfusion equally distributed between the operated and nonoperated lungs.

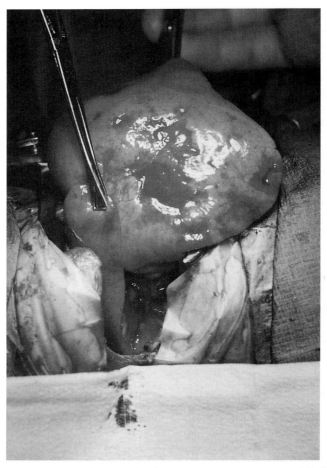

Figure 71–3. *Operative photograph, showing emphysematous middle lobe ballooning out of thoracotomy incision. Forceps hold edge of collapsed right upper lobe. After middle lobectomy, the right lower and upper lobes reexpanded normally. (See also color plate).*

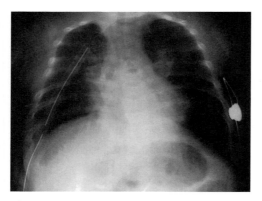

Figure 71–4. *Postoperative chest x-ray showing mediastinum and trachea back in midline position. A chest tube is present on the right. Emphysema is still present in both lungs.*

FOLLOW-UP The operation performed was a right thoracotomy and middle lobectomy. When the chest retractor was inserted between the ribs, the middle lobe (Figure 71–3; see also color plate) ballooned out of the incision. After middle lobectomy, the collapsed right upper and right lower lobes expanded normally. The infant made a rapid recovery, and he was extubated on the morning after operation. His postoperative chest x-ray was improved (Figure 71–4). He was discharged on the sixth postoperative day, and he had no further respiratory problems.

BIBLIOGRAPHY

de Lorimier AA. Respiratory problems related to the airway and lung. In: O'Neill JA Jr, Rowe MI, Grosfeld JL, et al. eds. *Pediatric Surgery.* 5th ed. St. Louis: Mosby-Year Book; 1998:873–897.

Gilbert EF, Opitz JM. Malformations and genetic disorders of the respiratory tract. In: Stocker JT, ed. *Pediatric Pulmonary Disease.* New York: Hemisphere Publishing Corporation; 1989:29–100.

Oldham KT. Lung. In: Oldham KT, Colombani PM, Foglia RP, eds. *Surgery of Infants and Children: Scientific Principles and Practice.* Philadelphia: Lippincott-Raven; 1997:935–970.

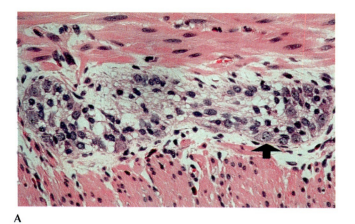
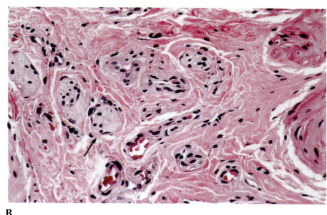

A

B

Figure 1–4. A. This is a high power hematoxylin and eosin (H&E) stain of normal colon. Longitudinal smooth muscle is at the top of the image and circular smooth muscle at the bottom. The nerve plexus in between the muscle layers shows multiple ganglion cells (arrow points to one). These are large cells with complex nuclei. **B.** This is a neural plexus in a patient with Hirschsprung disease. Ganglion cells are absent and multiple areas of hypertrophied nerve fibers are seen (arrow).

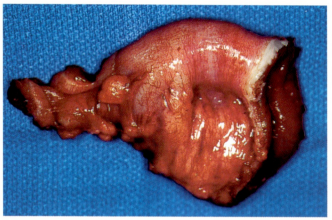

Figure 1–5. This is a resected segment of sigmoid colon at the level of the transition zone. The collapsed bowel (on left) is aganglionic bowel distal to the transition zone. The dilated bowel (on right) has normal ganglion cells and is chronically distended due to the distal functional obstruction.

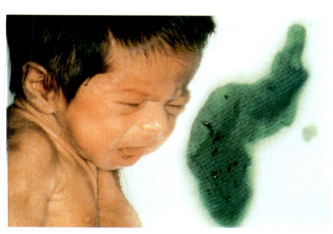

Figure 2–1. Appearance of a 1-week-old baby who began vomiting yesterday.

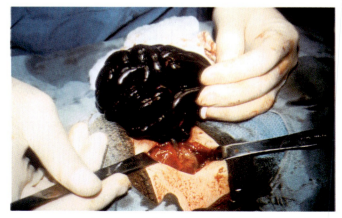

Figure 2–4. Malrotation with midgut volvulus. The bowel in this case (different from the one discussed in Case 2) is clearly necrotic. In cases where intestinal viability is uncertain, the bowel is returned to the abdomen, and a second-look laparotomy is done in 24 to 48 hours.

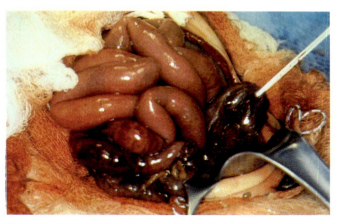

Figure 7–3. Operative photograph of infant with necrotizing enterocolitis, showing gangrenous loops of ileum and colon in the foreground. There is a perforation of the ileum. The jejunum (in the background) is viable.

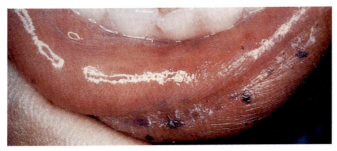

Figure 9–1. *Appearance of the lower lip in a 6-year-old boy with abdominal pain and vomiting. (From Misiewicz JJ et al. Atlas of Clinical Gastroenterology. 2nd ed. London, Wolfe-Mosby; 1994.)*

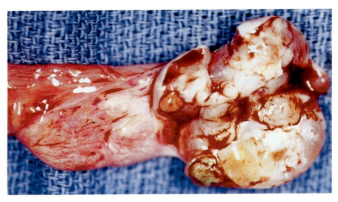

Figure 13–2. *Tumor on cut section demonstrates fat and cartilage consistent with mature teratoma.*

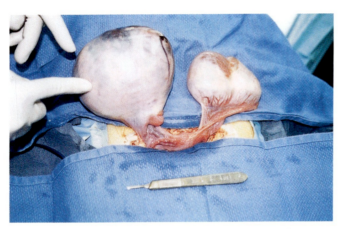

Figure 15–2. *Findings at laparotomy revealed bilateral ovarian teratomas.*

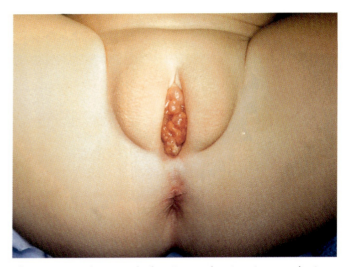

Figure 18–1. *Photograph showing prolapsing tissue at the introitus.*

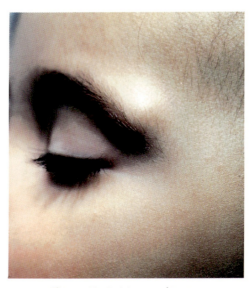

Figure 19–1. *Mass on brow.*

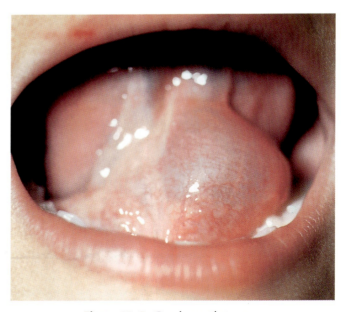

Figure 19–2. *Cyst beneath tongue.*

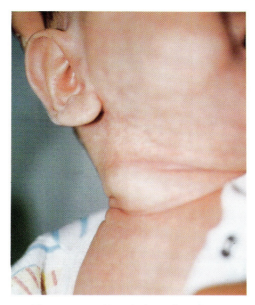

Figure 19–3. *Mass in lateral neck.*

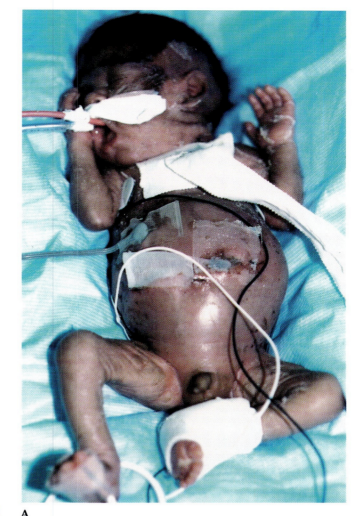

A

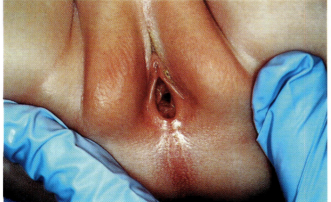

Figure 22–1. *Appearance of the perineum in a newborn girl with imperforate anus.*

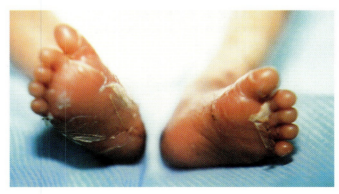

B

Figure 23–2. A. *Premature infant (650 g) with* Staphylococcus epidermidis *sepsis and necrotizing enterocolitis (NEC). Portals of entry for infection are thin, cracked skin and catheters in vascular, urinary, gastrointestinal (GI), and respiratory systems.* **B.** *The rash, with peeling of the skin of the hands and feet, is a manifestation of a staphyloccal toxin.*

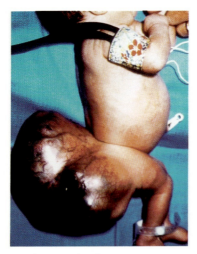

Figure 24–3. *Newborn with a large sacrococcygeal teratoma.*

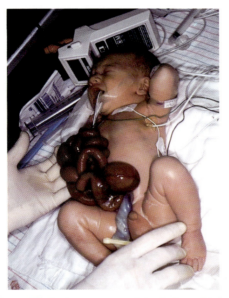

Figure 27–1. *Appearance of the baby at birth.*

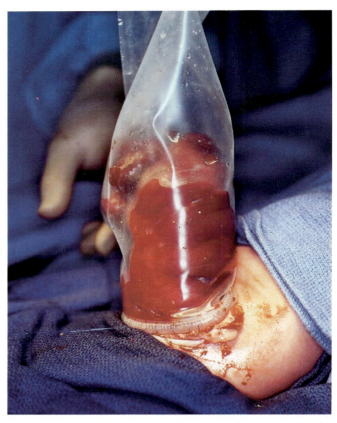

Figure 27–2. *Baby with gastroschisis in an abdominal silo. The top of the silo will be serially compressed in order to reduce the bowel into the abdominal cavity gradually. At a second operation, the silo will be removed, and the abdomen closed.*

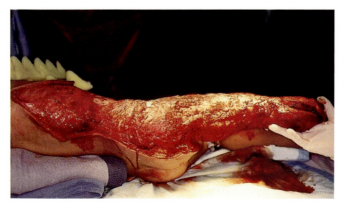

Figure 28–2. *This patient required five operative debridements and amputation of his right foot in order to control the infection. He required excision of all skin and subcutaneous tissue of 35% of his body surface area. He is shown here prior to skin grafting. This patient survived and is doing well.*

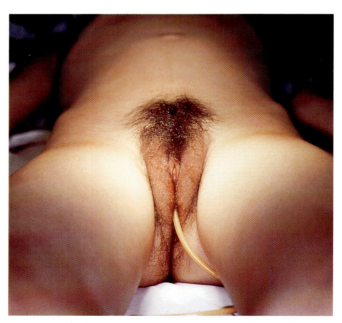

Figure 32–1. *The appearance of this 5-year-old girl with marked clitoromegaly and pubic hair.*

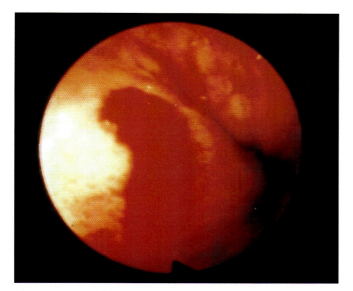

Figure 33–1. *Endoscopic appearance of an actively bleeding esophageal varix.*

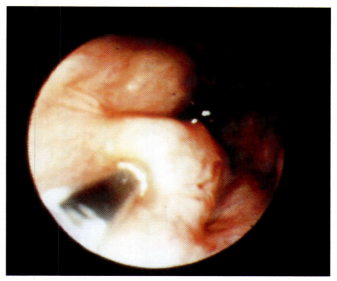

Figure 33–2. *Intravariceal sclerotherapy achieves arrest of hemorrhage.*

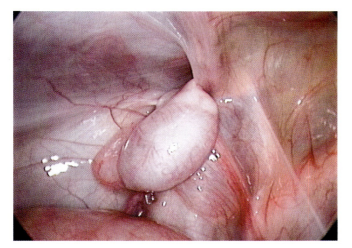

Figure 34–3. *Laparoscopic appearance of a left intra-abdominal testis. The testis is just inside the internal ring. This child underwent immediate orchiopexy via a groin approach and the testis was successfully mobilized into the scrotum.*

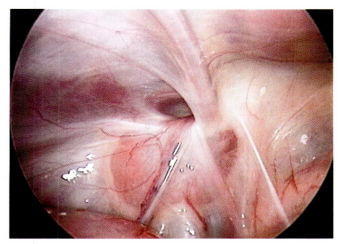

Figure 34–4. *Laparoscopic appearance of a vas and vessels exiting an open internal inguinal ring suggesting the presence of a testicle within the inguinal canal.*

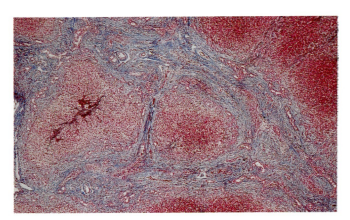

Figure 36–2. *This is the histologic appearance of a liver biopsy taken from a 12-week-old baby with extrahepatic biliary atresia. It is shown at 15 × magnification and has been stained with trichrome. Collagen (fibrous tissue) appears blue. Portal triads are surrounded by fibrosis, and trails of fibrous tissue "bridging" to other parts of the liver are seen. Nodule formation suggests that the patient is progressing from bridging fibrosis to cirrhosis.*

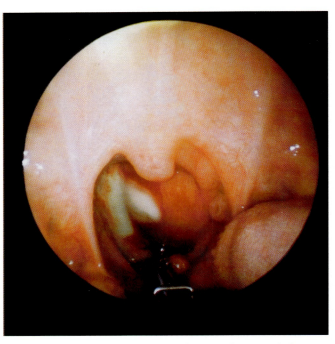

Figure 37–2. *Transoral drainage of a retropharyngeal abscess.*

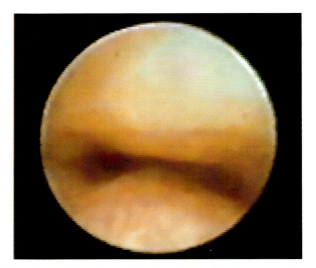

Figure 39–1. *Bronchoscopic photograph showing severe tracheomalacia.*

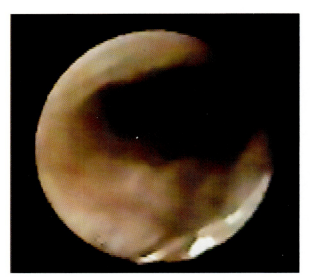

Figure 39–2. *Bronchoscopic photograph after aortopexy.*

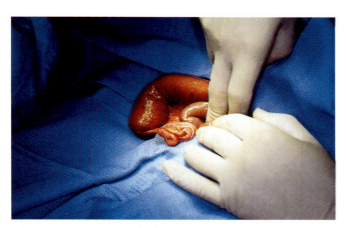

Figure 45–2. *Operative findings showing dilated proximal bowel and contracted distal bowel connected by a fibrous cord. A considerable caliber discrepancy between proximal and distal bowel is typical of jejunal atresia.*

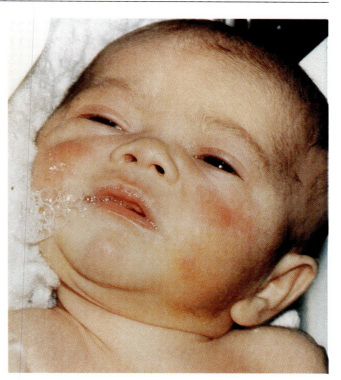

Figure 46–1. *Appearance of a newborn infant with excessive salivation.*

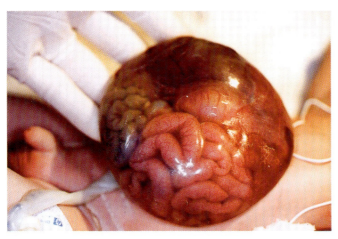

Figure 47–1. *Giant omphalocele with intact amnion containing all hollow and solid viscera. Primary closure was impossible, and placement of a prosthetic silo was necessary to achieve gradual reduction of herniated viscera.*

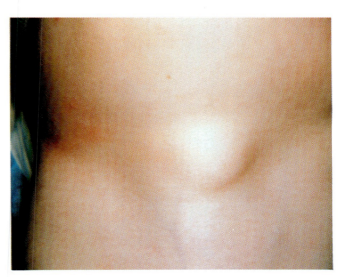

Figure 53–1. *Midline anterior cervical mass overlying the hyoid bone.*

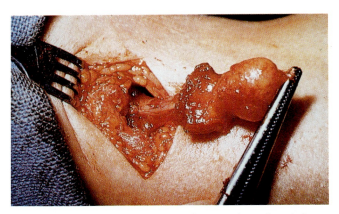

Figure 53–2. *Operative specimen showing thyroglossal duct cyst, middle one-third of the hyoid bone, and suprahyoid tract.*

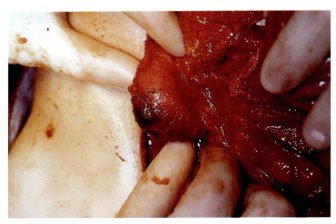

Figure 56–2. *Appearance of a traumatic duodenal hematoma at operation. The duodenum has been mobilized out of the retroperitoneum. The hematoma is at the bottom of the C-loop in the third portion.*

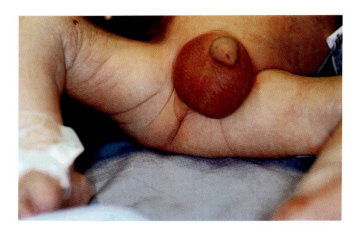

Figure 58–1. *Appearance of this newborn boy's perineum 4 hours after birth.*

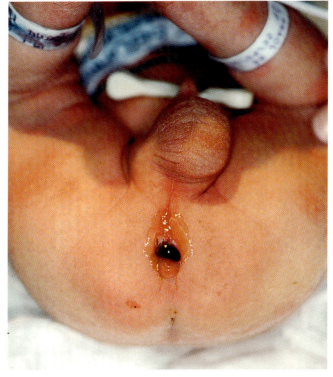

Figure 58–3. *Appearance of the perineum of a different patient at 24 hours of life. A small fistula is seen on the perineum anterior to the location of a normal anal opening. Frequently, these fistulae are not evident immediately after birth and only become apparent when colorectal peristalsis forces meconium through the tiny opening. The presence of a perineal opening correlates very strongly with a low lesion.*

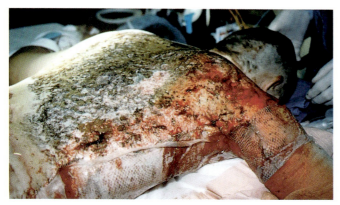

Figure 60–1. *Patient with extensive full thickness burn to back.*

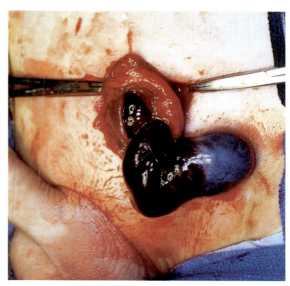

Figure 61–2. *This is a photograph (from a different patient) showing a clearly necrotic testicle due to torsion. This patient was explored via an inguinal incision because of diagnostic concern regarding testicular tumor.*

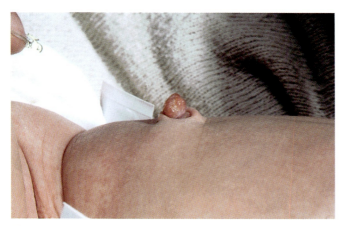

Figure 62–1. *A 2-month-old girl with an umbilical mass.*

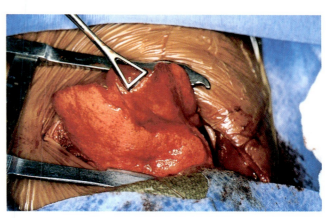

Figure 65–3. *Operative photograph, right lower lobe, showing intralobar sequestration well demarcated from normal lung.*

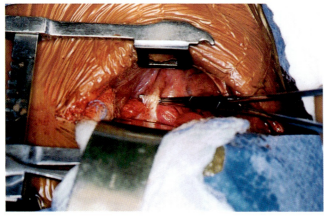

Figure 65–4. *Operative photograph showing inferior pulmonary ligament containing large artery that supplies sequestration.*

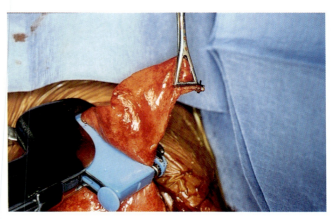

Figure 65–5. *Operative photograph, intralobar sequestration showing stapled wedge resection.*

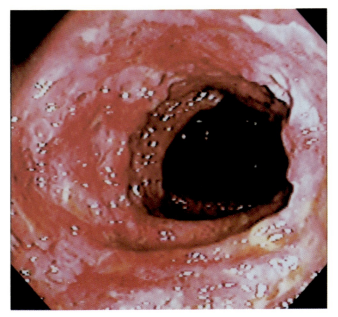

Figure 69–2. *Endoscopic appearance of the transverse colon. The mucosa is severly inflamed with exudative, bloody mucus, and ulcerations. The folds appear thickened and nondistensible from swelling and spasm. No pseudomembranes are present. These changes are nonspecific, and could be seen in acute infectious colitis or inflammatory bowel disease.*

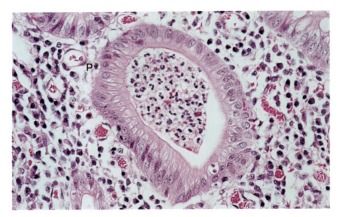

Figure 69–3. *High-powered cross-section through a colonic gland demonstrating pus in the lumen, with occasional polymorphs (P) near the basement membrane, consistent with a crypt abscess.*

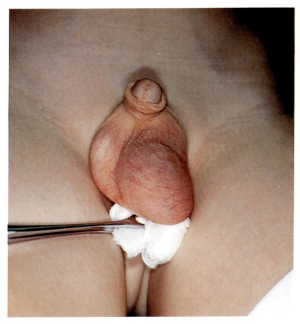

Figure 72–1. *Appearance of the groin of a 3-year-old healthy boy with a scrotal mass.*

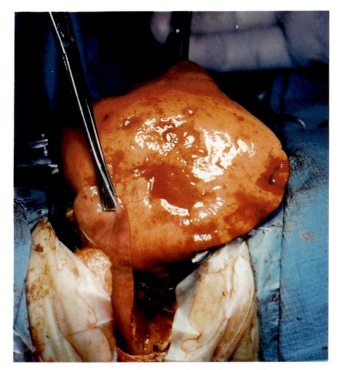

Figure 71–3. *Operative photograph of lobar emphysema in (right) middle lobe .*

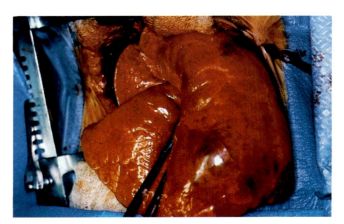

Figure 73–5. *Operative photograph showing large cyst in left lower lobe and normal left upper lobe.*

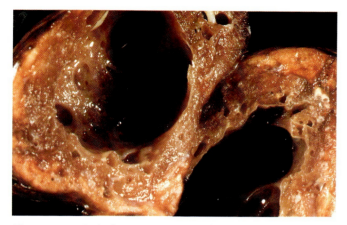

Figure 73–6. *Pathologic specimen. Left lower lobe showing single dominant cyst with multiple satellites. Specimen has been opened (bivalved) for examination.*

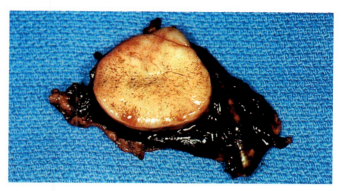

Figure 74–2. *Cut section of a pheochromocytoma. The fleshy yellow appearance is typical of these tumors. Malignancy is best determined by biologic behavior rather than histologic appearance.*

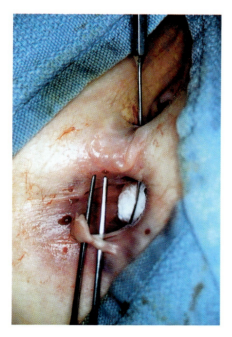

Figure 75–1. *Appearance of the perineum of a 13-year-old girl with history of multiple perianal abscesses. Probes are in fistulous tracts and in a recto vaginal fistula.*

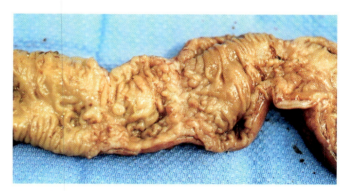

Figure 75–4. *Pathologic appearance of the resected ileum in Crohn's disease. The mucosa is deeply ulcerated. Islands of mucosa among these deep ulcerations appear to be polyps and are referred to as pseudopolyps.*

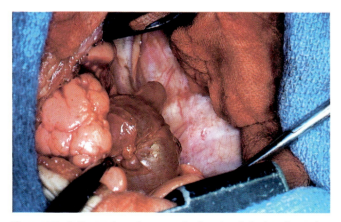

Figure 76–4 *Operative photograph showing lobulated cyst beneath arch of aorta.*

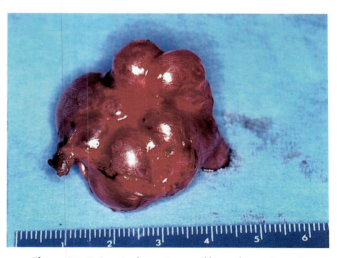

Figure 76–5 *Surgical specimen of bronchogenic cyst.*

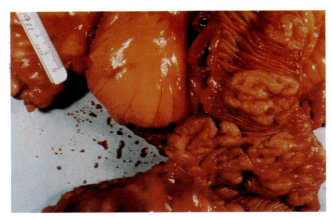

Figure 77–2. *Gross appearance of the resected specimen. The cauliflower-shaped tumor masses are arising from the submucosa. With permission from Lin KM, David GP, Mahmaud A, et al. Advantage of surgery and adjutant chemotherapy in the treatment of primary gastrointestinal lymphoma. J Surg Oncol. 1997;64(3):237–241.*

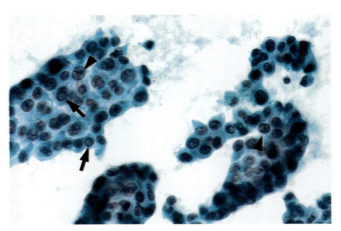

Figure 78–1. *Fine needle aspiration (FNA) preparation of papillary carcinoma showing finger-like papillae containing cells with dense metaplastic cytoplasm, occasional intranuclear inclusions (arrows), and nuclei with longitudinal grooves (arrowheads). (Papanicolaou × 600)*

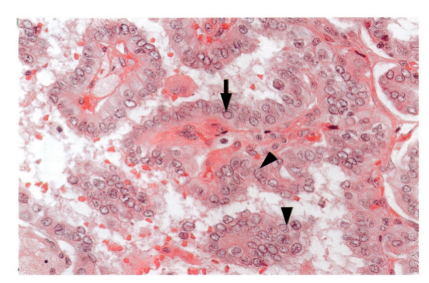

Figure 78–2. *High power magnification from resection specimen showing papillary carcinoma. The delicate papillae are lined by cuboidal-to-columnar cells with vesicular nuclei, occasional intranuclear inclusions (arrow), and conspicuous nuclear grooves (arrowheads). (Hematoxylin and eosin × 400.)*

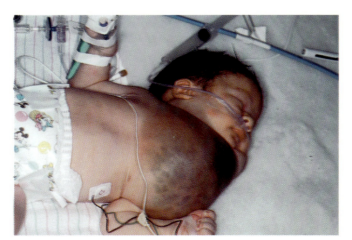

Figure 80–1. *A newborn boy with a neck mass. The baby is otherwise healthy.*

A 3-YEAR-OLD BOY WITH A SWOLLEN TESTIS

HISTORY A 3-year-old boy is brought to the pediatrician by his mother because of a swelling in the left scrotum. His mother has noticed the enlargement for around a week. The boy has been otherwise entirely healthy and active. He has never complained of pain or discomfort in the affected testicle. The pediatrician asks you to see the patient because he cannot reduce the scrotal swelling.

EXAMINATION The boy is well developed and well nourished. His vital signs are normal. Heart and lung examination is unremarkable. There is a vague abdominal fullness on the left, but examination is limited because the patient is very ticklish. The appearance of his groin is seen in Figure 72–1 (see also color plate). The left hemiscrotum has a dark bluish cast. Palpation of the swelling reveals a soft, mushy, wormlike consistency unlike any hydrocele you have felt. The underlying testis is not tender and seems to be of normal size. The mass is not reducible.

Please answer all questions before proceeding to discussion section.

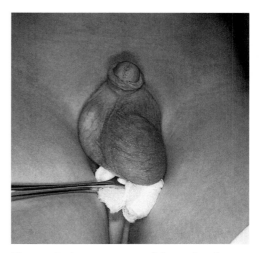

Figure 72–1. *appearance of the groin of a 3-year-old healthy boy with a scrotal mass. (See also color plate.)*

✓ QUESTIONS

1. Which of the following diagnoses is most likely?
   A. Incarcerated hernia
   B. Hydrocele of the spermatic cord
   C. Germ cell tumor of the testis
   D. Wilms' tumor
   E. Acute testicular torsion

HOSPITAL COURSE Based on your initial impression, you obtain an ultrasound examination of the abdomen. This reveals a large left-sided retroperitoneal mass. The mass appears to be in the kidney. The renal vein and vena cava are well seen and are normal.

2. Your next move is to:
   A. Order a computed tomography (CT) scan of the abdomen
   B. Send urine for catecholamine studies
   C. Operate immediately to remove the mass
   D. Obtain a CT-scan guided percutaneous needle biopsy for diagnosis
   E. Ask the oncologist to begin chemotherapy with vincristine and actinomycin-D

3. Which of the following is the most important prognostic factor following excision of a renal tumor in childhood?
   A. Size of the tumor
   B. Presence or absence of periaortic lymph nodes containing tumor
   C. Tumor histology
   D. Age of the patient
   E. Whether or not the tumor was ruptured at the time of resection

4. Wilms' tumor occurs with increased frequency in which of the following?
   A. Beckwith-Wiedemann syndrome
   B. Denys-Drash syndrome
   C. Aniridia
   D. Hemihypertrophy
   E. All of the above

5. Which genetic factors have been shown to contribute to the development of Wilms' tumor?
   A. Mutation in the WT1 tumor supressor gene on chromosome 11
   B. Mutation in the p53 tumor supressor gene
   C. Duplication of genetic material at the 11p15 locus
   D. All of the above
   E. None of the above

6. Wilms' tumor may invade the renal vein and subsequently the inferior vena cava (IVC). What is the correct management of a child with a large tumor thrombus extending up the IVC into the right atrium?
   A. Resection via the abdominal approach with careful extraction of the tumor thrombus as the renal vein is opened
   B. Resection of the intracardiac portion of the tumor using cardiopulmonary bypass followed by resection of the abdominal tumor within 2 weeks
   C. Combined *en bloc* resection of the abdominal tumor and excision of the intracardiac tumor using cardiopulmonary bypass
   D. Combined resection of the abdominal tumor and excision of the intracardiac tumor without cardiopulmonary bypass
   E. Administration of preoperative chemotherapy

7. Management of the child with bilateral Wilms' tumor includes:
   A. A generous transabdominal incision
   B. Biopsy of all abnormal areas in both kidneys
   C. Partial nephrectomy if preservation of two thirds of renal parenchyma is possible
   D. Postoperative chemotherapy based on the most unfavorable histology from all specimens
   E. All of the above

8. Which patients with Wilms' tumor should have abdominal irradiation?
   A. Patients with unresectable disease prior to excision
   B. All patients with bilateral Wilms' tumors
   C. Patients with stage III or greater disease and unfavorable histology
   D. Patients with stage III or greater disease regardless of histology or patients with unfavorable histology and stage II or greater disease
   E. Patients with stage IV (metastatic disease)

9. Which of the following are correct regarding surgical excision of Wilms' tumor?
   A. Gerota's fascia on the contralateral side must not be opened to avoid tumor spillage
   B. The tumor should be removed *en bloc* with as many enlarged lymph nodes as feasible
   C. The renal vein must be ligated before significant manipulation of the tumor to avoid tumor spread
   D. The adrenal gland must be preserved or postoperative steroid administration will be necessary
   E. All of the above

ANSWERS AND DISCUSSION

1. **D** This child has a varicocele of the left testis. Varicocele results from dilation of the testicular veins and may occur for unknown reasons in adults, but are extremely uncommon in children. A varicocele in a child is usually an indicator of renal vein obstruction due to a tumor. The most common abdominal tumor, which would cause a varicocele in a child of this age, is a nephroblastoma or Wilms' tumor. An incarcerated hernia (**A**) is associated with pain and tenderness in the groin. Furthermore, on physical examination the swelling extends up through the external inguinal ring and is not confined to the scrotum as it is in this case. An incarcerated hernia is firm rather than soft and mushy. A hydrocele of the spermatic cord presents as a firm mass in the spermatic cord, which is separate from the testis. A germ cell tumor of the testis is the most common testicular tumor that would occur in this age group. These tumors, however, present as firm testicular masses. Acute testicular torsion is quite rare in a 3-year-old child. Testicular torsion presents with acute and severe testicular pain and results in an abnormal lie of the affected testis.

2. **A** The ultrasound examination is quite reliable in determining whether or not a mass is within the renal substance. The ultrasound examination confirms your suspicion that this child indeed does have a Wilms' tumor. Part of the preoperative evaluation includes an assessment of the renal vein and vena cava to determine whether or not there is tumor thrombus present in these vessels. Ultrasound provides an excellent means of answering this question. A CT scan of the abdomen is necessary for two important reasons. First, it allows the surgeon to determine the extent of the tumor (Figure 72–2). The vast majority of Wilms' tumors are readily resectable. Occasionally a very large tumor can cross the midline, however, and block access to the retroperitoneal vessels. Many experts believe that preoperative

chemotherapy in order to shrink the tumor is appropriate in such cases. The second reason for obtaining an abdominal CT scan is to evaluate fully the opposite kidney for the presence of any synchronous masses. About 5% to 10% of Wilms' tumors are bilateral.

Urine catecholemine studies (**B**) may be useful in the evaluation of the patient with neuroblastoma. Neuroblastoma can occasionally be confused with Wilms' tumor. It occurs in the adrenal gland, and the mass pushes the normal kidney inferiorly rather than invades it. While operation is indicated for this patient, it certainly need not be done as an emergency. Adequate preoperative preparation usually includes a mechanical bowel preparation and obtainment of blood for type and cross-match. Percutaneous needle biopsy is not useful in the management of renal tumors in children. Because all tumors require resection, histologic examination prior to resection is not necessary. Furthermore, there can be considerable histologic variation between one area and another in a given Wilms' tumor. For this reason, a small sample of cells may not be indicative of the tumor's overall histology. Chemotherapy for Wilms' tumor generally includes vincristine and actinomycin-D. Chemotherapy, however, is only used preoperatively if the tumor is believed to be unresectable. Doxorubicin is added to the regimen for tumors with positive lymph nodes or unfavorable histology.

3. **C** Histology is the most important tumor characteristic predicting prognosis in children with renal tumors. The presence of anaplasia in a Wilms' tumor, clear cell sarcoma, or rhabdoid tumor of the kidney is a highly negative prognostic factor. Anaplastic Wilms' tumors are characterized by nuclei that are two to three times larger than normal and are hyperchromatic with abnormal mitotic figures. Anaplasia is rarely seen in tumors of patients younger than 2 years of age and has an overall incidence of 3% to 7%. Reports have found that anaplastic tumors commonly have mutations in the tumor suppressor gene p53. Patients with stage I anaplastic Wilms' tumors have a reasonably good outcome following resection. Survival for children with stages II through V anaplastic tumor, however, is only 30% to 40%. Anaplasia within a Wilms' tumor is an indication for treatment within more aggressive chemotherapy, including doxorubocin.

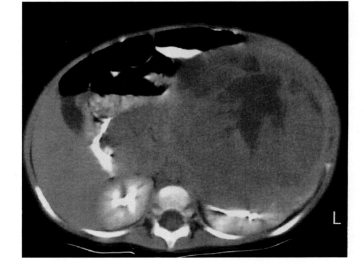

Figure 72–2. *A computed tomography (CT) scan of a patient with a large left-sided Wilms' tumor. This very large tumor crosses the midline and deviates the major branches of the aorta. A markedly distorted renal collecting system containing contrast is seen posterior to the tumor. The section of right kidney appears normal.*

TABLE 72–1   WILMS' TUMOR: NWTS-4 STAGING SYSTEM

Stage I
The tumor is limited to the kidney and is completely excised. The surface of the renal capsule is intact. The tumor was not ruptured before or during removal. No residual tumor is apparent beyond the margins of resection.

Stage II
The tumor extends beyond the kidney but is completely excised. Regional extension of the tumor (through the outer surface of the renal capsule) may exist into the perirenal soft tissues. Blood vessels outside the kidney may be infiltrated by or contain tumor thrombus. The tumor may have been biopsied or local spillage may be present, which is confined to the ipsilateral flank. No residual tumor is apparent at or beyond the margins of resection.

Stage III
Residual nonhematogenous tumor remains within the abdomen. Any one or more of the following may be observed: lymph node metastases, diffuse peritoneal contamination, tumor penetration through the peritoneal surface, peritoneal implants, gross or microscopic residual tumor remains postoperatively, or an incompletely resected tumor.

Stage IV
Hematogenous metastases are observed.

Stage V
Bilateral disease is present at diagnosis.

NWTS, National Wilms' Tumor Study.

Clear cell sarcoma of the kidney and rhabdoid tumor of the kidney were previously considered Wilms' tumors with unfavorable histology. Improved histologic, immunochemical, and molecular characterization of these tumors, however, have shown that they are indeed distinct from Wilms' tumor. Both of these tumors have poor prognoses following resection despite aggressive postoperative chemotherapy. Clear cell sarcoma of the kidney is particularly likely to metastasize to bone. Rhabdoid tumor of the kidney has the worst prognosis of any pediatric renal tumor; survival at 3 years is less than 20%. Metastases frequently arise in multiple sites with pulmonary lesions being the most common (70%), and brain metastasis occurring in 14% of patients.

The size of the tumor is less important than the tumor stage (Table 72–1). The presence of periaortic lymph nodes containing tumor is one of the criteria for stage III disease. Age of the patient does not appear to be a particularly important prognostic variable. Tumor rupture at the time of resection was previously felt to alter prognosis. Data suggest, however, that this may not be the case.

4. **E** Many factors point to the importance of genetic predisposition in the development of Wilms' tumors. The marked increase in incidence of Wilms' tumor in certain genetic syndromes provides supporting evidence for this. Beckwith-Wiedemann syndrome is associated with hyperinsulinemic hypoglycemia, visceromegaly, omphalocele, macroglossia, and umbilical defects (Figure 72–3). Children with Beckwith-Wiedemann syndrome have a markedly increased incidence of abdominal tumors, including Wilms' tumor, hepatoblastoma, neuroblastoma, and adrenocortical carcinoma.

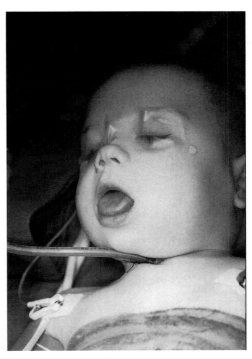

Figure 72–3. A child with Beckwith-Weidemann syndrome. Note the protrusion of the large tongue. These children have an increased incidence of Wilms' tumor, hepatoblastoma, neuroblastoma, and adrenocortical carcinoma.

Denys-Drash syndrome results in intersex disorders, nephropathy, and an increased incidence of Wilms' tumor. Aniridia is a congenital disorder of the iris that is associated with an increase in the incidence of Wilms' tumor. Aniridia is often a component of the WAGR syndrome, which includes Wilms' tumor, aniridia, genitourinary malformations, and mental retardation. Hemihypertrophy results in the enlargement of extremities on one side in comparison to the contralateral side. These children have an increased incidence of Wilms' and other abdominal tumors.

Management of children known to have these syndromes includes frequent imaging studies of the abdomen in order to lead to earlier detection of associated tumors. One report recommends that children with syndromes, such as Beckwith-Wiedermann syndrome, undergo an abdominal ultrasound every 3 months throughout childhood.

5. **D** The genetics of Wilms' tumor formation is a slowly unraveling mystery. The gene most closely associated with the development of Wilms' tumor is the WT1 gene. This gene seems to be directly related to the development of Wilms' tumor in the rare WAGR syndrome mentioned in answer 4. More than 30% of children with this syndrome develop Wilms' tumor. Karyotypic analysis of these children reveals a deletion in the short arm of one copy of chromosome 11 at band 13. This important genetic area includes the WT1 Wilms' tumor suppressor gene. Usually inactivation of both copies of a tumor suppressor gene is necessary for tumorigenesis. The specific alterations in a single copy of tumor suppressor gene may, however, convert that gene into a dominant negative oncogene.

Mutations of the p53 tumor suppressor gene on chromosome 17 have been found frequently in a variety of malignant tumors in adults. Mutations in the p53 suppressor gene have been found in Wilms' tumors with anaplastic features. p53 abnormalities have also been reported in favorable histology Wilms' tumors.

The WT2 Wilms' tumor suppressor gene is located at the 11p15 locus. Beckwith-Wiedemann syndrome is thought to result from an overexpression of a gene at this location.

The genetic basis of Wilms' tumor has been clearly documented in patients with a syndromic tendency toward the development of these tumors. The genetic basis of the more common, sporadically occurring Wilms' tumors remains to be elucidated. It is important that the surgeon ensure that fresh tissue is sent for cytogenetic analysis in all resected Wilms' tumors so that this mystery may continue to be unraveled.

6. **E** Traditional management of tumor thrombus extending into the atrium included a combined procedure including removal of the abdominal tumor along with resection of the cardiac tumor on cardiopulmonary bypass. The excellent response of Wilms' tumor to preoperative chemotherapy has now made this procedure unnecessary. A review of data from the National Wilms' Tumor Study of 30 children with inferior vena cava or atrial extension of tumor reported an excellent response to preoperative chemotherapy in all. None of the children required cardiopulmonary bypass. In seven children, the tumor thrombus had completely disappeared by the time of operation.

7. **E** Bilateral Wilms' tumor occurs in 5% to 10% of all patients with Wilms' tumor. Girls are affected twice as frequently as boys, and pa-

tients tend to be younger at diagnosis than those with unilateral tumors (25 months versus 44 months). For many years, the management of bilateral Wilms' tumor varied depending on the institution treating the child. Efforts by the National Wilms' Tumor Study Group have standardized care. Recommendations include wide exploration of both kidneys with a biopsy of nephroblastomatosis (a condition of uncertain etiology but associated with Wilms' tumor), nephrogenic rests (a precursor to Wilms' tumor), or Wilms' tumor of unfavorable histology. Nephrectomy of either kidney should not be performed at the initial procedure unless greater than two thirds of that kidney's renal parenchyma can be preserved. The major goal of therapy for bilateral Wilms' tumor should be to preserve as much renal parenchyma as possible. For this reason, most patients are best treated by preoperative chemotherapy to provide maximal tumor shrinkage followed by limited resection of the remaining tumor. Data suggest that survival following the occurrence of bilateral Wilms' tumor is greater than 75%.

8. **D** Abdominal irradiation is recommended for patients with stage III or greater disease of any histology or for patients with unfavorable histology and stage II or greater disease. Patients with "unresectable" disease are usually treated with vincristine and actinomycin-D prior to resection. Their postoperative chemotherapy and radiation therapy is then determined by tumor stage at the time of excision. Patients with bilateral Wilms' tumors are treated based on the least favorable histology from all of the specimens obtained. Abdominal irradiation includes 2000 cGy to the flank and abdomen and is remarkably well-tolerated. The incidence of radiation-related complications is very low.

9. **B** Removal of a Wilms' tumor involves dissection of the retroperitoneal vessels. Dissection should proceed along the aorta and vena cava and include all enlarged lymph nodes up to and including those at the renal hilum. Figure 72–4 shows an example of a resected specimen. The contralateral kidney absolutely must be explored for evi-

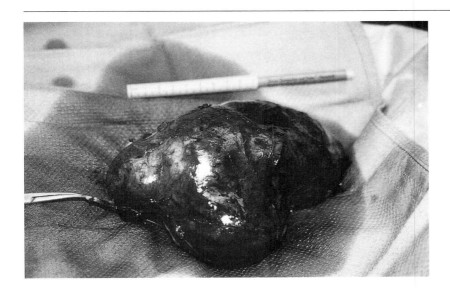

Figure 72–4. *Resected specimen from this patient. The child was tolerating a regular diet on postoperative day 4 and began chemotherapy.*

dence of contralateral disease that may not have been seen on preoperative imaging studies. The protocol of the National Wilms' Tumor Study calls for the surgeon to open Gerota's fascia on the contralateral side and palpate that kidney. It is not necessary to ligate the renal vein to avoid tumor spread. In fact, early ligation of the vein can result in considerable swelling of the tumor from arterial inflow with resultant bleeding or rupture. The adrenal gland is often removed *en bloc* with particularly large tumors. If this is necessary, it should be done. Postoperative steroid therapy is not likely to be necessary as the contralateral adrenal should provide adequate function.

BIBLIOGRAPHY

Bardeesy N, Falkoff D, Petruzzi MJ, et al. Anaplastic Wilms' tumour, a subtype displaying poor prognosis, harbours p53 gene mutations. *Nat Genet.* 1994;7:91–97.

Beckwith JB. Nephrogenic rests in the pathogenesis of Wilms' tumor: developmental and clinical considerations. *Am J Med Genet.* 1993;79:268–273.

Coppes MJ, Egeler RM. Genetics of Wilms' tumor. *Sem Urol Oncol.* 1999;17:2–10.

de Kraker J, Voute PA, Lemerle J. Preoperative chemotherapy in Wilms' tumour: results of clinical trials and studies on nephroblastomas conducted by the International Society of Paediatric Oncology (SIOP). *Prog Clin Biol Res.* 1982;100:131–144.

Herskowitz I. Functional inactivation of genes by dominant negative mutations. *Nature.* 1987;329:219–222.

Othersen HB, Tagge EP, Garvin AJ. Wilms' tumor. In: O'Neill JA Jr, Rowe MI, Grosfeld JL, et al. eds. *Pediatric Surgery.* 5th ed. St. Louis: Mosby-Year Book; 1998:391–404.

Ritchey ML, Kelalis PP, Haase GM, et al. Preoperative therapy for intracaval and atrial extension of Wilms' tumor. *Cancer.* 1993;71:4104–4110.

Shamberger RC. Pediatric renal tumors. *Semin Surg Oncol.* 1999;16:105–120.

A FETUS/NEONATE WITH A CYSTIC MASS IN THE LEFT CHEST

HISTORY   A cystic structure is identified on prenatal ultrasound (Figures 73–1 and 73–2) in the left hemithorax of a fetus. Close prenatal supervision is carried out. No evidence of polyhydramnios or pre-eclampsia develops; both mother and fetus remain healthy. At 38 weeks, spontaneous labor begins, and progresses well. Fourteen hours later (just after midnight), a healthy appearing male infant is delivered. He is suctioned in the delivery room and breathes spontaneously. Apgars are 9 and 10 at (1 minute and 5 minutes, respectively.) Nasal oxygen is administered. He is transported to the neonatal intensive care unit.

EXAMINATION   The patient is an active male infant in no respiratory distress. He is not cyanotic. Blood pressure is 76/52, pulse 140, temperature 37.5°C. Weight is 3.5 kg. There are no abnormalities of the head or neck. The chest is symmetric. There are no retractions. Breath sounds are diminished over the left hemithorax and slightly increased over the right hemithorax. The cardiac impulse is maximal just to the right of the sternum. A faint, grade I/VI midsystolic murmur is heard. The abdomen is not distended. It is soft with no enlarged organs or masses. The extremities are well perfused. Peripheral pulses are good.

LABORATORY   Hemoglobin, hematocrit, white blood cell count, and differential are all normal. The oxygen saturation is 98% on 30% oxygen. The chest x-ray is shown in Figure 73–3.

Please answer all questions before proceeding to discussion section.

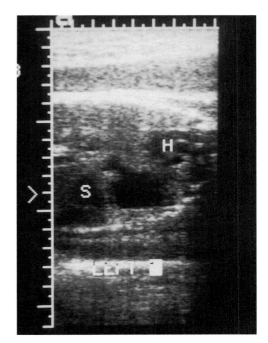

Figure 73–1. *Prenatal ultrasonogram, longitudinal view, showing cystic mass located cephalad to stomach. (H, heart; S, stomach.)*

✓ QUESTIONS

1. The procedure of choice now is:
    A. Immediate left thoracotomy
    B. Immediate laparotomy

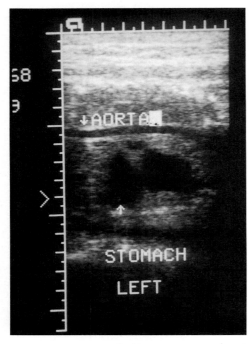

Figure 73–2. *Prenatal ultrasonogram, coronal view, showing cystic mass (arrow) located cephalad to stomach.*

C. A computed tomography (CT) scan of chest and abdomen with double (intravenous and gastrointestinal) contrast
D. Upper gastrointestinal (GI) contrast study
E. Diagnostic pneumoperitoneum

2. Which of the following is true regarding congenital cystic adenomatoid malformation (CCAM)?
A. Type I typically contains multiple large cysts or occasionally a single dominant cyst with smaller satellite cysts
B. The upper lobes are most commonly affected
C. Blood supply is usually from systemic vessels arising from the descending aorta or abdominal aorta
D. The cysts in all types are lined with glandular epithelium, hence the term "adenomatoid"
E. Thirty percent to 40% of cases of CCAM have associated cystic renal disease

3. All of the following statements regarding CCAM are true *except:*
A. Polyhydramnios is a sign of danger during pregnancy in which CCAM has been identified
B. Lobectomy is usually curative for CCAM
C. Rhabdomyosarcoma and carcinoma in childhood have been described as originating in cystic adenomatoid malformations
D. Angiography plays an important role in preoperative evaluation of CCAM
E. Fatal mediastinal shift is a complication of infant pneumonectomy for CCAM

HOSPITAL COURSE A nasogastric tube is placed, and contrast material is injected (Figure 73–4). The infant remains stable without respiratory difficulty. The following morning, he is taken to the operating room where left thoracotomy is performed. The operative findings (Figure 73–5; see also color plate) and pathologic specimen (Figure 73–6; see also color plate) are shown.

ANSWERS AND DISCUSSION

1. **D** An upper GI contrast study will differentiate congenital cystic adenomatoid malformation (CCAM) from congenital diaphragmatic hernia. The distinction is crucial because different operations are required for these two conditions. Upper GI can be performed more expeditiously than CT scan with double contrast (**C**), which will also make the diagnosis. Since the infant is in no respiratory distress, the corrective operation, either left thoracotomy (**A**) or laparotomy (**B**), can then be performed within a few hours as an urgent, but not emergent, procedure. Pneumoperitoneum (**E**) might produce respiratory embarrassment and is not recommended in this situation.

2. **A** CCAM has been classified into three different categories. Type I is characterized by multiple large cysts greater than 2 cm in diameter or by a single dominant cyst with small satellites. Type II is chacterized by multiple evenly spaced cysts that rarely exceed 1.2 cm in diameter and are separated by intervening dilated alveolar struc-

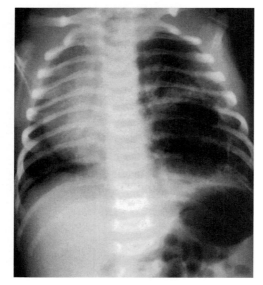

Figure 73–3. *Chest x-ray showing cystic mass in left hemithorax. Mediastinum is shifted to the right.*

tures. In type III, the entire lobe is inflitrated with bronchiole-like structures usually smaller than 0.5 cm in diameter. The lobe of type III is bulky and produces mediastinal shift in all cases. An alternative classification considers the anomaly as a macrocystic or microcystic type. All of the other statements are false. Congenital cystic adenomatoid malformation (CCAM) has a slight predilection for the lower lobes, not the upper lobes (**B**). Location of the lesion in a composite series was as follows: left lower lobe, 25%; left upper lobe, 20%; right lower lobe, 19%; right upper lobe, 10%; bilateral, 2%; more than one lobe, the remainder. The blood supply of CCAM usually comes from pulmonary, not systemic (**C**), vessels, although cases of "hybrid" lesions that display the pathologic appearance of CCAM and the vascular supply of pulmonary sequestration have been reported. The cysts of CCAM are typically lined with respiratory epithelium, usually of the ciliated columnar or ciliated cuboidal type. Only type I contains mucogenic cells that resemble glandular epithelium (**D**). Congenital cystic adenomatoid malformation (CCAM) is rarely associated with cystic renal disease (**E**). The *total* of anomalies associated with CCAM is about 20%, the most common of which are cardiac malformations.

3. **D** Preoperative angiography has little or no role in the diagnosis of CCAM or, for that matter, other pediatric lung anomalies in the modern environment. The information formerly derived from angiography is now available by less invasive means. All of the other statements are true. The appearance of polyhydramnios (**A**) may signal fetal mediastinal compression by the CCAM in utero. This may be followed by hydrops fetalis and fetal death. Close observation of such a pregnancy is mandatory. The onset of fetal hydrops may be an indication for transfer to a fetal treatment center for prenatal intervention. Cyst aspiration, shunting, and even pulmonary lobectomy have been performed for the fetus with CCAM. Fortunately, CCAM is usually confined to a single lobe, and it is curable (**B**) by lobectomy. Malignancy (eg, rhabdomyosarcoma and carcinoma [**C**]) has been reported as originating in CCAM; thus, there is no role for

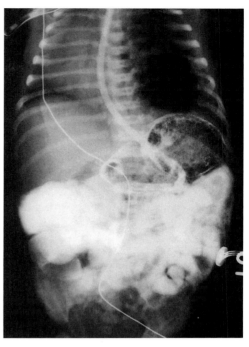

Figure 73–4. *Upper gastrointestinal (GI) contrast study confirming location of stomach below diaphragm. Contrast does not enter cystic mass above diaphragm.*

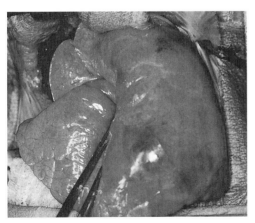

Figure 73–5. *Operative photograph showing large cyst in left lower lobe and normal left upper lobe. (See also color plate.)*

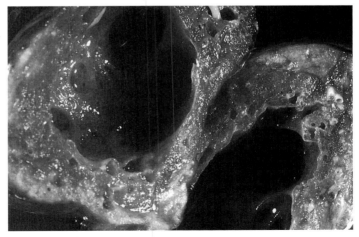

Figure 73–6. *Pathologic specimen. Left lower lobe showing single dominant cyst with multiple satellites. Specimen has been opened (bivalved) for examination. (See also color plate.)*

watchful waiting in this condition. Fatal mediastinal shift (**E**) is a dreaded complication that may occur after infant pneumonectomy, especially right pneumonectomy. Although rarely necessary in infants, pneumonectomy is occasionally required for CCAM involving an entire lung. Insertion of a prosthesis into the thoracic cavity may prevent the mediastinal shift. The author has reported successful placement of an expandable prosthesis (a tissue expander) following pneumonectomy in a 3-week-old infant with CCAM.

BIBLIOGRAPHY

Adzick NS, Harrison MR, Flake AW, et al. Fetal surgery for cystic adenomatoid malformation of the lung. *J Pediatr Surg.* 1993;28:806–812.

de Lorimier AA. Respiratory problems related to the airway and lung. In: O'Neill JA Jr, Rowe MI, Grosfeld JL, et al. eds. *Pediatric Surgery.* 5th ed. St. Louis: Mosby-Year Book; 1998:873–897.

Gilbert EF, Opitz JM. Malformations and genetic disorders of the respiratory tract. In: Stocker JT, ed. *Pediatric Pulmonary Disease.* New York: Hemisphere Publishing Corporation; 1989:29–100.

Kosloske AM, Williamson SL. An expandable prosthesis for stabilization of the infant mediastinum following pneumonectomy. *J Pediatr Surg.* 1992;27:1521–1522.

Oldham KT. Lung. In: Oldham KT, Colombani PM, Foglia RP, eds. *Surgery of Infants and Children: Scientific Principles and Practice.* Philadelphia: Lippincott-Raven; 1997:935–970.

A 9-YEAR-OLD BOY
WITH HEADACHES

HISTORY   You are asked to evaluate a 9-year-old boy with a history of headaches. He had never experienced headaches in his life until the past several months. He describes the headaches as "pounding," and they are particularly severe during times of exertion or stress. The boy's mother believes that he is sweating a lot and describes removing soaked sheets from his bed every night. The child has had a voracious appetite, but his weight has decreased 5 pounds in the past couple of months.

EXAMINATION   The child appears well but a bit thin. Temperature 37.0°C, heart rate 92, blood pressure 165/95, respiratory rate 24. The lungs are clear to auscultation, the heart has a regular rate and rhythm without murmur. The abdomen is soft and flat with no masses or hepatosplenomegaly. Neck examination reveals several 1-cm cervical nodes that are fairly soft and mobile.

Please answer all questions before proceeding to discussion section.

✓ QUESTIONS

1. Important diagnostic maneuvers include:
   A. Measuring blood pressure in all four extremities
   B. Serum electrolytes
   C. Urinalysis
   D. Urine for catecholamines
   E. All of the above

2. You see the child again after you learn that his 24-hour urine collection revealed a vanillylmandelic acid of 17 mg. Your next move is to:
   A. Arrange for immediate operation to remove a pheochromocytoma
   B. Treat his hypertension with hydralazine, and order a computed tomography (CT) scan of the abdomen

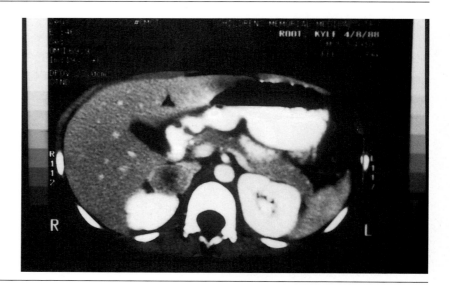

Figure 74–1. *A computed tomography (CT) scan of a child with a right adrenal pheochromocytoma.*

C. Admit him to the intensive care unit for invasive monitoring
D. Start him on phenoxybenzamine
E. Obtain a CT scan of his head

3. A CT scan of the abdomen reveals a right adrenal mass (Figure 74–1). Which is true regarding imaging of these tumors?
A. A CT scan will identify the tumor in 95% of children
B. Metiodobenzylguanidine (MIBG) scan is the initial study of choice
C. A magnetic resonance imaging (MRI) scan is unlikely to show the lesion
D. An ultrasound study must be done to look for vascular invasion prior to operation
E. All of the above

4. Pheochromocytoma in children differs from adults in which of the following respects?
A. More are bilateral
B. Hypertension is usually sustained rather than episodic
C. Less are malignant
D. More are extra-adrenal
E. All of the above

5. When you speak with the parents prior to operation, what do you tell them is the greatest risk to their child?
A. Bleeding from the vena cava
B. Unresectability due to malignant disease
C. Postoperative renal failure
D. Hemodynamic instability during the operation
E. Malignant hyperthermia related to the anesthetic

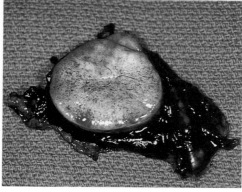

Figure 74–2. *Cut section of a pheochromocytoma. The fleshy yellow appearance (see also color plate) is typical of these tumors. Malignancy is best determined by biologic behavior rather than histologic appearance.*

6. The tumor is resected without incident and is shown in Figure 74–2 (see also color plate). You now tell the family:
A. Blood pressure should normalize in the next 24 to 48 hours
B. Determination as to whether the tumor is benign or malignant may take several days as immunohistochemical analysis is necessary

    C. The patient's siblings should be screened for hypertension
    D. The patient will require postoperative radiotherapy
    E. Postoperative MIBG scan should be done in 1 month

ANSWERS AND DISCUSSION

1. **E** This 9-year-old child has a marked elevation in his blood pressure. Hypertension is very unusual in this age group. In a 9-year-old child, hypertension is more likely due to a secondary cause than to essential hypertension. Therefore, the preliminary work-up should be directed toward potential secondary causes. Coarctation of the aorta can present late and would cause a marked differential in blood pressure between the upper and lower extremities. Abnormal serum electrolytes can often be the key to endocrine causes of hypertension, such as Cushing disease. Renal abnormalities are responsible for secondary hypertension in 75% of children. Urinary tract infection is a common finding. Additional findings on urinalysis may suggest the presence of glomerulonephritis or other renal parenchymal disease. Pheochromocytoma is a cause of sustained hypertension in childhood. Examination of a 24-hour urine collection for catecholamine levels is a sensitive test for this disorder.

2. **D** This child has a phenochromocytoma. The most important diagnostic test for pheochromocytoma in childhood is the measurement of urinary catecholamine levels. Epinephrine and norepinephrine are secreted by adrenal pheochromocytomas. These hormones, however, are extensively metabolized in the blood stream and only 2% to 4% of them are excreted free in the urine. Therefore, measurement of metabolites of these catecholamines in the urine is most useful. Metanephrine and vanillylmandelic acid (VMA) are the most readily identifiable metabolites of epinephrine. Norepinephrine is converted to normetanephrine and then VMA. Homovanillic acid (HVA) is a metabolite of dopamine.

   Once a pheochromocytoma is diagnosed, efforts should be made to treat the pateint with alpha-blocking medications and to localize the tumor. Phenoxybenzamine is an alpha-receptor antagonist that will both lower blood pressure preoperatively and significantly reduce the likelihood of catecholine storm at the time of operation. Treatment should be started at least 3 to 5 days prior to anticipated resection of the tumor. Normalization of blood pressure on alpha-blocking medications correlates highly with successful intra- and postoperative results. Hydralazine is an inappropriate medication to treat this patient's hypertension. Admission to the intensive care unit with invasive monitoring is not necessary. Many surgeons, however, recommend admission to the hospital for close monitoring of blood pressure as alpha blockade is started. A CT scan of the head is not indicated.

3. **A** A CT scan of the abdomen is a highly reliable test in localizing pheochromocytomas during childhood. Most series report successful localization of the tumor in over 95% of children. An MIBG scan involves administration of I^{131}-labeled MIBG. The active agent is a guanethidine analog that inhibits the uptake of catecholamines by chromaffin cells and blocks adrenergic neurons. After MIBG is ad-

ministered, a small amount is concentrated by the tumor and can be seen on scintigraphy. Results of this test are highly variable, depending on the experience of the center. An MIBG scan is considered a secondary test, which is useful when normal measures of localization fail or when it is necessary to identify recurrent or metastatic disease. An MRI scan is also an excellent means of evaluating adrenal and retroperitoneal lesions. This is likely to visualize most pheochromocytomas. An ultrasound study to look for vascular invasion is not necessary. These tumors rarely invade blood vessels.

4. **E** Seven percent of pheochromocytomas have been reported to be bilateral in the adult population. When children are followed for many years, the incidence of bilateral disease is as high as 70%. Children with pheochromocytoma more likely have a genetic predisposition to the disease from disorders such as multiple endocrine neoplasia type II. The hypertension that occurs in children with pheochromocytoma is typically sustained in comparison to the episodic hypertension seen in adults. Adult pheochromocytomas are malignant 10% to 15% of the time, while roughly 5% of childhood tumors are malignant. Thirty percent of children with pheochromocytoma have extra-adrenal disease, which is roughly twice the rate of that seen in adults.

   Pheochromocytomas originate from chromaffin cells, which are migratory catecholamine-producing cells that are precursors to the sympathetic ganglia, the adrenal medulla, and the paraganglia. Chromaffin cells typcially migrate along the aorta and its major branches. Extra-adrenal pheochromocytomas typically occur along the aorta or near the aortic bifurcation.

5. **D** The greatest risk to any child undergoing resection of pheochromocytoma is hemodynamic instability due to the wide swings in catecholamine levels, which can occur during resection of the tumor. Simply touching the tumor can cause a massive release of catecholamines into the blood stream. This may require aggressive treatment with drugs that lower the blood pressure. As catecholamine levels fall rapidly, the patient may experience hypotension. Anesthetic management of children during resection of pheochromocytoma is extremely important and has been the subject of much literature. Induction of general anesthesia is especially critical because inadequate sedation can result in extremely severe hypertension. Excessive alpha blockade without the necessary expansion in blood volume can result in hypotension.

   Enflurane or isofluorane are the anesthetic agents of choice, although the depth of anesthesia appears to be much more important than the particular agent used. Enflurane is selected because it does not sensitize the myocardium to exogenous catecholamines as halothane does, and it does not stimulate the reduction of catecholamines. Episodes of hypotension, which may occur immediately following tumor removal, are treated with either volume expansion or norepinephrine.

   Bleeding from the vena cava is no more likely during resection of a pheochromocytoma than any other adrenal tumor. These tumors are rarely unresectable even when they are malignant. Postoperative renal failure should not be a problem as long as renal perfusion is maintained during the operation. Malignant hyperthermia is a severe anesthetic complication that does not occur with increased frequency in patients with pheochromocytoma.

6. **C** There is a high incidence of familial pheochromocytoma in children; therefore, all siblings and parents should be screened for hypertension. Blood pressure frequently does not normalize for several weeks following tumor resection and continued antihypertensive therapy may be necessary during this interval. Determination as to whether the tumor is benign or malignant is based more on biologic behavior than on histologic characteristics. It is quite common for childhood pheochromocytomas to display lymphatic, vascular, and capillary invasive characteristics, as well as cellular pleomorphism. The majority of these tumors will prove to be benign on long-term follow-up. Postoperative radiotherapy is rarely necessary or recommended. An MIBG scan may be useful in a patient suspected of having metastatic or recurrent disease. In the normal postoperative patient who is clinically well without hypertension, however, an MIBG scan is not indicated.

BIBLIOGRAPHY

Ein SH, Weitzman S, Thorner P, et al. Pediatric maligant pheochromocytomas. *J Pediatr Surg.* 1994;29:1197–1201.

Fonkalsrud EW, Dunn J. Adrenal glands. In: O'Neill JA Jr, Rowe MI, Grosfeld JL, et al. eds. *Pediatric Surgery.* 5th ed. St. Louis: Mosby-Year Book; 1998:1555–1573.

Galfand MJ. Meta-iodobenzylguanidine in children. *Sem Nucl Med.* 1993;23:231–242.

Kaplan RA, Hellerstein S, Alon U. Evaluation of the hypertensive child. *Child Nephrol Urol.* 1992;12:106–112.

Stringle G, Ein SH, Creighton R, et al. Pheochromocytoma in children—an update. *J Pediatr Surg.* 1980;15(4):496–500.

A 13-YEAR-OLD GIRL WITH RECURRENT PERIANAL INFECTIONS

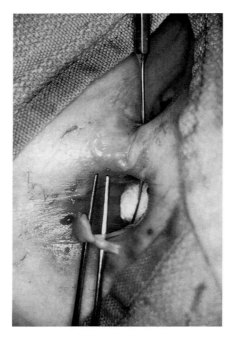

Figure 75–1. *Appearance of the perineum of a 13-year-old girl with history of multiple perianal abscesses. Probes are in fistulous tracts and in a recto vaginal fistula. (See also color plate.)*

HISTORY   A general surgeon calls you to discuss a patient she has treated for the past 6 months with recurrent perianal abscesses. The patient is a 13-year-old girl who was well until 6 months ago when she developed a right-sided perianal abscess. This was drained, but the wound had failed to heal 6 weeks later. Subsequently, she developed a left-sided perianal abscess, and 2 months later, a third abscess developed in the posterior midline. All three of these wounds have remained open and continue to drain mucus and pus.

Her treating physician obtained a barium enema that was reported to be normal. When you seen this young woman in your office you are surprised to find that she appears entirely healthy. She is well nourished and complains only of her annoying perianal disease. She otherwise feels entirely well.

EXAMINATION   Vital signs are normal. Lungs are clear, and there is no cardiac murmur. Her abdomen is soft, flat, nondistended, and nontender with no masses or hepatosplenomegaly. Her perianal region is badly excorated due to chronic drainage. Multiple fistulous tracts are seen (Figure 75–1; see also color plate).

LABORATORY   White blood count, hemoglobin, and hematocrit are normal. Electrolytes, transaminase levels, and amylase are normal.

Please answer all questions before proceeding to discussion section.

✓ QUESTIONS

1. What is the most likely diagnosis?
   A. Chronic granulomatous disease
   B. Recurrent perianal abscesses in the absence of any underlying disorder
   C. Villous adenoma of the rectum

358

   D. Ulcerative colitis
   E. Crohn's disease

2. Clinical trials in children have proven which of the following agents to be most effective for this patient?
   A. Oral metronidazole
   B. Intravenous metronidazole
   C. 6-mercaptopurine
   D. Corticosteroids
   E. None of the above

3. At this point, which of the following might you recommend?
   A. Immediate wide debridement of the perianal area in the operating room
   B. Sigmoid colostomy
   C. Ileostomy
   D. Barium enema
   E. Upper gastrointestinal series

4. You elect to start this patient on a course of oral metronidazole. Following this, she has an excellent response, and all wounds are healed within 4 weeks. The upper gastrointestinal series is normal. You should now:
   A. Continue metronidazole for 3 months
   B. Continue metronidazole for 6 months
   C. Discontinue therapy, and instruct her to return if the perianal problems or any other gastrointestinal symptoms occur
   D. Start her on corticosteroids every other day
   E. Obtain a computed tomography (CT) scan of the abdomen

FOLLOW-UP COURSE   The patient returns to see you in 1 year, and she does not look well. She has been having abdominal pain for the last 3 months. Her appetite is very poor, and she vomits three to four time per week. She appears very pale. Abdominal examination reveals a moderately distended abdomen with fullness in the right lower quadrant that is tender. You obtain a barium study of the small intestine that is shown in part in Figure 75–2.

5. Which of the following treatment plans are appropriate?
   A. Ileostomy
   B. Sigmoid colostomy
   C. Immediate resection of the involved ileum with primary anastomosis
   D. Start treatment with oral steroids and sulfasalazine
   E. Start treatment with cyclosporine A

6. The patient is treated by an excellent pediatric gastroenterologist for the next 6 months. She is treated with a variety of drug combinations, but none of them seem to work. She has lost an additional 15 pounds during this time. Repeat upper gastrointestinal series shows very severe disease in the terminal ileum, but the remainder of the intestine appears normal. Which of the following are relative indications for operation in Crohn's disease in children?
   A. Significant growth delay
   B. Delayed onset of puberty
   C. Severe disease localized to a single area

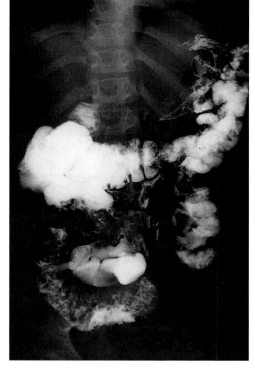

Figure 75–2. *Upper gastrointestinal series shows stricture of the terminal ileum with moderate dilation of bowel loops above the stricture.*

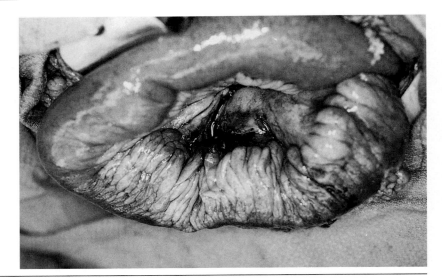

Figure 75–3. *Appearance the terminal ileum in a patient with Crohn's disease. Note the marked thickening of the bowel wall and "creeping mesenteric fat" that completely surrounds the serosa of the affected bowel. This is in contrast to the normal unaffected loops of ileum in the background.*

    D. Enterocolic fistula
    E. All of the above

7. You elect to operate on this patient. At laparotomy, you find a severely diseased terminal ileum shown in Figure 75–3. The remainder of the small and large intestine are not remarkable. Which operation should you do?
    A. Resection of the grossly involved bowel with ileostomy and plans for reanastomosis in 6 weeks
    B. Wide resection of the involved bowel with 7-cm margins of normal bowel on either side of the resected area and primary anastomosis
    C. Resection of the area with frozen section examination of the margins to ensure that all the diseased bowel is removed
    D. Resection of gross disease only with primary anastomosis
    E. Bypass of the affected area with side-to-side anastomosis

8. The cause of Crohn's disease is:
    A. Genetic abnormality
    B. Infectious
    C. Immune mediated
    D. Environmental
    E. Unknown

ANSWERS AND DISCUSSION

1. **E** The presence of recalcitrant perianal abscesses and fistulae is often the first sign of Crohn's disease. Healthy patients without inflammatory bowel disease should heal rapidly following drainage of perianal abscess. Multiple recurrent abscesses are almost always indicative of an underlying disorder. Perianal disease has been reported to be the presenting feature in up to 25% of patients with Crohn's disease. Often, perianal disease may precede the intestinal manifestations by several years. A survey of pediatric tertiary care centers found that 14% to 62% of patients with Crohn's disease have perianal manifestations. These lesions include anal fissures and tags, fistulas, ab-

scesses, and highly destructive perianal disease, including cavitating ulceration.

Chronic granulomatous disease is a defect in white blood cell function that results in multiple subcutaneous abscesses, usually with staphylococcus. Villous adenoma of the rectum is highly unusual in this age group and would tend to present with rectal bleeding or mucus production. Ulcerative colitis always affects the colon, but it rarely causes significant perianal disease.

2. **E** Despite the fact that 25% of patients with Crohn's disease are children, there is little hard evidence regarding the best therapy in this population. Most clinical trials have excluded children and adolescents. All of the choices, **A** through **D**, have been used with varying success to treat perianal disease in the pediatric population. One uncontrolled study reported a good response in 70% to 75% of patients treated with oral metrondiazole. Other centers suggest that this drug be given intravenously. Several patients with serious intestinal disease who were treated with 6-mercaptopurine experienced significant healing of their perianal disease. Corticosteroids have been reported as successful in other centers. The bottom line is that all of these agents are moderately effective, but none of them have been shown to be superior to the others.

Other reports using an elemental diet as primary treatment documented healing of perianal fistulas in 67% to 85% of patients. There was, however, a significant relapse rate in this series. One small study used hyperbaric oxygen therapy and produced complete healing in 70% of patients without recurrence after 18 months.

3. **E** The role of surgical therapy for perianal manifestations of Crohn's disease is limited. Aggressive surgical debridement or drainage frequently produces large, nonhealing or even ulcerating wounds. Surgical treatment may be appropriate for simple low fistulas or for incision and drainage of large collections of pus. In general, in a patient who does not have evidence of acute infection or undrained pus, surgical therapy is best reserved until a course of medical treatment has been instituted. Diverting colostomy is often necessary for patients with the most severe perianal problems. Colostomy, however, would not be indicated in this patient. She is generally doing well and has never had a trial of medical therapy. Ileostomy should never be necessary to treat perianal disease and is contraindicated in Crohn's disease because peristomal manifestations of Crohn's disease frequently develop.

A barium enema has already been done and has been normal. Upper gastrointestinal series is indicated in order to determine whether or not the patient has any intestinal manifestations of Crohn's disease. This will help in selecting the most appropriate course of medical therapy.

4. **C** This patient probably has Crohn's disease but has yet to develop intestinal manifestations. She has healed her perianal disease, and no further treatment is indicated. There is no evidence to suggest that long-term treatment with metronidazole has any role in preventing recurrence. Corticosteriods are not indicated as she has responded well to a far less toxic medication. A CT scan of the abdomen has no role.

This patient will almost certainly return with either recurrent perianal disease, intestinal manifestations of Crohn's disease, or both. In the interim, no treatment is necessary.

5. **D** This patient has evidence of Crohn's disease in the terminal ileum as manifested by narrowing and bowel wall thickening in this location. Any type of surgical therapy would be premature as the patient has yet to be treated medically. There are a variety of potential medical regimens, including steroids, metronidazole, 5-ASA preparations, and immunosuppressive drugs, such as azathioprine, methotrexate, and cyclosporin A.

The mainstay of initial medical therapy is treatment with corticosteroids. Cyclosporin A is a drug with strong immunosuppressive effects that should only be used in extreme circumstances after primary treatment has failed.

If it becomes necessary to resect the terminal ileum, primary anastomosis is usually well tolerated. Ileostomy is rarely necessary for ileal Crohn's disease. Sigmoid colostomy would be of no benefit.

6. **E** As a general rule, surgical therapy should be considered as a last resort for young patients with Crohn's disease. This is because patients are likely to require frequent operations throughout their lifetime. Each of these operations results in resection of additional intestine. Many patients with Crohn's disease develop short gut syndrome by midadulthood. A study followed 68 patients with juvenile-onset Crohn's disease. Seventy percent has required operation within 2 years, 50% within 6 years, and 85% within 14 years.

Operation should be considered based on all of the indications mentioned. Children with Crohn's disease are at significant risk of delayed growth and maturaton due to both the chronic disease and the high levels of steroid therapy necessary to treat it. If growth delay is not treated aggressively, the patient's epiphyses will close, and the patient will never achieve full stature.

Patients with severe disease localized to a single area, most commonly the terminal ileum, may benefit greatly from surgical therapy. If the majority of disease can be removed by resecting a short segment of intestine and the remainder of the intestine is relatively unaffected, patients may do well for a long period of time. A fistula between the small bowel and the colon is generally considered an indication for operation. In isolated circumstances, these fistulae will respond to medical therapy.

7. **D** Bowel resection in Crohn's disease should involve the gross disease only; there is no advantage to obtaining wide surgical margin. This will neither reduce the complication nor recurrence rates. Primary anastomosis is appropriate in this case. Stomas should be avoided at all costs in patients with Crohn's disease. This is because there is a high incidence of peristomal complications, and the creation of stomas results in the need for resection of additional lengths of intestine. Frozen-section examination of the resection margins, while theoretically appealing, has not been shown to correlate with good outcome. Microscopic features of Crohn's disease may extend well beyond the gross disease (Figure 75–4; see also color plate). This bowel does not need to be resected. Bypass of an affected segment is inappropriate.

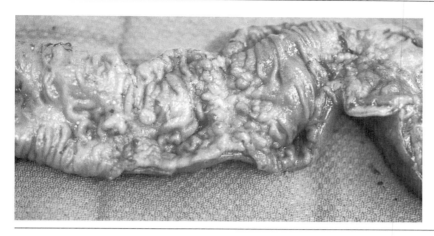

Figure 75–4. *Pathologic appearance of the resected ileum in Crohn's disease. The mucosa is deeply ulcerated. Islands of mucosa among these deep ulcerations appear to be polyps and are referred to as pseudopolyps. (See also color plate.)*

Outcome after this procedure is typically quite good. In patients with isolated disease of the terminal ileum, 40% to 60% will be disease-free and off all medical therapy 5 years later. Unfortunately, effective surgical treatment of the ileal disease does not necessarily result in improvement in perianal manifestations of Crohn's disease.

8. **E** Despite many years of extensive research, the cause of Crohn's disease remains unknown. One multidisciplinary panel concluded, "The available evidence suggests that Crohn's disease results from a genetically conditioned susceptibility to immune-mediated bowel injury which is triggered by one or more environmental factors." It would be difficult to be more vague than this. Clearly, genetic susceptibility is important in the pathogenesis of Crohn's disease. A family history of a first-degree relative with inflammatory bowel disease is the most important risk factor for Crohn's disease. In contrast, Crohn's disease has rarely been described in spouses. There is a much higher rate of concordance for Crohn's disease among monozygotic twins as compared to dizygotic twins. There is also substantial clincal and experimental evidence that suggests that Crohn's disease may be due to an abnormally heightened immune response to normal bacterial flora. The strongest evidence for this is the fact that chronic gastrointestinal and joint inflammation is absent when experimental models of inflammatory bowel disease are induced in germ-free animals. Other investigators contend that a "priming" event occurs early in life, perhaps in infancy, which causes the patient to be susceptible to the development of later Crohn's disease. Another body of evidence entirely supports the autoimmune basis disease.

The bottom line is that the cause remains unknown. It is not likely that there will be an uniformly successful treatment for Crohn's disease until the cause is elucidated.

BIBLIOGRAPHY

Cohen MB, Seidman E, Winter H, et al. Controversies in pediatric inflammatory bowel disease. *Inflam Bowel Dis.* 1998;4:203–227.

Ekbom A, Adami HO, Helmick CG, et al. Prenatal risk factors for inflammatory bowel disease: a case-controlled study. *Am J Epidemiol.* 1990; 132:1111–1119.

Elson CO, Sartor RB, Tennyson GS, et al. Experimental models of inflammatory bowel disease. *Gastroenterol.* 1995;109:1344–1367.

Grand RJ, Ramakrishna J, Calenda KA. Inflammatory bowel disease in the pediatric patient. *Gastroenterol Clin North Am.* 1995;24:613–632.

Hyams JS. Crohn's's disease in children. *Pediatr Clin North Am.* 1996;43:255–277.

Mack DR. Ongoing advances in inflammatory bowel diseases, including maintenance therapies, biologic agents, and biology of disease. *Curr Opin Pediatr.* 1998;10:499–506.

McCartney S, Ballinger A. Growth failure in inflammatory bowel disease. *Nutrition.* 1999;15:169–171.

Peeters M, Nevens H, Baert F, et al. Familial aggregations in Crohn's disease: increased age-adjusted risk and concordance in clinical characteristics. *Gastroenterol.* 1996;111:597–603.

Sartor RB. Current concepts of the etiology and pathogenesis of ulcerative colitis and Crohn's disease. *Gastroenterol Clin North Am.* 1995; 24:475–507.

A 14-MONTH-OLD BOY WITH LEFT LUNG ATELECTASIS

HISTORY A 14-month-old boy is transferred to the children's hospital with left lung atelectasis. Six weeks previously, he was treated for pneumonia and left lower lobe atelectasis at a local hospital. He recovered after treatment with antibiotics and bronchodilators. His cough and respiratory distress recurred 6 weeks later, however, and it did not resolve in spite of treatment with antibiotics, bronchodilators, and chest physiotherapy. Steroids were given without improvement. He was referred for further diagnosis and therapy.

EXAMINATION He is a well-developed, well-nourished toddler who is (surprisingly) in minimal respiratory distress at admission. His blood pressure is 79/54, pulse 130, temperature 36.8°C. Weight is 8.6 kg. His trachea is in the midline. There is hyperresonance to percussion over the right hemithorax and dullness to percussion over the left. Breath sounds are bronchial. They are increased on the right and markedly diminished on the left. Heart tones are maximal at the left anterior axillary line. No cardiac murmur is heard. The abdomen is soft and nontender without masses or hernias. The remainder of the examination is unremarkable.

LABORATORY Hemoglobin 11.9 gm%, hematocrit 36%, white blood cell count 14.9/mm^3. Platelets are 600,000/mm^3. Urinalysis is normal. A chest x-ray is shown in Figure 76–1. A computed tomography (CT) scan of the chest is shown in Figure 76–2.

HOSPITAL COURSE Bronchoscopy is performed. The left mainstem bronchus appears to be occluded (Figure 76–3), but the Storz 3.5-mm bronchoscope is gently advanced through the collapsed area into a normal appearing bronchus distally. The left upper lobe orifice, lower lobe bronchus, and segmental bronchi are normal.

Please answer all questions before proceeding to discussion section.

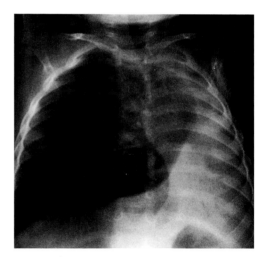

Figure 76–1. *Chest x-ray showing atelectasis of left lung with herniation of right lung across the midline.*

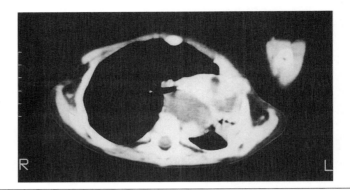

Figure 76–2. *A computed tomography (CT) scan of the chest showing cystic mediastinal mass above left mainstem bronchus.*

✓ QUESTIONS

1. The most likely diagnosis is:
   A. Congenital lobar emphysema
   B. Bronchogenic cyst
   C. Congenital cystic adenomatoid malformation (CCAM)
   D. Pulmonary sequestration
   E. Pericardial cyst

2. The operation of choice for this infant is:
   A. Lobectomy
   B. Pneumonectomy
   C. Segmental resection
   D. Cystectomy
   E. Marsupialization

HOSPITAL COURSE (CONT.)   Left thoracotomy is performed, and a 4-cm, lobulated cyst is resected from beneath the arch of the aorta (Figures 76–4 and 76–5; see also color plates). The recurrent laryngeal nerve is carefully preserved. The left mainstem bronchus is compressed and soft at the site of attachment of the cyst. Positive pressure ventilation reexpands the atelectatic left lung, but as closure of the chest begins, the left lung becomes emphysematous and rigid. These changes, attributed to severe acute bronchomalacia, improve after bronchopexy is performed. Repeat bronchoscopy after closure of the chest shows a patent left mainstem bronchus (Figure 76–6). The patient makes an uneventful recovery. The technique of bronchopexy is reported.

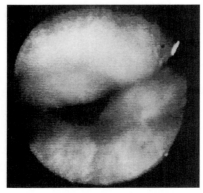

Figure 76–3. *Bronchoscopic view showing left mainstem bronchus collapsed.*

3. A 2.5-cm solitary cyst is found on the chest x-ray obtained in a 2-year-old girl who was a restrained passenger in a minor automobile accident. There was no direct trauma to her chest. The cyst is located at the pulmonary hilum adjacent to the mediastinum. She has no history of pulmonary problems and never had x-rays previously. Her chest examination is normal, and she remains healthy. On follow-up film 6 weeks later, the cyst is unchanged. Your advice to the parents is:
   A. Immediate thoracotomy, excision
   B. Elective thoracotomy, excision
   C. Thoracoscopic biopsy, drainage of the cyst
   D. Watchful waiting, yearly chest films, excision only if complications (eg, infection, bronchial compression) develop
   E. Reassurance that the cyst is benign, no specific follow-up

ANSWERS AND DISCUSSION

1. **B** Bronchogenic cyst is the most likely diagnosis. These cysts are usually found at the pulmonary hilum or in the subcarinal area. This one, typically, is located atop the left mainstem bronchus (Figure 76–2). The infant's symptoms worsened gradually, as the cyst grew. Enlargement occurs because of mucous production from the bronchial mucosa lining the cyst. The diagnosis may be delayed until the cyst causes compression of the airway or becomes infected. In this infant, the initial manifestation was left lower lobe atelectasis; collapse of the entire left lung followed 6 weeks later. Congenital lobar emphysema (**A**) usually presents in the neonatal period. Rapid and progressive respiratory failure may occur from hyperinflation of the affected lobe, collapse of adjacent lobes, and mediastinal shift. Congenital cystic adenomatoid malformation (CCAM) (**C**) also presents with respiratory distress in the neonatal period. Sequestrations (**D**) are usually located in lower lobes, and they are most often diagnosed after they become infected. An infiltrate on x-ray fails to clear with antibiotic treatment for suspected pneumonia. Pericardial cysts (**E**) are extremely rare, and they are not reported to cause bronchial compression.

2. **D** Cystectomy is the treatment of choice for a bronchogenic cyst. The cyst usually can be "shelled out" of the mediastinum or hilar portion of the lung without sacrificing normal lung tissue. The surgeon should make every effort to avoid removal of normal lung in a pediatric patient; thus, lobectomy (**A**) or pneumonectomy (**B**) is not indicated. Segmental resection (**C**), which requires removal of an anatomic bronchopulmonary segment, is associated with postoperative air leaks, and it is rarely performed in children. Cystectomy is usually done via thoracotomy, although a thoracoscopic approach has been described for selected patients. Marsupilization (**E**) is a rare option that should be used if a portion of the cyst wall is so adherent to a vital structure that it cannot be safely dissected; however, the surgeon should strip out any mucosa from the cyst wall that is left behind.

3. **B** Elective thoracotomy and excision of the cyst, most likely a bronchogenic cyst, is the safest management of this patient. It is not a dire emergency (**A**), but there is *no* evidence to support watchful waiting until complications (**D**) develop. Infection or bronchial compression, which eventually develop in virtually *all* bronchogenic cysts, may require a more extensive operation than simple excision prior to complications. Pneumatoceles are pseudocysts without an epithelial lining that may occur following pneumonia or direct trauma to the chest. They may rupture (creating a pneumothorax), enlarge (compressing normal lung), or resolve spontaneously. Since this patient had neither pneumonia nor direct trauma, bronchogenic cyst is a more likely diagnosis than pneumatocele. Thoracoscopic drainage and biopsy (**C**) are not curative for a bronchogenic cyst, which will fill up again with mucus if its epithelial lining remains. Reassurance about possible malignancy (**E**) is not appropriate, since there are reports of pulmonary sarcoma and carcinoma presenting as a solitary lung cyst in pediatric patients.

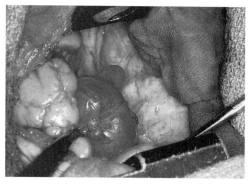

Figure 76–4. *Operative photograph showing lobulated cyst beneath arch of aorta. (See also color plate.)*

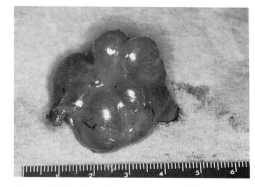

Figure 76–5. *Surgical specimen of bronchogenic cyst. (See also color plate.)*

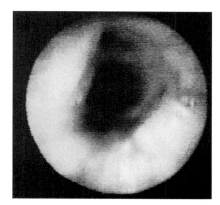

Figure 76–6. *Bronchoscopic view showing left mainstem bronchus widely patent after cyst resection and bronchopexy.*

BIBLIOGRAPHY

de Lorimier AA. Respiratory problems related to the airway and lung. In: O'Neill JA Jr, Rowe MI, Grosfeld JL, et al. eds. *Pediatric Surgery.* 5th ed. St. Louis: Mosby-Year Book; 1998:873–897.

Gilbert EF, Opitz JM. Malformations and genetic disorders of the respiratory tract. In: Stocker JT, ed. *Pediatric Pulmonary Disease.* New York: Publishing Corporation; 1989:29–100.

Goldthorn JF, Duncan MH, Kosloske AM, et al. Cavitating pulmonary fibrosarcoma in a child. *J Thorac Cardiovasc Surg.* 1986;91:932–934.

Kosloske AM. Left mainstem bronchopexy for severe bronchomalacia. *J Pediatr Surg.* 1991;26:260–262.

Oldham KT. Lung. In: Oldham KT, Colombani PM, Foglia RP, eds. *Surgery of Infants and Children: Scientific Principles and Practice.* Philadelphia: Lippincott-Raven; 1997:935–970.

Phillippart AI, Farmer DL. Benign mediastinal cysts and tumors. In: O'Neill JA Jr, Rowe MI, Grosfeld JL, et al., eds. *Pediatric Surgery.* 5th ed. St. Louis: Mosby-Year Book; 1998:839–851.

A 7-YEAR-OLD BOY WITH ABDOMINAL PAIN AND VOMITING

HISTORY A 7-year-old boy is brought to the emergency department with a 2-day history of crampy abdominal pain and vomiting. Today, his vomiting has become bilious, and he has passed a bloody, mucousy stool. He was well previously, and has no history of prior abdominal surgery.

PHYSICAL EXAMINATION The examination reveals a young boy in obvious abdominal distress. He has no fever, but is tachycardiac and appears dehydrated. His abdomen is distended and mildly tender, and a mass is palpable in the right upper quadrant. His groins are clear. Rectal examination demonstrates fresh blood, but no stool. A nasogastric tube is placed for bilious returns, and intravenous resuscitation is commenced. Abdominal plain films are obtained, which demonstrate a distal intestinal obstruction, but no free air.

Please answer all questions before proceeding to discussion section.

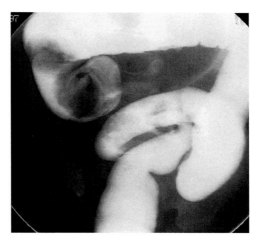

Figure 77–1. *Contrast enema demonstrating a nonreducible ileocolic intussusception. The patient's age raises the likelihood that the lead point is pathologic.*

✓ QUESTIONS

1. At this point, you would:
   A. Proceed directly to laparotomy
   B. Scan obtain an air or contrast enema
   C. Obtain an abdominal computer tomography (CT)
   D. Obtain an abdominal ultrasound

2. A contrast enema demonstrates nonreducible ileocolic intussusception (Figure 77–1). Candidates for the "lead point" include:
   A. Meckel's diverticulum
   B. Ileal duplication
   C. Peyer's patch lymph nodes
   D. All of the above

3. Following appropriate fluid resuscitation and administration of antibiotics, the patient is brought to the operating room and explored through a transverse right lower abdominal incision. The intussuscepiens is delivered, and attempts at reduction of the intussusceptum are unsuccessful. In addition to apparent submucosal ileal tumor (Figure 77–2; see also color plate), note is made of a firm, 3-cm lobular mass in the root of the ileal mesentery. At this point, you would:
   A. Proceed with ileocolic resection with primary anastomosis and biopsy of the mesenteric mass with frozen section
   B. Attempt *en bloc* resection of mesenteric mass with ileocolon, with primary intestinal anastomosis, provided all gross intra-abdominal disease is resectable without extensive enterectomy
   C. Perform staging laparotomy for presumed non-Hodgkin's lymphoma
   D. Proceed with ileocolic resection with ileostomy and biopsy of mesenteric mass with frozen section

4. The frozen section biopsy from the mass in the mesentery returns as "small round blue cell" tumor. Which of the following diagnostic or prognostic variables is *not* relevant to this particular tumor type?
   A. Urinary vanillylmandelic acid (VMA) and homovanillic acid (HVA)
   B. C-*myc* proto-oncogene translocation
   C. Alpha-fetoprotein levels in serum
   D. Alveolar histology

5. The most likely identity of this tumor is:
   A. Neuroblastoma
   B. Lymphoblastic lymphoma
   C. Hodgkin lymphoma
   D. Burkitt lymphoma

6. Which of the following statements regarding the role of surgery in non-Hodgkin's lymphoma is false?
   A. Completeness of resection is the strongest predictor of outcome
   B. Mechanical ureteral obstruction by retroperitoneal tumor requires stenting prior to institution of chemotherapy, to minimize the risk of renal shutdown from tumor lysis syndrome

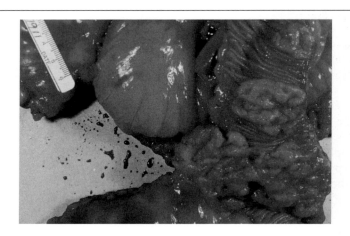

Figure 77–2. *Gross appearance of the resected specimen. The cauliflower-shaped tumor masses are arising from the submucosa. With permission from Lin KM, David GP, Mahmaud A, et al. Advantage of surgery and adjutant chemotherapy in the treatment of primary gastrointestinal lymphoma. J Surg Oncol. 1997;64(3):237–241. (See also color plate.)*

C. Attempts at massive complete resection in patients with extensive abdominal disease are associated with increased rates of complication, and lead to delay in institution of essential chemotherapy

D. Patients with gastrointestinal lymphoma that are not resectable for cure, should have the involved segment of bowel resected in an effort to reduce the likelihood of bleeding and/or perforation associated with intensive chemo or radiation therapy

ANSWERS AND DISCUSSION

1. **C** Although many surgeons would proceed directly to laparotomy, an abdominal CT scan with intravenous and enteral contrast would likely offer the most diagnostic information in this child, in whom a malignant cause of obstruction must be seriously considered. The symptoms of crampy abdominal pain, bilious vomiting, and mucousy, bloody (currant jelly) stool are typical for intussusception, which would be distinctly unusual at this age, but if present, would likely be nonreducible and associated with a pathologic lead point.

2. **D** In most cases of intussusception occurring in the "physiologic" age range of 3 months to 3 years, the intussusceptum (lead point) is an enlarged Peyer's patch lymph node. Pathologic lead points are the usual initiators of intussusception occurring outside the usual age range, and include Meckel's diverticula, polyps, duplication cysts, and abnormal mural or mesenteric masses such as gastrointestinal lymphomas or appendiceal carcinoid tumors. Henoch-Schoenlein purpura can result in intestinal wall edema or intramural hemorrhage that may serve as a lead point for intussusception.

3. **B** The finding of a nonreducible ileocolic intussusception in conjunction with a pathologic mesenteric nodal mass makes for a likely diagnosis of gastrointestinal lymphoma. If after abdominal exploration, it appears that the tumor bearing tissue is completely resectable without significant morbidity, then complete excision should be undertaken. Palliative resection and biopsy is appropriate for those patients with extensive retroperitoneal or hepatic disease. Staging laparotomy has no role to play in non-Hodgkin's lymphoma, since essentially all patients will receive chemotherapy.

4. **C** Small round blue cell tumor is the cytologic description given to tumors composed of round cells which are smaller than macrophages and possess large- or medium-sized nuclei and basophilic cytoplasm. The list of small round blue cell tumors includes lymphoma, neuroblastoma, rhabdomyosarcoma, Ewing sarcoma, and primitive neuroectodermal tumor (PNET). Urinary screening for VMA and HVA is part of the workup for neuroblastoma, C-*myc* proto-oncogene translocation between chromosomes 8 and 14 is associated with Burkitt lymphoma, and alveolar histology rhabdomyosarcoma is considered an unfavorable histologic subtype. None of the small round blue cell tumors are associated with increased serum production of alpha-fetoprotein.

5. **D** Lymphoma is by far the most common primary intestinal malignancy of childhood. Almost all intestinal lymphomas are non-Hodgkin's type, and of these, most are undifferentiated, small non-cleaved (SNC) cell, or Burkitt histology. Burkitt lymphoma in western equatorial Africa usually arises in the mandible, and is endemic in nature because of its association with Epstein-Barr virus (EBV). American (nonendemic) Burkitt lymphoma occurs almost exclusively within the abdomen, arising in the germinal centers of the bowel wall, or in mesenteric or retroperitoneal lymph nodes. Lymphoblastic lymphomas occur predominantly in the anterior mediastinum, and account for approximately 30% of all childhood non-Hodgkin's lymphomas.

6. **A** It is now realized that childhood non-Hodgkin's lymphoma is, in virtually all cases, a disseminated disease at diagnosis and that chemotherapy is essential for long-term, disease-free survival. Although some authors have claimed a direct relationship between surgical resectability and outcome, therefore advocating aggressive, complete resection (often at the expense of delayed initiation of chemotherapy), the question of whether tumor bulk determined resectability and ultimate prognosis, or whether surgical resection alone had a primary effect on outcome has been a frequently contested issue. A report form the Children's Cancer Study Group (CCG) put this specific question to multivariate analysis and concluded that the most important predictor of event-free survival in abdominal non-Hodgkin's disease is extent of disease at diagnosis, and not surgical resectability.

Recognition of ureteral obstruction causing hydroureteronephrosis should prompt attempts to decompress the kidney before starting chemotherapy, since the high uric acid load superimposed on a partially obstructed kidney may incite complete renal shutdown.

When feasible, diseased bowel should be resected as this may reduce the risks of subsequent intestinal perforation and hemorrhage during chemotherapy or radiation therapy.

BIBLIOGRAPHY

Crump M, Gospodarowicz M, Shepherd FA. Lymphoma of the gastrointestinal tract. *Semin Oncol.* 1999;26:324–337.

LaQuaglia MO, Stolar CJH, Krailo M, et al. The role of surgery in abdominal non-Hodgkin's lymphoma: Experience from the Children's Cancer Study Group. *J Pediatr Surg.* 1992;27:230–235.

Law MM, Williams SB, Wong JH. Role of surgery in the management of primary lymphoma of the gastrointestinal tract. *J Surg Oncol.* 1996; 61:199–204.

A 15-YEAR-OLD GIRL WITH A PAINLESS NECK MASS

HISTORY   A 15-year-old girl is referred for outpatient evaluation of a right of midline, lower neck mass. The mass is painless and has doubled in size since she first noticed it 6 months earlier. She has no other symptoms. There is no family history of thyroid cancer.

EXAMINATION   No abnormal facies are noted. There is a nontender 2.5-cm nodule in the lower pole of the right thyroid lobe. The remainder of the thyroid gland feels normal, and there is no cerivcal lymphadenopathy.

Please answer all questions before proceeding to discussion section.

✔ QUESTIONS

1. The next most appropriate step is:
   A. A 3-month trial of suppressive thyroid hormone therapy
   B. Thyroid scintigraphy to determine whether the nodule is "hot" or "cold"
   C. Fine needle aspiration biopsy
   D. Thyroid lobectomy

2. You opt for a fine needle aspiration biopsy. The cytology is "consistent with papillary carcinoma" (Figure 78–1; see also color plate). Recommended therapeutic options include:
   A. Right thyroid lobectomy
   B. Right thyroid lobectomy and ipsilateral cervical lymph node sampling
   C. Total thyroidectomy and ipsilateral lymph node sampling
   D. Preoperative I^{131} scanning

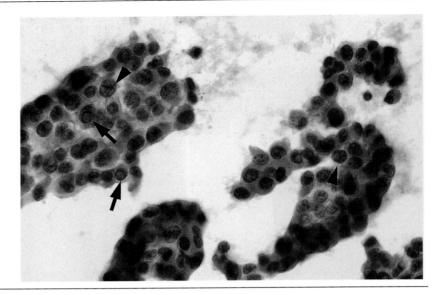

Figure 78–1. *Fine needle aspiration (FNA) preparation of papillary carcinoma showing finger-like papillae containing cells with dense metaplastic cytoplasm, occasional intranuclear inclusions (arrows), and nuclei with longitudinal grooves (arrowheads). (Papanicolaou × 600.) (See also color plate.)*

3. The pathology on her surgical specimen demonstrated multicenteric papillary carcinoma with metastases present in two lymph nodes (Figure 78–2; see also color plate). Your next step would be:
   A. Ipsilateral modified radical or "functional" neck dissection
   B. I^{131} scanning in 6 weeks without thyroid hormone replacement and with radioiodine ablation of any residual functioning thyroid tissue
   C. Adjuvant chemotherapy
   D. None of the above

4. A solitary thyroid nodule is more likely to be malignant in a child than an adult:
   A. True
   B. False

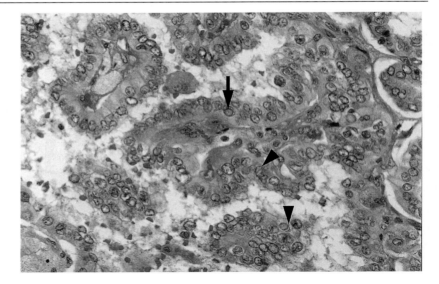

Figure 78–2. *High power magnification from resection specimen showing papillary carcinoma. The delicate papillae are lined by cuboidal-to-columnar cells with vesicular nuclei, occasional intranuclear inclusions (arrow), and conspicuous nuclear grooves (arrowheads). (Hematoxylin and eosin × 400.) (See also color plate.)*

5. Which of the following is *not* a component of the multiple endocrine neoplasia (MEN) IIA syndrome?
   A. Medullary carcinoma of the thyroid
   B. Pituitary adenoma
   C. Pheochromocytoma
   D. Hyperparathyroidism

6. A missense mutation in the ret proto-oncogene is 100% predictive of the development of medullary carcinoma of the thyroid and justifies prophylactic thyroidectomy in early childhood:
   A. True
   B. False

ANSWERS AND DISCUSSION

1. **C** The likelihood that this nodule represents thyroid cancer is high, in the range of 30% to 50%. Fine needle aspiration is very likely to provide a cytologic diagnosis of cancer if the cells are papillary, but it cannot differentiate benign from malignant neoplasms of follicular or Hurthle cell origin. Any patient with malignant or suspicious cytology on fine needle aspiration should proceed to surgery. Suppressive therapy should be considered only after benign histology has been proven, and continued growth or failure to involute should lead one to question the cytologic diagnosis and, thus, to prompt excision. Thyroid scintigraphy usually points toward neoplasia, if the nodule is "cold," although occasionally, cancers can appear as "hot" nodules. In instances where cytology is unavailable or unreliable, it is appropriate to proceed directly to surgical excision.

2. **C** There is significant controversy over what represents adequate surgical treatment for patients with papillary thyroid cancer. Based on the tendency of papillary cancer to be multicentric throughout the gland, there is little argument among thyroid surgeons that except for the very smallest papillary tumors (< 1 cm), surgery should consist of nothing less than "near total" thyroidectomy (which intentionally leaves a little normal thyroid tissue along the branches of the superior and inferior thyroid arteries in an effort to protect the parathyroid glands). Those who advocate near total thyroidectomy argue that total thyroidectomy does not reduce mortality rate, yet does increase the risks of permanent hypoparathyroidism and injury to the recurrent laryngeal nerve. Those who favor total thyroidectomy argue that the incidence of hypoparathyroidism and recurrent laryngeal nerve injury is extremely low and that removal of all thyroid tissue faciliates detection and treatment of metastases with I^{131}, which otherwise must compete with normal thyroid for uptake. Another advantage of total thyroidectomy is that it allows monitoring of thyroglobulin levels as a means of detecting persistent or recurrent disease. Lymph nodes are routinely sampled from suspicious areas, but lymph node dissections, such as those undertaken with squamous head and neck cancers are not usually performed.

3. **B** I^{131} is an important adjuvant to the surgical treatment of well-differentiated thyroid cancers (papillary and follicular). Six weeks following total or near total thyroidectomy, patients are scanned

with I^{131}, and if there are areas of uptake corresponding to residual thyroid tissue or metastases, then a therapeutic dose of I^{131} is administered. It is important that no thyroid hormone be administered during that time so as to maximize iodine uptake during scanning.

4. **A** Solitary thyroid nodules in children are rare in comparison to adults (present in 4% of persons age 30 to 60), but when present, they are more likely to be malignant. It is estimated that a palpable thyroid nodule in a child carries a 25% to 55% risk of malignancy, versus approximately 20% for adults. Most childhood thyroid cancers are well-differentiated papillary cancers, and they occur most frequently in the 15 to 19 year old age group. Girls are affected two to three times more often than boys, and approximately 50% have cervical lymph node metastases at presentation. Two important factors that increase the risk that a solitary nodule is malignant are a history of head and neck irradiation and a family history of endocrine tumors, suggesting multiple endocrine neoplasia (MEN) type II and medullary carcinoma of the thyroid (MCT).

5. **B**

6. **A** Mutations in the ret protooncogene on chromosome 10 are present in patients with MEN IIA (medullary carcinoma of the thyroid [MTC], pheochromocytoma, and hyperparathyroidism from parathyroid hyperplasia), and IIB (MTC, pheochromocytoma, mucosal ganglioneuromatosis, typical facies, marfanoid body habitus). A MTC associated with MEN IIB seems to be more aggressive and occurs at an earlier age. Children with a family history of endocrine tumors should be screened for the ret mutation, and if present, they should undergo prophylactic thyroidectomy by age 5 if MEN IIA, and by age 1 if MEN IIB.

BIBLIOGRAPHY

Geiger JD, Thompson NW. Thyroid tumors in children. *Otolaryngol Clin North Am.* 1996;29:711–719.

La Quaglia MP, Telander RL. Differentiated and medullary thyroid cancer in childhood and adolescence. *Semin Pediatr Surg.* 1997;6:42–49.

A 15-YEAR-OLD GIRL WITH RIGHT UPPER QUADRANT ABDOMINAL PAIN

HISTORY   A 15-year-old Vietnamese girl is referred for evaluation of intermittent upper abdominal pain and vomiting. The pain is typically postprandial and localized to the right upper quadrant, lasting 1 to 2 hours. The girl notes that for the last 2 to 3 days her urine has appeared concentrated. There is no history of fever or chills and no infectious exposure risks.

EXAMINATION   Physical examination reveals a moderately obese female with scleral icterus. Her abdomen is soft, but she does have mild right upper quadrant tenderness to deep palpation without hepatomegaly. You order an abdominal ultrasound (Figure 79–1) and liver function tests. Her liver function test results are as follows: total bilirubin 3.2 (0.6 to 1.4 mg/dL), direct bilirubin 2.1 (0 to 0.3 mg/dL), aspartate amino transferase (AST) 88 (13 to 44 IU/I), alanine amino transferase (ALT) 74 (10 to 25 IU/L), alkaline phosphatase 560 (150 to 380 IU/dL).

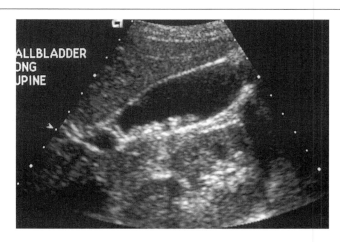

Figure 79–1. *Ultrasound image of the gallbladder in a 15-year-old girl with abdominal pain.*

377

Please answer all questions before proceeding to discussion section.

✓ QUESTIONS

1. The most likely diagnosis is:
   A. Hepatitis A infection
   B. Choledochal cyst with cholangitis
   C. Cholelithiasis and choldedocholithiasis
   D. Oriental cholangitis

2. The next most indicated test or procedure would be:
   A. Hepatitis serology
   B. Hepato-iminodiacetic acid (HIDA) scan
   C. Laparoscopic cholecystectomy
   D. Endoscopic retrograde cholangiopancreatography (ERCP)

3. The pertinent finding of this procedure is shown in Figure 79–2. The treatment options at this point include all of the following *except:*
   A. Laparoscopic cholecystectomy with common bile duct exploration
   B. Laparoscopic cholecystectomy with follow-up ultrasound in 2 weeks
   C. Endoscopic papillotomy followed by laparoscopic cholecystectomy
   D. Open cholecystectomy with common bile duct exploration

4. Inadvertent common bile duct injury during laparoscopic cholecystectomy can be best avoided by:
   A. Routine use of operative cholangiography
   B. Sufficient dissection and structure identification within the triangle of Calot
   C. Avoiding cautery dissection within the triangle of Calot
   D. Mobilizing the gallbladder prior to dissecting the triangle of Calot

5. One week after laparoscopic cholecystectomy, the girl returns with abdominal pain, fever, and recurrent scleral icterus. Presuming that a preoperative ERCP following papillotomy and stone retrieval demonstrated a clear common bile duct, the most likely cause of these symptoms is:
   A. Retained common bile duct stones
   B. Post-ERCP pancreatitis
   C. Biloma formation from a cystic duct stump leak
   D. Common bile duct injury

6. You obtain an abdominal ultrasound that shows a subhepatic fluid collection and nondilated intra- and extrahepatic bile ducts. The most appropriate next step would be:
   A. An ERCP and nasobiliary drain placement with percutaneous pigtail catheter drainage of the subhepatic collection
   B. Percutaneous transhepatic cholangiography (PTC) with catheter placement for external biliary drainage and percutaneous pigtail catheter drainage of the subhepatic collection

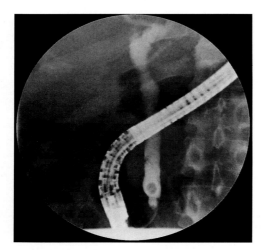

Figure 79–2. *ERCP image of a patient with cholelithiasis and direct hyperbilirubinemia.*

C. A HIDA scan and percutaneous pigtail catheter drainage of the subhepatic collection

D. Laparoscopic exploration with intraoperative cholangiography

ANSWERS AND DISCUSSION

1. **C** This patient gives a history consistent with biliary colic. The ultrasound study shows multiple round densities within the lumen of the gallbladder confirming cholelithiasis. The recent onset of direct hyperbilirubinemia with a predominantly obstructive liver biochemistry profile is highly suggestive of choledocholithiasis, which can often be seen directly on ultrasound or can certainly be inferred by the observation of dilated extrahepatic ducts. Choledochal cysts occasionally present in adolescence with the classic triad of abdominal pain, jaundice, and a palpable abdominal mass. Oriental cholangiohepatitis is a frequent cause of obstructive biliary disease in southeast Asia, in which parasitic biliary infestation leads to secondary cholangitis and duct dilation with the formation of intraductal pigment stones.

2. **D** Endoscopic retrograde pancreatography (ERCP) is now widely available, and with smaller side viewing endoscopes, it can be performed even in very young children. It has become an essential diagnostic tool in the evaluation of obstructive pancreatiobiliary disease, and it offers the added therapeutic benefit of papillotomy and stone retrieval.

3. **B** The ERCP image shows a spherical filling defect in the distal common bile duct. The duct is moderately dilated. These findings are diagnostic of a common bile duct stone. The documentation of common duct stones associated with cholelithiasis mandates their removal in conjunction with cholecystectomy to avoid the potentially life-threatening complications of ascending cholangitis or biliary pancreatitis. In this era of endoscopy and minimally invasive surgery, this can be accomplished in one of two ways. A preoperative ERCP that documents the presence of common duct stones and then removes them following endoscopic papillotomy obviates the need for cholangiography and stone retrieval during subsequent laparoscopic cholecystectomy. On the other hand, skilled laparoscopists with the appropriate equipment can perform intraoperative cholangiography and laparoscopic common bile duct exploration at the time of cholecystectomy, which makes preoperative ERCP unnecessary.

4. **B** Common bile duct injury during laparoscopic cholecystectomy is best avoided by precise low-cautery dissection and identification of the cystic artery, the cystic duct, and its junction with the gallbladder before any structures are clipped or divided. Major bile duct injuries occur in approximately 0.5% of cases of laparoscopic cholecystectomy, which is not different from the historic rate reported for open cholecystectomy. In most cases, recognition of injury does not occur at the time of surgery, but in retrospective video review is the result of incomplete dissection of the medial aspect of the triangle of Calot. The question of whether routine operative cholangiography during laparoscopic cholecystectomy reduces the risk of iatrogenic bile duct injury is frequently debated but remains unanswered.

5. **C** Retained common duct stone, pancreatitis, cystic duct stump leak, and unrecognized bile duct injury could all account for the symptoms of abdominal pain, fever, and jaundice following laparoscopic cholecystectomy. In this case, however, the delay in onset of symptoms and the comparative frequency of postoperative bile leaks (2.5%) versus major bile duct injuries (0.5%) favor the diagnosis of a bile leak from either the hepatic parenchyma, an accessory duct of Luschka, or from the cystic duct. Pancreatitis after ERCP does not typically cause obstructive jaundice, and a retained stone is unlikely if the duct was cleared preoperatively by ERCP, unless one slipped out of the gallbladder and into the duct before or during cholecystectomy. To limit the number of unnecessary ERCP examinations and minimize the risk of retained stones resulting from a stone passing into the bile duct after a preoperative ERCP, some authors are recommending that ERCP be done under the same anesthesia as laparoscopic cholecsytectomy, either immediately before or after.

6. **A** Even though the bile ducts are not dilated, an ERCP is essential to exclude duct obstruction from retained stones or a bile duct injury and to identify, if possible, the site of the leak. Small leaks from the gallbladder bed will likely close spontaneously, but they may require percutaneous drainage of the accumulated bile for resolution of symptoms. Larger leaks from the cystic duct stump are more likely to close if the resistance to distal bile flow is diminished by internal stenting or nasobiliary drainage.

BIBLIOGRAPHY

Holcomb GW 3rd, Morgan WM 3rd, Neblett WW 3rd, et al. Laparoscopic cholecystectomy in children: lessons learned from the first 100 patients. *J Pediatr Surg.* 1999;34:1236–1240.

Holcomb GW 3rd, Peitsch JB. Gallbladder disease and hepatic infections. In: O'Neill JA, Rowe MI, Grosfeld JG, et al. eds. *Pediatric Surgery.* St. Louis: Mosby-Year Book; 1998.

MacFadyeb BV Jr, Passi RB. The role of endoscopic retrograde cholangiopancreatography in the era of laparoscopic cholecystectomy. *Semin Laparosc Surg.* 1997;4:18–22.

A NEWBORN BOY
WITH A NECK MASS

HISTORY   You are called to the neonatal intensive care unit to evaluate a newborn boy with a large neck mass. The baby is shown in Figure 80–1 (see also color plate). He is not in any respiratory distress.

EXAMINATION   The baby is alert and active. Vital signs are normal. This mass is soft and balottable. It does not seem tender. The lungs are clear with equal breath sounds on both sides. The remainder of the physical examination is normal.

STUDIES   A chest x-ray was obtained upon arrival to the NICU and is shown in Figure 80–2.

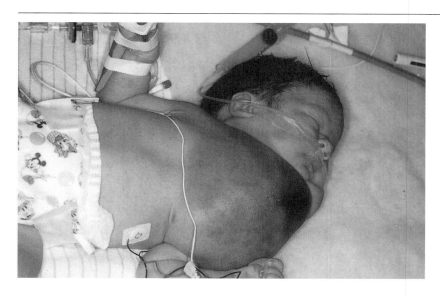

Figure 80–1. *A newborn boy with a neck mass. The baby is otherwise healthy. (See also color plate.)*

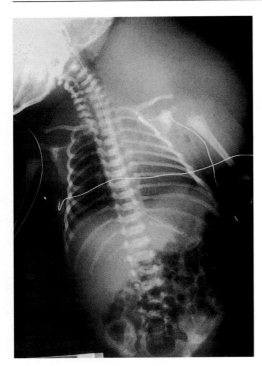

Figure 80–2. *Chest x-ray of a newborn boy with a neck mass.*

Please answer all questions before proceeding to discussion section.

✓ QUESTIONS

1. What is the most likely diagnosis?
   A. Hematoma secondary to birth trauma
   B. Cystic hygroma
   C. Teratoma
   D. Hemangioma
   E. None of the above

2. These lesions most commonly occur in the:
   A. Cervical region
   B. Axillae
   C. Groin
   D. Mediastinum
   E. Retroperitoneum ·

3. Appropriate management options at this point include:
   A. Surgical excision
   B. Needle aspiration
   C. Drain placement
   D. Administration of antibiotics
   E. Observation until the child is 4 years old since many of these lesions spontaneously regress

4. Which of the following is true of radiation therapy for these lesions?
   A. It is the first line treatment of choice
   B. It provides effective shrinkage but surgical resection is necessary following radiation
   C. It is more effective when administered with radiation sensitizing agents such as 5-FU
   D. A and C
   E. It has no role

5. During surgical excision of cystic hygromas:
   A. *En bloc* excision of adjacent organs is necessary to prevent recurrence
   B. Preoperative cyst aspiration will decrease the size of the necessary incision and facilitate removal
   C. Invaded vascular structures should be excised but nerves should not be transected
   D. Vital structures should be preserved even if this means incomplete resection
   E. Destruction of adjacent organs is frequently found

6. You are asked to see the family of a 17-week-gestation fetus found to have a large nuchal cystic hygroma on screening prenatal ultrasound examination. Which is true?
   A. Screening for associated renal defects is most important
   B. The presence of other anomalies is unlikely
   C. The baby is not likely to survive to term
   D. Chromosomal analysis will likely be normal
   E. All of the above

7. If you had seen the parents of this patient 2 weeks prior to the mother's due date, you would have told them:
   A. Cesarean delivery to prevent dystocia is necessary
   B. Umbilical cord compression during delivery places the baby at increased risk
   C. Rupture of the lesion in utero can occur late in gestation; early delivery is indicated
   D. Airway compromise in the delivery room may require complex management
   E. All of the above

ANSWERS AND DISCUSSION

1. **B** The history and physical findings are consistent with a cystic hygroma. Cystic hygromas are multiloculated cystic spaces caused by malformations of the lymphatic spaces. They are lined by a single-cell layer of endothelial cells and often segmented by fine walls and septae. Cystic hygromas occur in about 1 in 12,000 live births. Just slightly over half are visible in the newborn, while 80% to 90% appear by the second year of life. They present as large, soft, fluid-filled masses, which may distort, but do not invade, anatomic structures. The chest x-ray in Figure 80–2 shows simply a large, soft-tissue mass, which is not particularly helpful in confirming the diagnosis.

   Teratomas can produce large neck masses in newborns. Typically, they are firmer and more irregular. They often contain calcium, which would be visible on the x-ray film. Hematoma secondary to birth trauma of this size would result in severe hypovolemia or exsanguination. A hemangioma or vascular malformation can be found in newborns. Vascular malformations rarely attain this size and typically have a characteristic vascular pattern over the skin.

2. **A** Cystic hygromas most commonly are found in the cervical region of the neck. They have a predilection for the posterior triangle on the left side. About 75% of all cystic hygromas are in this region. The next most common region is the axillae, accounting for 20% of cystic hygromas. The remainder occur in the mediastinum, retroperitoneum, and the groin.

   Cystic hygromas result from abnormal development of the embryologic origin of the lymphatic system. When part or all of the structures fail to develop drainage into the venous system, cystic hygroma results. When a soft, ballotable mass is found in these locations, the diagnosis usually is not in doubt. If there is diagnostic uncertainty, however, ultrasound examination is quite useful. Since these lesions are fluid-filled, they have distinct ultrasonographic characteristics. Evaluation of lesions in the mediastinum or in the retroperitoneum may be facilitated by CT scan or MRI.

3. **A** Large cystic hygromas are generally best treated by surgical excision. Needle aspiration is ineffective as fluid within the hygroma will rapidly reaccumulate. Furthermore, needle aspiration may introduce infection into the large cystic space. Drain placement is not indicated for similar reasons. Fluid within cystic hygromas is secreted by

the endothelial cells lining the wall. Unless these cells are removed, fluid will continue to drain.

Antibiotics are not indicated unless there is infection. It is certainly not warranted to observe a mass of this size. Vascular malformations frequently undergo spontaneous involution. Lymphatic malformations, on the other hand, either remain stable or increase in size with time.

An alternative management strategy has gained popularity in Japan. This includes injection of a sclerosing substance (OK-432) into the lesion. OK-432 is produced by incubating *Streptococcus pyogenes* and seems to produce inflammation, which results in scarification and shrinking of the lesion. Results following OK-432 injection are variable. This therapy has yet to be compared with surgical excision in a clinical trial.

4. **E** Radiation therapy was used in an attempt to treat these lesions many years ago. Currently, it has no role in the treatment of cystic hygroma. Radiation therapy is contraindicated in any growing patient, especially a newborn baby, as it can interfere with growth and development.

5. **D** Cystic hygromas are not neoplasms and they do not invade tissue. Rather, they tend to insinuate themselves in and around vital structures. For this reason, vital structures such as nerves and major vascular structures should *not* be sacrificed during excision of a cystic hygroma, even when this means that the lesion is only partially excised. For example, during excision of the large hygroma in this patient, small amounts of cyst wall were left adherent to the vagus, spinal accessory, phrenic, and marginal mandibular nerves. Additional tumor was left along the wall of the carotid artery.

Such an approach will result in a slightly higher recurrence rate, but is preferable to the sacrifice of vital structures. *En bloc* resection of other tissue is never indicated during removal of cystic hygromas. Preoperative aspiration of the cyst fluid is a big mistake and will make excision much more difficult. The surgeon should make every effort to avoid entry into the cyst(s) during dissection. Once the

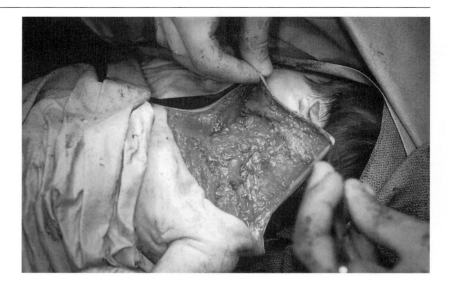

Figure 80–3. *Appearance of the neck during surgical excision. The baby's head is to the right. Note the large skin flaps created. Dissection must proceed cautiously taking care to identify all the major nerves and vascular structures of the neck.*

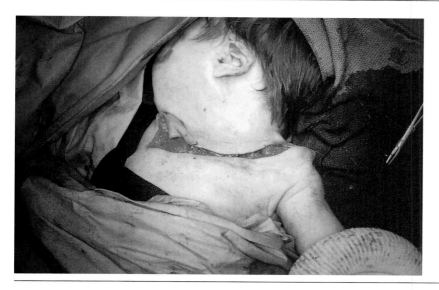

Figure 80–4. *Appearance at the time of wound closure. The incision should be placed such that the suture line is low in the neck and follows a skin crease.*

fluid is out of the lesion and it collapses, it is extremely difficult to excise from the surrounding tissue and the recurrence rate is much higher. Cystic hygromas are fed by many tiny lymphatic channels; it is rare to find a single or very few major feeding channels that can be ligated.

Figure 80–3 shows the appearance of the child's neck during removal of this lesion. Large skin flaps are created superiorly and inferiorly. Care should be taken to place the incision such that the suture line for the wound closure will lie in a cosmetically acceptable location. Figure 80–4 shows the skin flaps as they are being laid together for closure.

This child had an excellent postoperative result and is seen on his third birthday in Figure 80–5.

6. **C** Cystic hygroma diagnosed early in gestation is highly associated with major chromosomal anomalies, fetal loss, and a poor prognosis. Clearly, the cystic hygromas seen in healthy newborns represent a subset of a broader population. Chromosomal anomalies are very unlikely to be found in liveborn patients with cystic hygroma. Presence of cystic hygroma in the nuchal region carries a particularly negative prognosis. Fetal intervention has not proven to be necessary or successful for cystic hygroma. Spontaneous regression of the cystic hygroma during gestation is very unlikely.

7. **D** Very large midline neck masses may compress the trachea and prevent spontaneous ventilation from occurring at the time of delivery. Endotracheal intubation can be extremely difficult or even impossible in this setting. Management of these difficult patients has been facilitated by the delivery of the infant via cesarean section with maintenance of the intact placenta and umbilical cord. In this way, the baby can be maintained on placental support while the airway is manipulated bronchoscopically to secure adequate access. A number of these procedures have been successfully done with good postnatal outcome.

Rupture of the hygroma with hemorrhage is virtually unheard of. Arrested labor secondary to dystocia does not occur since the mass is

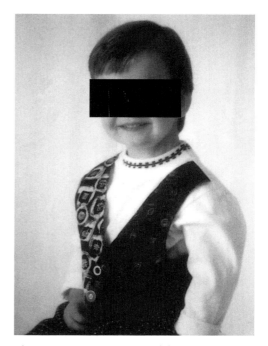

Figure 80–5. *Appearance of this patient on his third birthday.*

soft and deformable. Compression of the umbilical cord during delivery has not been reported.

BIBLIOGRAPHY

Anderson NG, Kennedy JC. Prognosis in fetal cystic hygroma. *Aust N Z J Obstet Gynaecol.* 1992;32:36–39.

Edwards MJ, Graham JM. Posterior nuchal cystic hygroma. *Clin Perinatol.* 1990;17:611–640.

Filston HC. Hemangiomas, cystic hygromas, and teratomas of the head and neck. *Semin Pediatr Surg.* 1994;3:147–159.

Fonkalsrud EW. Congenital malformations of the lymphatic system. *Semin Pediatr Surg.* 1994;3:62–69.

Koeller KK, Alamo L, Adair CF, et al. Congenital cystic masses of the neck: radiologic pathologic correlation. *Radiographics.* 1999;19:121–146.

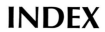

INDEX

Please note: *f* following a page reference indicates a figure, *t* indicates a table, and CP indicates a color plate.

Thalassemia, overwhelming postsplenectomy infection and, 67
Thal fundoplication, for gastroesophageal reflux, 305
Thalidomide, two vessel umbilical cord and, 315
Third degree burns, 286–287
Thoracoscopy
  bronchogenic cysts and, 367
  for empyema, 272
Thoracostomy tube
  acquired lobar emphysema and, 339
  for chylothorax, 325
  for tension pneumothorax, 65
Thoracotomy
  for bronchogenic cyst, 367
  for cardiac tamponade, 158
  for chylothorax, 326
  for congenital diaphragmatic hernia, 212
  for cystic mass in chest, 350
  for empyema, 271
  for esophageal atresia, 16
  for lobar emphysema, 340, 340f, CP
  for patent ductus arteriosus, 298–299
  for tracheomalacia, 191–192
Thrombocytopenia, indomethacin and, 297
Thrombosis
  cholestasis and, 154
  chylothorax and, 326
  extrahepatic portal vein, 165
  necrotizing enterocolitis and, 35
Thyroglossal duct cyst, 101, 256f, 256–257, CP
Thyroid
  cancer of, 373–376, 374f
    in children vs. adults, 376
    papillary, 374f, 375, CP
  lateral aberrant, 257
  lingual, thyroglossal duct cyst and, 256–257
  midline ectopic, 257
Thyroidectomy, for thyroid cancer, 375
Thyroid gland, cysts on, 256–257
Todandi, 223
Tolazoline, in ventilation, 212
Tongue, cyst beneath, 99–100, 100f, 101, CP
Tonsillitis, 184
TORCH infections, differential diagnosis, 180
Torticollis, 100, 101f, 101–102, 260, CP
Toxic megacolon, risks for, 330
Tracheal occlusion, 242, 242f
Tracheobronchoscopy, for esophageal atresia, 15
Tracheoesophageal fistula (TEF)
  diagnosis of, 228
  esophageal atresia with, 15–19, 227
  H-type, 15–17
    diagnosis of, 228
    differential diagnosis, 192

  recurrent, 17–18
  tracheomalacia and, 191
Tracheomalacia, 191–192, 192f, CP
Traction nerve injuries, eventration of hemidiaphragm and, 280
Transfer of patient, principles of, 212
Transillumination, for hydrocele, 202
Transition zone, Hirschsprung disease and, 3
Transperitoneal drainage, of perforated appendix, 44
Transplantation, of liver
  for biliary atresia, 181–182
  for hepatoblastoma, 335–336
Trauma
  bicycle accidents, 266–268
  bronchogenic cysts and, 367
  car accidents, 63–67, 89–93, 243–247
  explosion, 283–287
  nonaccidental, differential diagnosis, 101
  pleural effusion and, 325
Triple therapy
  for appendicitis, 105
  for perforated appendix, 43
Trisomies
  omphalocele and, 232
  two vessel umbilical cord and, 315
Trisomy 9, 214
Trisomy 13, 214
Trisomy 18, 214
  congenital diaphragmatic hernia and, 241
  esophageal atresia and, 17
Trisomy 21, atresia and, 223
Trochlars, for empyema, 271
Tuberculosis, differential diagnosis, 271
Tuberculous adenitis, differential diagnosis, 264
Tumor(s)
  abdominal, 72–78, 332f–333f
  adrenocortical, 160
  appendiceal carcinoid, ileocolic intussusception and, 371
  endodermal sinus, 69–70
  epithelial ovarian, 83
  estrogen-producing ovarian, 160
  germ cell
    ovarian, 82–83
    of testis, 343
  gonadal stromal, 70
  intestinal, with Peutz-Jeghers syndrome, 49
  Leydig cell, 70
  liver, 334–336
  metastatic, differential diagnosis, 264
  ovarian, 82–83
  pelvic, 133
  primitive neuroectodermal, 128, 371
  renal, 344–345
  round blue cell, 128

INFORMATION FOR READERS INTERESTED IN OBTAINING CONTINUING MEDICAL EDUCATION CREDIT

The reader may review the material as often as he or she wishes. Credit will be granted based on the number of chapters read, and will be granted one time only. Evidence of the reader's efforts will be by means of a written narrative describing the most salient feature of each chapter, which the participant reviewed.

The purpose of the book is to increase the reader's knowledge and clinical judgment in the management of children with surgical problems. The reader of the book is presented with eighty common clinical problems in pediatric surgery and is asked to manage these problems by means of a series of multiple-choice questions. The questions were carefully designed to address common pitfalls and misconceptions in the management of these patients. The reader will be exposed to relevant x-rays, histologic material, and photographs showing physical and intra-operative findings. We anticipate that successful completion of this book will significantly increase the readers' knowledge and competence in caring for children with surgical problems.

As evidence of completion of the material, the reader is asked to describe the single clinical issue learned from each chapter that is most relevant to his or her practice. The authors believe that this type of activity will be a far better indicator of the reader's engagement with the material than simply providing the CME office with correct answers to the questions. The correct answers are already given in the discussion section of each chapter.

The Stanford University School of Medicine is accredited by the Accreditation Council for Continuing Medical Education to sponsor continuing medical education for physicians. The Division of Pediatric Surgery and Department of Surgery at Stanford University School of Medicine takes responsibility for the content, quality, and scientific integrity of this CME activity.

The Stanford University School of Medicine designates this educational activity for up to 40.0 hours in category 1 credit towards the AMA Physician's Recognition Award. Each physician should claim only those hours of credit that he or she actually spent in the educational activity.

This activity was planned and produced in accordance with the ACCME Essentials.

Procedure for obtaining CME credit:

1. Thoroughly review each chapter for which you would like to obtain credit including a review of the references where relevant to your needs.

2. Determine the issues you have learned which are most relevant to the care of your patients.

3. Write down the single most relevant issue on the form that follows. Return the form along with a check payable for $40.00 per participant seeking CME. The check should be made payable to: Stanford University School of Medicine and mailed to:

   Attn: CME Department
   Stanford University School of Medicine
   251 Campus Dr., MSOB X341
   Stanford, CA 94305-5423

4. Once the CME office has verified your eligibility for credit you will receive a certificate of completion.

5. Please direct questions to: Stanford University School of Medicine CME Department (650) 723-7188 or 1-800-305-2436

CASE STUDIES IN PEDIATRIC SURGERY:
Application for CME credit

NAME (FIRST, MIDDLE, AND LAST NAME) _____

TITLE (EXAMPLE: MD, PhD, RN, ...) _____

ADDRESS (STREET, CITY, STATE, ZIP)

_____

_____

_____

MEDICAL LICENSE NUMBER AND STATE_____

DAY TIME PHONE NUMBER _____

FAX NUMBER _____

E-MAIL ADDRESS _____

NUMBER OF CREDIT HOURS REQUESTED _____

SIGNATURE _____

Remember to include check for $40 payable to Stanford University School of Medicine and send to:

> ATTN: CME DEPARTMENT
> STANFORD UNIVERSITY SCHOOL OF MEDICINE
> 251 CAMPUS DR., MSOB X341
> STANFORD, CA 95305-5423

Please list the issues learned from each chapter that is most relevant to the care of your patients.

1.

2.

3.

4.

5.

6.

7.

8.

9.

10.

11.

12.

13.

14.

15.

16.

17.

18.

19.

20.

21.

22.

23.

24.

25.

26.

27.

28.

29.

30.

31.

32.

33.

34.

35.

36.

37.

38.

39.

40.

41.

42.

43.

44.

45.

46.

47.

48.

49.

50.

51.

52.

53.

54.

55.

56.

57.

58.

59.

60.

61.

62.

63.

64.

65.

66.

67.

68.

69.

70.

71.

72.

73.

74.

75.

76.

77.

78.

79.

80.